Disasters and
Mental Health

Disasters and Mental Health

Edited by

Juan José López-Ibor
Complutense University of Madrid, Spain

George Christodoulou
University of Athens, Greece

Mario Maj
University of Naples, Italy

Norman Sartorius
University of Geneva, Switzerland

and

Ahmed Okasha
Ain Shams University, Cairo, Egypt

WILEY

Other Wiley Editorial Offices

John Wiley & Sons Inc., 111 River Street, Hoboken, NJ 07030, USA

Jossey-Bass, 989 Market Street, San Francisco, CA 94103-1741, USA

Wiley-VCH Verlag GmbH, Boschstr. 12, D-69469 Weinheim, Germany

John Wiley & Sons Australia Ltd, 33 Park Road, Milton, Queensland 4064, Australia

John Wiley & Sons (Asia) Pte Ltd, 2 Clementi Loop #02-01, Jin Xing Distripark, Singapore 129809

John Wiley & Sons Canada Ltd, 22 Worcester Road, Etobicoke, Ontario, Canada M9W 1L1

Wiley also publishes its books in a variety of electronic formats. Some content that appears in print may not be available in electronic books.

Library of Congress Cataloging-in-Publication Data

Disasters and mental health / edited by Juan José López-Ibor ... [et al.].
    p. ; cm.
  Includes bibliographical references and index.
  ISBN 0-470-02123-3 (alk. paper)
  1. Disasters–Psychological aspects. 2. Disasters–Psychological aspects–Case studies.
  3. Disaster victims–Mental health. 4. Post-traumatic stress disorder. I. López-Ibor Aliño, J. J. (Juan José). 1941-
    [DNLM: 1. Disasters. 2. Stress Disorders, Traumatic–pscychology. WM 172 D611 2005]
  RC451.4.D57D55 2005
  616.85′210651–dc22
                                                                                    2004055304

British Library Cataloguing in Publication Data

A catalogue record for this book is available from the British Library

ISBN 0-470-02123-3

Typeset in 10/12pt Palatino by Dobbie Typesetting Ltd, Tavistock, Devon

Contents

Mental Health Consequences of Disasters: Experiences in Various Regions of the World

List of Contributors

Mordechai Benyakar   University of Buenos Aires, Avenida Libertador 4944 9B, Capital Federal, Buenos Aires 1426, Argentina

Linda M. Bierer   Bronx Veterans Affairs Medical Center, Mental Health Patient Care Center, 130 West Kingsbridge Road, Bronx, New York, NY 10468-3904, USA

Evelyn J. Bromet   Department of Psychiatry and Preventive Medicine, State University of New York at Stony Brook, Putnam Hall, South Campus, Stony Brook, NY 11793-8790, USA

José Miguel Caldas de Almeida   Mental Health Unit, Pan American Health Organization, 525 23rd Street NW, Washington, DC 20037, USA

Alain Chiapello   Croix-Rouge Ecoute, Croix-Rouge Française, 1 Place Henry Dunante, 75008 Paris, France

George N. Christodoulou   Department of Psychiatry, Athens University Medical School, Eginition Hospital, 72-74 Vas. Sofias Avenue, 11528 Athens, Greece

Carlos R. Collazo   University of El Salvador, Avenida Pueyredon 1625, Buenos Aires 1118, Argentina

Louis Crocq   Cellule d'Urgence Médico-Psychologique, SAMU de Paris, Hôpital Necker, 149 rue de Sèvres, 75015 Paris, France

Marc-Antoine Crocq   Centre Hospitalier de Rouffach, 27 rue du 4ème RSM – BP 29, 68250 Rouffach, France

Carole Damiani   Association "Paris Aide aux Victimes", 4–14 rue Ferrus, 75014 Paris, France

Lynn E. DeLisi   Department of Psychiatry, New York University, 650 First Avenue, New York, NY 10016, USA

Saveta Draganic-Gajic   Institute of Mental Health, School of Medicine, University of Belgrade, Palmoticeva 37, 11000 Belgrade, Serbia and Montenegro

Eyad El Sarraj   Gaza Community Mental Health Programme, PO Box 1049, Gaza Strip, Palestine

Carol S. Fullerton   Department of Psychiatry, Uniformed Services University of the Health Sciences, 4301 Jones Bridge Road, Bethesda, MD 20814, USA

Peykan G. Gökalp   Anxiety Disorders (Neurosis) Department, Bakirkoy Training and Research Hospital for Psychiatry and Neurology, Istanbul, Turkey

Johan M. Havenaar   Altrecht Institute for Mental Health Care, Lange Nieuwstraat 119, 3512 PZ Utrecht, The Netherlands

Syed Arshad Husain   Department of Psychiatry, Division of Child and Adolescent Psychiatry, University of Missouri, Columbia, MO 65212, USA

Dusica Lecic-Tosevski   Institute of Mental Health, School of Medicine, University of Belgrade, Palmoticeva 37, 11000 Belgrade, Serbia and Montenegro

Juan José Lopez-Ibor   Department of Psychiatry and Medical Psychology, Complutense University of Madrid, Spain

Alexander C. McFarlane   Department of Psychiatry, University of Adelaide, Queen Elizabeth Hospital, 28 Woodville Road, Woodville South, SA 5011, Australia

R. Srinivasa Murthy   National Institute of Mental Health and Neurosciences, Department of Psychiatry, Hosur Road, Bangalore 560029, Karnataka, India

Frank Njenga   Upperhill Medical Center, PO Box 73749, 00200 Nairobi, Kenya

Caroline Nyamai   Upperhill Medical Center, PO Box 73749, 00200 Nairobi, Kenya

Thomas J. Paparrigopoulos   Department of Psychiatry, Athens University Medical School, Eginition Hospital, 72–74 Vas. Sofias Avenue, 11528 Athens, Greece

Samir Qouta   Gaza Community Mental Health Programme, PO Box 1049, Gaza Strip, Palestine

Jorge Rodríguez   Mental Health Unit, Pan American Health Organization, 525 23rd Street NW, Washington, DC 20037, USA

Arieh Y. Shalev   Department of Psychiatry, Hadassah University Hospital, Jerusalem 91120, Israel

Naotaka Shinfuku   International Center for Medical Research, University School of Medicine, Kusunoki-Cho, 7-Chome, Chuo-ku, Kobe 650-0017, Japan

Vera Folnegović Šmalc   Vrapče Psychiatric Hospital, Bolnička Cesta 32, 10 090 Zagreb, Croatia

Constantin R. Soldatos   Department of Psychiatry, Athens University Medical School, Eginition Hospital, 72–74 Vas. Sofias Avenue, 11528 Athens, Greece

Robert J. Ursano   Department of Psychiatry, Uniformed Services University of the Health Sciences, 4301 Jones Bridge Road, Bethesda, MD 20814, USA

Rachel Yehuda   Bronx Veterans Affairs Medical Center, Mental Health Patient Care Center, 130 West Kingsbridge Road, Bronx, New York, NY 10468-3904, USA

Preface

The mental health consequences of disasters have been the subject of a rapidly growing research literature in the last few decades. Moreover, they have aroused an increasing public interest, due to the dramatic impact and the wide media coverage of many recent disastrous events—from earthquakes to hurricanes, from technological disasters to terrorist attacks and war bombings.

The World Psychiatric Association has had for a long time a great interest and commitment in this area, especially through the work of the Section on Military and Disaster Psychiatry and the Program on Disasters and Mental Health. Several sessions on this topic have taken place in past World Congresses of Psychiatry, and other scientific meetings organized by the Association have dealt exclusively with disaster psychiatry.

Several research and practical issues remain open in this area. Among them, those of the boundary between "normal" and "pathological" responses to disasters; of the early predictors of subsequent significant mental disorders; of the range of psychological and psychosocial problems that mental health services should be prepared to address; of the efficacy of the psychological interventions which are currently available; of the nature and weight of risk and protective factors in the general population; of the feasibility, effectiveness and cost-effectiveness of the preventive programs which have been proposed at the international and national level. Moreover, wherever disasters strike, policy and service organization issues that plague the mental health field worldwide receive even more prominence: the detection and management of mental health problems are assigned less priority than care for physical problems; trained personnel is lacking; community resources for mental health care are poor; a vast proportion of people in need hesitate to ask for or accept mental health care.

However, it is clear that the field is progressing rapidly from the scientific viewpoint (with a refinement of early diagnostic concepts and treatment strategies, and a deeper understanding of resilience factors at the individual and community level) and that in a (slowly) growing number of countries concrete steps have been taken concerning training of personnel, education of the population, and the development of a network of services prepared to deal with psychological emergencies.

This volume aims to portray this evolutionary phase, by providing an overview of current knowledge and controversies about the mental health consequences of disasters and their management, and by offering a selection of first-hand accounts of experiences in several regions of the world. We were impressed by the liveliness of some of the reports, and particularly touched by some of the chapters dealing with the mental health consequences of armed conflicts, especially on children and adolescents. The authors of these chapters have accepted our advice to be as objective as possible in their descriptions. However, despite the intentions of the authors and the editors, some traces of their unavoidable emotional involvement may have been left in their chapters.

Neither the research overview nor the selection of experiences presented in this volume should be seen as being comprehensive. We hope, however, that the book will throw more light on the issue of mental health consequences of disasters, stimulate acquisition of more knowledge through research, enhance our sensitivity, and contribute to a more effective prevention and management of the behavioural effects of disasters. Disasters have been happening since time immemorial and will continue to happen. We must be prepared to face them and deal with their consequences.

Juan José López-Ibor
George Christodoulou
Mario Maj
Norman Sartorius
Ahmed Okasha

This volume is based in part on presentations delivered at the 12th World Congress of Psychiatry (Yokohama, Japan, 24–29 August, 2002).

1

What is a Disaster?

Juan José López-Ibor

Complutense University of Madrid, Spain

INTRODUCTION

It is almost impossible to find an acceptable definition of what a disaster is. Nevertheless, a definition is unavoidable if we want to be able to face disasters and their consequences. Quarantelli [1] states that, if the experts do not reach an agreement whether a disaster is a physical event or a social construct, the field will have serious intellectual problems, and that defining what a disaster is does not mean becoming involved in a futile academic exercise. On the contrary, it means delving into what are the significant characteristics of the phenomenon, the conditions that lead to it and its consequences. On the other hand, a definition is also needed to guide the interventions following a natural event, for instance, when a government declares a region devastated by a flooding as a "catastrophe area". Furthermore, a definition is needed for understanding, because any concrete disaster poses the question of its meaning.

A danger is an event or a natural characteristic that implies a risk for human beings, i.e., it is the agent that, at a certain moment, produces individual or collective harm. A danger is therefore something potential. A risk is the degree of exposure to the danger, it is therefore something probable. A reef shown on a nautical map is a danger; but it is a risk only for those who sail in waters nearby. A disaster is the consequence of a danger, the actualisation of the risk.

The literature on disasters offers several definitions from different perspectives, as summarised in the following sections.

THE MAGNITUDE OF THE DAMAGE PRODUCED BY THE EVENT

Human losses, number of injured persons, material and economic losses and the harm produced to the environment are often considered in order to

Disasters and Mental Health. Edited by Juan José López-Ibor, George Christodoulou, Mario Maj, Norman Sartorius and Ahmed Okasha.
©2005 John Wiley & Sons Ltd. ISBN 0-470-02123-3.

define a disaster. For some authors (e.g., 2) the number of 25 deceased has to be exceeded; for others (e.g., 3) this figure has to be higher, more than 100 deceased and more than 100 injured or losses worth more than one million US dollars; or even higher (e.g., 4), an event leading to 500 deaths or 10 million US dollars in damages. According to Wright [5], experience shows that when an event affects more than 120 persons, except for cases of war, non-routine interventions and coordination between different organisations are needed, something which is already pointing out another important characteristic of a disaster. For German insurance companies, damages greater than one million marks or more than 1,000 deceased are needed [2]: these figures are obviously given in order to limit responsibilities of insurance policies.

To define a disaster by the magnitude of the damage caused has many inconveniences. First, it may be difficult to evaluate the damages, especially in the initial stages. Second, such definitions are of no use for comparative studies in different countries or social situations and are affected by inflation [6]. Third, disasters have a different impact in different environments: an earthquake of an intensity to cause a fright in California nowadays would have been a catastrophe before 1989 and would be a catastrophe in many developing countries at present. There may even exist disasters with zero harm. The best example of this was the broadcast in 1935 by Orson Welles of *The War of the Worlds* [7]: more than one million persons showed intense panic reactions because of what they believed to be a Martian invasion. But, what is more important, these definitions fail to capture what is essential in a disaster.

EXCEPTIONAL EXTERNAL AGENT

Disasters are often considered as events from the physical environment which are harmful for human beings and are caused by forces which are unfamiliar to them [8,9]. Disasters are normally unforeseen and catch the populations and administrations affected off-guard. However, there are disasters that repeat themselves, for example in areas affected by flooding, and others which are persistent, as in many forms of terrorism. In these cases a culture of adaptation and resignation to disasters develops.

Disasters are normally considered as events that occur "by chance" and therefore unavoidable. In the past they were ascribed to divine punishment, and even nowadays it is not unusual to read that an event "reached Biblical proportions", or that nature's powers have been unchained as they were when God had to punish the evildoing of human beings with the Flood. In fact, the etymology of disaster, from Latin (*dis* "lack" or "ill-", *astrum* "heavenly body", "star"), indicates bad luck or fortune.

An important characteristic of disasters is their centrality [10]. Catastrophes are disasters of a great centrality. A total breakdown of everyday functioning takes place in them, with the disappearance of normal social functioning, loss of immediate leaderships, and the insufficiency of the health and emergency systems, in such a way that the survivors do not know where to go to receive help.

THE NATURE OF THE AGENT

Human-made disasters are normally distinguished from those which are consequences of the inclemency of nature. Among the first sort, some are not intended, i.e., they are the consequence of human error. In this case, the responsibility is considered to be institutional, and compensations from insurance companies are granted.

There are also human-made disasters that are the consequence of a clear intention, as in the case of conventional war. In these cases, individuals are able to start up more or less legitimate or efficient coping or defence mechanisms to confront the aggression. The First World War was a war of fronts that affected little the rearguard, while in the Spanish Civil War and in the Second World War there were as many victims due to combat actions in the rearguard as in the front (settling of scores, bombing of the civil population, and so on). Therefore the psychological and psychopathological reactions were different. During the First World War, those evacuated from the front came to a safe rearguard, in which they were assisted in an attentive way, favouring the appearance of very dramatic conversion symptoms. During the Spanish Civil War [11,12], those evacuated came to a rearguard which was also affected and they presented more psychosomatic symptoms, i.e., more internalised ones. The same happened during the Second World War.

On other occasions, violence is due to terrorist attacks, assaults by rapists or similar events. This is an anonymous violence whose goal is to cause harm to whomever, something that prevents the people affected from developing any kind of defence. This kind of violence may affect any person, in any place of the world, at any time.

In disasters produced by the inclemency of nature, the kind of disaster normally determines the way the pain is perceived and the quantum of guilt. Some are more foreseeable, as for example in hurricane areas, volcano eruptions or floodings, and other are not so foreseeable, as in some earthquakes or massive fires.

However, it is not possible to accept that there are purely natural disasters, since the human hand is always present. This is the thesis of Steinberg [13], who studied a large series of disasters in the USA. It has to be taken into account that the degree of development of a community is a determinant fact. Between 1960 and 1987, 41 out of the 109 worst natural disasters took place in developing countries, with the death of 758,850 persons, while the remaining 59% of disasters took place in developed countries, with the death of 11,441 persons [14]. It is curious enough that these proportions are similar to those in famine, HIV infection or refugee status [15].

THREAT TO THE SOCIAL SYSTEM

Definitions of disasters based on the idea of an exceptional agent are not fully satisfying. In fact, when reviewing them, other elements appear which are related to social conditions. The flooding of an uninhabited non-cultivated plain with no ecological value is not a disaster; human presence is needed. Carr [16] was the first to point out the importance of the social aspects: "Not every windstorm, earth-tremor, or rush of water is a catastrophe. A catastrophe is known by its works; that is to say, by the occurrence of disaster. So long as the ship rides out the storm, so long as the city resists the earth-shocks, so long as the levees hold, there is no disaster. It is the collapse of the cultural protections that constitutes the disaster proper."

Therefore, the impact of an event on a social group is related to the adaptive mechanisms and abilities that the community has developed. If they are efficient, we can speak of an emergency, not of a disaster. For instance, a traffic accident with ten victims is a disaster in a little village, but not in a city [17]. Disasters have been defined from this perspective as external attacks which break social systems [8], which exert a disruptive effect on the social structure [18]. The social, political and economic environment is as determinant as the natural environment: it is what turns an event into a disaster [19]. Social disruption may create more difficulties than the physical consequences of the event [20].

The United Nations Coordinating Committee for Disasters [21] stipulates that a disaster, seen from a sociological point of view, is an event located in time and space, producing conditions under which the continuity of the structures and of the social processes becomes problematic. The American College of Emergency Medicine [22] points out that a disaster is a massive and speedy disproportion between hostile elements of any kind and the available survival resources. The same appears in a definition by the World Health Organization [23]: "A disaster is a severe psychological and psychosocial disruption, that largely exceeds the ability to cope of the affected community". In the United Nations glossary [24] we find the same: "A serious disruption of the functioning of society, causing widespread human, material, or environmental losses which exceed the ability of affected society to cope using only its own resources".

Crocq *et al.* [25] point out the importance of the loss of social organisation after a disaster. For them the most constant characteristic is the alteration of social systems that secure the harmonious functioning of a society (information systems, circulation of persons and goods, production and energy consumption, food and water distribution, health care, public order and security, as well as everything related to the corpses and funerary ceremonies in cemeteries).

In summary, disasters are events affecting a social group which produce such material and human losses that the resources of the community are overwhelmed and, therefore, the usual social mechanisms to cope with emergencies are insufficient.

The impact of the disaster can be cushioned by the ability of those affected to adapt psychologically, by the ability of the community structures to adapt to the event and its consequences or by the quantity and kind of external help.

Therefore, three levels of disaster have been described: level I (a localised event with few victims; with local health resources available, adequate to screen and treat; and with transportation means available for further diagnosis and treatment); level II (there are a lot of victims and resources are not enough; help coming from various organisms at a regional level is needed – the definition varies according to the size and kind of territorial organisation of the country); level III (the harm is massive; local and regional resources available are insufficient; and the deficiencies are so significant that national or international help is needed).

Thus, a disaster is something exceptional not only because of its magnitude. Mobilising more material and staff is not sufficient; unfamiliar tasks have to be carried out, changes in the organisation of the institutions are needed, new organisations appear, and persons and institutions which normally do not respond to emergencies are mobilised. Moreover, in some cases, the efficacy of teams and resources commonly utilised for emergencies decreases, and the normal processes aimed at coordinating the response of the community to the emergency may not adapt correctly to the situation.

Disasters induce huge social mobilisations and solidarity [26]. Sometimes a great part of this help is counterproductive, creating the so-called problems of the "second disaster", when excessive and unorganised help arrives causing a slowdown in recovery and interfering with the long-term evolution.

Several things are needed in order to produce a disaster: an extraordinary event capable of destroying material goods, of causing the death of persons or of producing injuries and suffering [27], or an event in the face of which the community lacks adequate social resources to react [28]. This leads to the need for intervention and external support, to a personal sensation of helplessness and threat, to tensions between social systems and individuals [29], and to a deterioration of the links that unite the population and that generate the sense of belonging to the community [30].

SOCIAL VULNERABILITY

Disasters do not only affect social functioning; they are also the consequence of a certain social vulnerability hardly perceived until they occur. They reveal previous failures.

Vulnerability decreases with the degree of development of civilisation, which in essence precisely aims to protect human beings from the negative consequences of their behaviour and from the forces unleashed by nature [31].

This social vulnerability is present even in the pathological reactions to disasters. Among the risk factors for post-traumatic stress disorder most often identified in the USA are: female sex; Hispanic ethnicity [32]; personal and family history of psychiatric disorders; experiences with previous traumas, especially during childhood; poor social stability; low intelligence; neurotic traits; low self-esteem; negative beliefs about oneself and the world and an external locus of control [33]. Curiously enough, there is a preventing factor which is political activism.

In the toxic oil syndrome catastrophe [34], social vulnerability was particularly evident since the toxin did not cross the haemato-encephalic (blood–brain) barrier and those affected did not suffer from symptoms due to a direct cerebral harm. The factors related to the appearance of psychopathological sequelae were female sex, low socio-economic level, low educational level, and the previous history of "nervous disorders" and of psychiatric consultations.

POST-MODERN PERSPECTIVE

Quarantelli [1] introduced a post-modern perspective considering disasters from the subjective perspective of those affected, including rescue staff and all those who have been involved in any way or even showed interest. Any disaster affects intimately and stirs up the foundations of the world everyone builds for his/her own and where he/she lives. Moreover, a disaster affects a community and is like a magnifying glass that increases the appreciation of the lack of social justice and equity. From this perspective, disasters are part of a social change; they are more an opportunity than an event; they are social crises which open new perspectives.

DISASTERS ARE POLITICAL EVENTS

If politics is an allocation of values, the link between politics and disasters is determined by the allocation of values by the authorities regarding security in the period previous to the event, the survival possibilities during the emergency stage and the opportunities to survive during recovery and reconstruction [35].

A disaster is also a political opportunity to develop innovative initiatives, essential to diminish the present and future consequences of the danger. However, not all events attract the same degree of attention and unleash a political reaction. Social vulnerability, as mentioned before, and politics play an important role here [36]. A thorough statistical study [37] on the relationship between the severity of a disaster and political stability showed that reactions to a disaster are affected by the repression exercised by an authoritarian regime or by a high level of development, but not by inequality of income.

There is also a political use of disasters, analysed by Edelman [38]. Governments usually behave in different ways when confronted with problems and with a crisis. In the case of problems they try to induce a systematic deflation of the attention to the inequality of the goods and services offered to the population. On the other hand, in the case of a crisis, they try to induce a systematic inflation of the attention to threats, allowing them to legitimise and demand an increase of authority. When a crisis occurs repeatedly, authoritarianism increases.

SCAPEGOATING IN DISASTERS

Disasters are a great opportunity to appoint scapegoats; efforts to lay the burden of guilt on a person or a group are constant. According to Allinson [39],

> Whenever a single cause for any event is sought in the human realm, it is thus very natural for one to look for who, as a singular agent, is responsible. If the event in question is a disaster, then the first inclination is to look for whose fault it is. Once blame can be assigned, the existence of the disaster will have been explained. Finding the guilty party or parties solves the disaster "problem". Of course it does not. What it does do, however, is to create the appearance of a solution, and this

appearance of a solution cannot assist one in the prevention of further disasters.

But scapegoating is not a means for finding and assigning responsibility. It is a means of avoiding finding and assigning true responsibility. Whenever the scapegoat mentality is at work, responsibility has been abrogated, not shouldered.

A DISASTER UNMASKS FALSE MYTHS

A disaster is an empirical falsification of human action, the proof of the incorrectness of human beings' conceptions on nature and culture [2] Not only structures and social functioning are affected; many mental schemes also break down. All of a sudden the loss of the sense of invulnerability becomes obvious [40]. Frankel [41], who survived a Nazi concentration camp, Brüll [42] and others have pointed out that, after such an experience, the vision of the world, of oneself, of the future, changes. Therefore, during the phase of overcoming the trauma, a process of re-adaptation to reality, a re-elaboration of the trauma [43], the establishment of new beliefs, and the overcoming of old and false beliefs ("the world is a safe place") and of new negative ones ("all the worst always happens to me") is needed.

VICTIMS OR DAMAGED?

The worst thing that can happen is the victimisation of those affected and here psychiatry can play an important role. Benyakar [18] has called attention to this. A "victim" is a person who remains trapped by the situation, petrified in that position, who passes from being an individual to becoming an object of the social reality, losing his/her subjectivity. "Damnified" is the person that has suffered a damage, prone to be repaired or irreparable, wholly or partly. The concept "damnified" connotes psychic mobility, as well as the preserving of the individual's subjectivity. Therefore, mental health services have to assist all those affected, not as victims but as damnified.

COMPENSATIONS IN DISASTERS

Reactions to disasters and their definition have always been marked by compensation. The literature on compensation neurosis is an old one [44]. In fact, the definitions that emphasise the presence of a stressing agent of great magnitude which would affect almost any person, such as that proposed by the DSM-III, turn even witnesses into victims. Since a disaster destroys social frameworks, it is obvious that any individual will turn to society to ask that the harm suffered be repaired. This is why there is a tendency of the victims to maximise "secondary benefits", perpetuating the psychic harm in order to receive a compensation, be it economic, affective or of any other kind. This is reinforced by the fact that the psychic harm usually affects persons who functioned normally before the disaster.

Compensations in disasters are indispensable and have to include psychic harms. However, the repercussion on the mental health of the damnified must also be evaluated. It is true that anybody has the right to change his/her lifestyle and, if the opportunity is given, to change it for another one in which he/she becomes a passive individual prone to the protection (and mending) of the government. But it is also true that mental health professionals are there to avoid iatrogenic effects and should help the damnified to overcome this situation, preventing the disability from becoming chronic. It is also true that society can impose limits to prevent any possible victimisation abuses.

Mental health professionals should participate in the allotting of indemnification and in the decision to include the damnified in a programme of reintegration into their everyday activities [18].

REFERENCES

1. Quarantelli E.L. (Ed.) (1998) *What is a Disaster?* Routledge, London.
2. Dombrowsky W.R. (1998) Again and again – is a disaster what we call a "disaster". In E.L. Quarantelli (Ed.), *What is a Disaster?*, pp. 241–254. Routledge, London.
3. Sheehan L., Hewitt H. (1969) Pilot survey of global natural disasters of the past twenty years. University of Toronto, Natural Hazard Research, Toronto.
4. Tobin G.A., Montz B.E. (1997) *Natural Hazards: Explanation and Integration.* Guilford, New York.
5. Wright S.B. (1997) Northridge Earthquake: Property Tax Relief. Disaster Legislation. White House, Washington, DC.
6. Dynes R.R. (1998) Coming to terms with community disaster. In E.L. Quarantelli (Ed.), *What is a Disaster?*, pp. 109–126. Routledge, London.
7. Holmsten B.Y., Lubertozz A. (2001) *The Complete War of the Worlds.* Sourcebooks, Napervill.
8. Burton I., Kates R.W. (1964) The perception of natural hazards in resource management. *Natural Resources J*, **3**: 412–441.
9. Burton I., Kates R., White G. (1993) *The Environment as Hazard*, 2nd edn. Guilford, New York.
10. Green B.L. (1982) Assessing levels of psychological impairment following disaster. *J Nerv Ment Dis*, **170**: 544–552.
11. López-Ibor J.J. (1942) *Neurosis de Guerra.* Científico-Médica, Madrid.

12. Rojas Ballesteros L. (1943) Alteraciones psíquicas de guerra. *Actas Luso-Españolas de Neurología y Psiquiatría*, **3**: 90–112.
13. Steinberg T. (2000) *The Acts of God: The Unnatural History of Disasters in America*. Oxford University Press, New York.
14. Benz G. (1989) List of major natural disasters. 1960–1987. *Earthquake and Volcanoes*, **20**: 226–228.
15. Easterly W. (2001) *The Elusive Quest for Growth, Economists' Adventures and Misadventures in the Tropics*. MIT Press, Cumberland.
16. Carr L. (1932) Disaster and the sequence-pattern concept of social change. *Am J Sociol*, **38**: 207–218.
17. Quarantelli E.L. (1997) Ten criteria for evaluating the management of community disasters. *Disasters*, **21**: 39–56.
18. Benyakar M. (2002) Salud mental en situaciones de desastres: nuevos desafíos. *Revista de Neurología Neurocirugía y Psiquiatría de Méjico*, **35**: 3–25.
19. Blaikie P., Cannon T., Davis I., Wisner B. (1994) *At Risk: Natural Hazards, People's Vulnerability, and Disasters*. Routledge, London.
20. Quarantelli E.L. (1988) Community and organizational preparations for and responses to acute chemical emergencies and disasters in the United States: research findings and their wider applicability. In H.B.F. Gow, R.W. Kay (Eds.), *Emergency Planning for Industrial Hazards*, pp. 251–273. Elsevier, Amsterdam.
21. United Nations Disaster Relief Coordinator Office (1984) *Disaster Prevention and Mitigation*, Vol. II: *Preparedness Aspects*. United Nations, New York.
22. American College of Emergency Physicians (1985) Disaster medical services. *Ann Emerg Med*, **14**: 1026.
23. World Health Organization (1991) *Psychosocial Consequences of Disasters – Prevention and Management*. World Health Organization, Geneva.
24. United Nations Department of Humanitarian Affairs (1992) *Internationally Agreed Glossary of Basic Terms Related to Disaster Management*. United Nations, Geneva.
25. Crocq L., Doutheau C., Salham M. (1987) Les réactions emotionnelles dans les catastrophes. In *Encyclopédie Médico-Chirurgicale*. Éditions Techniques, Paris, 37-113-D-10.
26. Blocker T.J., Rochford E.B., Sherkat D.E. (1991) Political responses to natural disaster: social movement participation following a flood disaster. *International Journal of Mass Emergencies and Disasters*, **9**: 367–382.
27. Cohen R. (1999) *Salud Mental para Víctimas de Desastres. Manual para Trabajadores*. Organización Panamericana de la Salud, Washington, DC.
28. Anderson, J.W. (1968) Cultural adaptation to threatened disaster. *Human Organizations*, **27**: 298–307.
29. Schulberg H.C. (1974) Disaster, crisis theory and intervention strategies. *Omega*, **5**: 77–87.
30. Erikson P., Drabek T.E., Key W.H., Crowe J.L. (1976) Families in disaster. *Mass Emergencies*, **1**: 206–213.
31. Gilbert J.E. (1958) Human behaviour under conditions of disaster. *Med Serv J Can*, **14**: 318–324.
32. Ruef A.M., Litz B.T., Schlenger W.E. (2000) Hispanic ethnicity and risk for combat-related posttraumatic stress disorder. *Cultur Divers Ethnic Minor Psychol*, **6**: 235–251.
33. Van Zelst W.H., de Beurs E., Beekman A.T., Deeg D.J., van Dyck R. (2003) Prevalence and risk factors of posttraumatic stress disorder in older adults. *Psychother Psychosom*, **72**: 333–342.

34. López-Ibor J.J. Jr, Soria J., Cañas F., Rodriguez-Gamazo M. (1985) Psycho-pathological aspects of the toxic oil syndrome catastrophe. *Br J Psychiatry*, **147**: 352–365.
35. Olson R.S. (2000) Toward a politics of disaster: losses, values, agendas, and blame. *International Journal of Mass Emergencies and Disasters*, **18**: 265–287.
36. Birkland T.A. (1997) *After Disaster*. Georgetown University Press, Washington, DC.
37. Drury A.C., Olson R.S. (1998) Disasters and political unrest: an empirical investigation. *Journal of Contingencies and Crisis Management*, **6**: 153–161.
38. Edelman M. (1977) *Political Language: Words that Succeed and Policies that Fail*. Academic Press, Boca Raton, FL.
39. Allinson R.E. (1993) *Global Disasters: Inquiries into Management Ethics*. Prentice Hall, New York.
40. Lifton R.J. (1979) *The Broken Connection*. Simon & Schuster, New York.
41. Frankel V. (1962) *Man's Search for Meaning*. Beacon Press, Boston.
42. Brüll F. (1969) The trauma – theoretical considerations. *Isr Am Psychiatr Relat Discip*, **7**: 96–108.
43. Horowitz M.J. (1993) Stress-response syndromes: a review of posttraumatic stress and adjustment disorders. In J.P. Wilson, B. Raphael (Eds.), *International Handbook of Traumatic Stress Syndromes*, pp. 145–155. Plenum Press, New York.
44. Kinzie J.D., Goetz R.R. (1996) A century of controversy surrounding posttraumatic stress stress-spectrum syndromes: the impact on DSM-III and DSM-IV. *J Trauma Stress*, **9**: 159–179.

2

Psychological and Psychopathological Consequences of Disasters

Carol S. Fullerton and Robert J. Ursano

Uniformed Services University of the Health Sciences,
Bethesda, MD, USA

INTRODUCTION

The majority of people exposed to trauma and disasters do well. However, some individuals experience distress, others have behavioral changes and some develop psychiatric illness post disaster. Such illnesses include those that are secondary to physical injury (e.g., organic brain disorders, psychological responses to physical disease) as well as specific trauma-related psychiatric disorders such as acute stress disorder (ASD), post-traumatic stress disorder (PTSD) and trauma-related depression [1]. The extent of the psychiatric morbidity depends on a number of factors, e.g., type of disaster, exposure, degree of injury, amount of life threat, and the duration of individual and community disruption. At times, traumatic events and disasters have beneficial effects by serving as organizing events and providing a sense of purpose and an opportunity for positive growth experiences [2,3]. The effects of trauma and disaster may be rekindled by new experiences that remind the person of the past traumatic event [4]. The effects of trauma and disaster also impact the community, the recovery environment for those affected by the traumatic event. In this chapter we examine the psychiatric responses to trauma and disasters including risk factors and mediators of the psychiatric, psychological and behavioral consequences of trauma and disaster.

Disasters and Mental Health. Edited by Juan José López-Ibor, George Christodoulou, Mario Maj, Norman Sartorius and Ahmed Okasha.
©2005 John Wiley & Sons Ltd. ISBN 0-470-02123-3.

HISTORY

The study of emotional reactions to disasters began with observations of the oldest human-made disaster, war. In the United States during the American Civil War, combat psychiatric casualties were thought to be suffering from "nostalgia", which was considered to be a type of melancholy, or mild type of insanity, caused by disappointment and longing for home [5]. This was also known as "soldier's heart". In World Wars I and II, terms such as "shell shock", "battle fatigue", and "war neuroses" were more common descriptors of the emotional responses to trauma [6,7]. The "thousand-mile stare" described the exhausted foot soldier on the verge of collapse. The symptoms of combat stress varied with the individual and the context but included anxiety, startle reactions and numbness [8] Some of the earliest descriptions of what is now referred to as PTSD came from traumatic injury. For example, in 1871 Rigler described the effects of injuries caused by railroad accidents as "compensation neurosis" [7]. In 1892 Sir William Osler [9], first Chief of Medicine at Johns Hopkins University, described the condition that followed an accident or shock as traumatic neurosis (also known as "railway brain", "railway spine", and "traumatic hysteria"). At the end of the nineteenth and beginning of the twentieth century, railway disasters, the World Wars, the Holocaust, and the atom bomb attacks on Hiroshima and Nagasaki prompted systematic descriptions of symptoms associated with traumatic stress. Labels included "fright neurosis", "survivor syndrome", "nuclearism", "operational fatigue" and "compensation neurosis". Charcot, Janet, Freud and Breurer suggested that psychological trauma caused hysterical symptoms; however, others at the time believed that a traumatic event was not sufficient to cause post-traumatic symptoms and organic causes were sought. This changed with the recognition that many veterans of the Vietnam War had long-term psychiatric and psychological problems and people without prior psychiatric difficulties could develop clinically significant psychiatric symptoms if they were exposed to horrific stressors. Following this the diagnosis of PTSD became a category in DSM-III [10].

Studies of the responses of various populations to traumatic experiences broadened our understanding of the psychiatric and psychological effects of trauma, e.g., concentration camp survivors [11–14], and rescue workers following the Hiroshima devastation [15]. The psychiatric and psychological consequences of several modern disasters have been studied in detail: the 1942 Coconut Grove Nightclub Fire [16,17], the 1972 Buffalo Creek Flood [18–20], the 1980 Mount St. Helens volcanic eruption [21,22], the Granville rail disaster, 1977 in a Sydney suburb [23], the imprisonment and torture of Norwegian sailors in Libya in 1984 [24], and the volcanic eruption in Colombia, 1985 that destroyed the town of Armero [25].

PSYCHIATRIC DISORDERS RELATED TO TRAUMA AND DISASTER

We are only in the infancy of understanding why some people exposed to traumatic events develop post-traumatic psychopathology and some people do not (for a meta-analysis of predictors of PTSD, see 26). Post-traumatic psychiatric disorders are most often seen in those directly exposed to the threat to life and the horror of a traumatic event. The greater the "dose" of traumatic stressors, the more likely an individual or group is to develop high rates of psychiatric morbidity. Certain groups, however, are at increased risk for psychiatric sequelae. Those at greatest risk are the primary victims, those who have significant attachments with the primary victims, first responders, and support providers [27]. Adults, children, and the elderly in particular who were in physical danger and who directly witnessed the events are at risk. Those who were psychologically vulnerable before exposure to a traumatic event may also be buffeted by the fears and realities of, for example, job losses, untenably longer commutes or eroded interpersonal and community support systems overtaxed now by increased demands. Persons who are injured are at higher risk, reflecting both their high level of exposure to life threat and the added persistent reminders and additional stress burden accompanying an injury. The Epidemiologic Catchment Area study of Vietnam veterans [28] documented a higher rate of PTSD in wounded than in non-wounded veterans. Similar findings were noted in the Veterans Affairs study [29,30].

Pre-existing psychiatric illness or symptoms are not necessary for psychiatric morbidity after a traumatic event, nor are they sufficient to account for it [31–34]. Nearly 40% of survivors of the Oklahoma City bombing with PTSD or depression had no previous history of psychiatric illness [35]. Therefore, those needing treatment will not all have the usually expected accompanying risk factors and coping strategies of other mental health populations. The less severe the disaster or traumatic event, the more important pre-disaster variables such as neuroticism or a history of psychiatric disorder appear to be [32,36–39]. The more severe the stressor, the less pre-existing psychiatric disorders predict outcome.

Overall, children and adolescents are at increased risk for psychiatric sequelae following trauma. Psychiatric disorders including PTSD, depression, and separation anxiety disorder [40] as well as the onset of a wide range of symptoms and behaviors [41,42] have been identified in children exposed to trauma. The re-experiencing symptoms common in ASD and PTSD may be evident in children through repetitive play with trauma themes, nightmares, and "trauma-specific reenactment" [43]. Children may also develop avoidant behavior to specific reminders of the tragedy (e.g., avoiding areas of the playground where someone has been killed) and the wish to stay home rather than be separated from family and loved ones. Other reactions commonly seen in children include fear of recurrence, worries about the safety of others, and guilt. Of special concern are increased risk-taking behaviors sometimes seen in adolescents following trauma [44]. The reactions of significant adults (e.g., parents and teachers) can greatly affect children's responses to trauma [45].

Media exposure is a part of nearly all community disaster events. Media exposure can be both reassuring and threatening. Limiting such exposure can minimize the disturbing effects especially in children [46]. Educating spouses and significant others of those distressed can assist in treatment as well as in identifying the worsening or persistence of symptoms.

Acute Stress Disorder and Post-Traumatic Stress Disorder

Exposure to a traumatic event, the essential element for development of ASD or PTSD, is a relatively common experience. Approximately 50–70% of the US population are exposed to a traumatic event sometime during their lifetime; however, only approximately 5–12% develop PTSD. In a nationally representative study of 5,877 people aged 15–45 in the US, the National Comorbidity Study (NCS) [47] found lifetime prevalence of exposure to trauma to be 60.7% in men and 51.2% in women. In a nationally representative sample of women in the US, the National Women's Study (NWS) [48] found that 69.0% of women were exposed to a traumatic event at some time in their lives. NCS found rates of PTSD to be 7.8%, while the NWS found rates of PTSD to be 12.3%. In an epidemiological study of people belonging to an urban health maintenance organization in the US, Breslau et al. [49] found the lifetime prevalence of PTSD to be 9.2% for adults. These studies used the DSM-III and DSM-III-R [50] Criterion A requiring only that the event be outside the range of human experience. In DSM-IV, this was replaced with Criterion A2, which requires that the response to the stressor be one of intense fear, helplessness, or horror.

PTSD has been widely studied following both natural and human-made disasters (for review, see 51). PTSD is not uncommon following many traumatic events, from terrorism to motor vehicle accidents to industrial explosions. In its acute form, PTSD may be more like the common cold, experienced at some time in one's life by nearly all. If it persists, it can be debilitating and require psychotherapeutic and/or pharmacological intervention.

Curiously absent from DSM-III and DSM-III-R was a diagnostic category for acute responses to trauma and disaster events. With the diagnosis of ASD, DSM-IV [52] acknowledged a broader spectrum of responses to traumatic events. Because ASD is a relatively new diagnosis, empirical investigations are just beginning to examine its course and outcome [53,54]. However, recent studies of war suggest that acute combat-related stress reactions (which could now be thought of as representing an ASD) predict an adverse outcome [32] and are associated with increased rates of somatic complaints [55–57]. Numerous investigations also document that acute symptoms of intrusion, avoidance, and dissociation [58], part of the symptom complex of ASD, predict the development of later psychiatric disorders, particularly PTSD [59–64]. Early symptoms usually respond to education, obtaining enough rest and maintaining biological rhythms (e.g. sleep at the same time, eat at the same time) [65].

The Traumatic Stressor Criterion: Criterion A

Recognizing that traumatic stressors are all too often a part of everyday life, DSM-IV [52] deleted the DSM-III-R [50] requirement that the stressor be "outside the range of usual human experience". An essential feature for ASD and PTSD in the DSM-IV is development of "intense fear, help-lessness, or horror" after exposure to a traumatic event that does not need to be outside the normal range of human experience (Criterion A) [43] (see Tables 2.1 and 2.2). Exposure can involve direct experience or witnessing or learning about a traumatic event that caused "actual or threatened death", "serious injury", or "threat to the physical integrity" of oneself or others. Both natural (e.g., tornadoes, earthquakes) and human-made traumatic events (e.g., accidents, rape, assault, war, terrorism) can evoke these symptoms. Some of these traumatic events occur only once while others involve chronic or repeated exposure.

In general, human-made traumatic events (as opposed to natural disasters) have been shown to cause more frequent and more persistent psychiatric symptoms and distress (for review see 66). However, this distinction is increasingly difficult to make. The etiology and consequences of natural disasters often are affected by human beings. For example, the damage and loss of life caused by an earthquake can be magnified by poor construction practices and high-density occupancy. Similarly, humans may cause or contribute to natural disasters through poor land-management practices that increase the probability of floods. Interpersonal violence between individuals (assault) or groups (war, terrorism) is perhaps the most disturbing traumatic experience. Technological disasters may bring specific psychiatric concerns about normal life events – for example, fear of flying after a plane crash or claustrophobia after a mine accident. Each of these requires evaluation and intervention to treat the specific phobia and limit generalization to other areas of life (e.g., "I cannot cook any more because the boiling water reminds me of the explosion").

TABLE 2.1   DSM-IV-TR diagnostic criteria for acute stress disorder (308.3)

A. The person has been exposed to a traumatic event in which both of the following were present:
   1. the person experienced, witnessed, or was confronted with an event or events that involved actual or threatened death or serious injury, or a threat to the physical integrity of self or others
   2. the person's response involved intense fear, helplessness, or horror
B. Either while experiencing or after experiencing the distressing event, the individual has three (or more) of the following dissociative symptoms:
   1. a subjective sense of numbing, detachment, or absence of emotional responsiveness
   2. a reduction in awareness of his or her surroundings (e.g., "being in a daze")
   3. derealization
   4. depersonalization
   5. dissociative amnesia (i.e., inability to recall an important aspect of the trauma)
C. The traumatic event is persistently re-experienced in at least one of the following ways: recurrent images, thoughts, dreams, illusions, flashback episodes, or a sense of reliving the experience; or distress on exposure to reminders of the traumatic event.
D. Marked avoidance of stimuli that arouse recollections of the trauma (e.g., thoughts, feelings, conversations, activities, places, people).
E. Marked symptoms of anxiety or increased arousal (e.g., difficulty sleeping, irritability, poor concentration, hypervigilance, exaggerated startle response, motor restlessness).
F. The disturbance causes clinically significant distress or impairment in social, occupational, or other important areas of functioning or impairs the individual's ability to pursue some necessary task, such as obtaining necessary assistance or mobilizing personal resources by telling family members about the traumatic experience.
G. The disturbance lasts for a minimum of 2 days and a maximum of 4 weeks and occurs within 4 weeks of the traumatic event.
H. The disturbance is not due to the direct physiological effects of a substance (e.g., a drug of abuse, a medication) or a general medical condition, is not better accounted for by Brief Psychotic Disorder, and is not merely an exacerbation of a preexisting Axis I or Axis II disorder.

Perhaps the best predictors of both the probability and the frequency of post-disaster psychiatric illness are the severity of the traumatic stressor and the degree of exposure. Shore et al. [21,22] found that psychiatric outcome was related to the intensity of disaster exposure following the Mount St. Helens volcanic eruption. They documented higher rates of post-disaster psychiatric illnesses, including PTSD, generalized anxiety disorder, and depression, in those who lived closer to the volcano. Additional evidence for the association of psychiatric illness and severity of the traumatic stressor is seen in the study of war trauma. Higher rates of PTSD, depression and alcohol abuse were significantly related to greater exposure

TABLE 2.2 DSM-IV-TR diagnostic criteria for post-traumatic stress disorder (309.81)

A. The person has been exposed to a traumatic event in which both of the following were present:
   1. the person experienced, witnessed, or was confronted with an event or events that involved actual or threatened death or serious injury, or a threat to the physical integrity of self or others
   2. the person's response involved intense fear, helplessness, or horror. Note: In children, this may be expressed instead by disorganized or agitated behavior
B. The traumatic event is persistently re-experienced in one (or more) of the following ways:
   1. recurrent and intrusive distressing recollections of the event, including images, thoughts, or perceptions. Note: In young children, repetitive play may occur in which themes or aspects of the trauma are expressed
   2. recurrent distressing dreams of the event. Note: In children, there may be frightening dreams without recognizable content
   3. acting or feeling as if the traumatic event were recurring (includes a sense of reliving the experience, illusions, hallucinations, and dissociative flashback episodes, including those that occur on awakening or when intoxicated). Note: In young children, trauma-specific reenactment may occur
   4. intense psychological distress at exposure to internal or external cues that symbolize or resemble an aspect of the traumatic event
   5. physiological reactivity on exposure to internal or external cues that symbolize or resemble an aspect of the traumatic event
C. Persistent avoidance of stimuli associated with the trauma and numbing of general responsiveness (not present before the trauma), as indicated by three (or more) of the following:
   1. efforts to avoid thoughts, feelings, or conversations associated with the trauma
   2. efforts to avoid activities, places, or people that arouse recollections of the trauma
   3. inability to recall an important aspect of the trauma
   4. markedly diminished interest or participation in significant activities
   5. feeling of detachment or estrangement from others
   6. restricted range of affect (e.g., unable to have loving feelings)
   7. sense of a foreshortened future (e.g., does not expect to have a career, marriage, children, or a normal life span)
D. Persistent symptoms of increased arousal (not present before the trauma), as indicated by two (or more) of the following:
   1. difficulty falling or staying asleep
   2. irritability or outbursts of anger
   3. difficulty concentrating
   4. hypervigilance
   5. exaggerated startle response
E. Duration of the disturbance (symptoms in Criteria B, C, and D) is more than 1 month.
F. The disturbance causes clinically significant distress or impairment in social, occupational, or other important areas of functioning.
Specify if:
   Acute: if duration of symptoms is less than 3 months.
   Chronic: if duration of symptoms is 3 months or more.
Specify if:
   With Delayed Onset: if onset of symptoms is at least 6 months after the stressor.

to combat in Vietnam [29]. In an interesting investigation of PTSD in monozygotic twins discordant for service in Vietnam, Goldberg *et al.* [31] found that PTSD was nine times as common in the twins who had been exposed to a high level of combat in Vietnam as it was in those who had not served in Southeast Asia.

Psychiatric morbidity is more likely to be engendered by some dimensions of traumatic events than others. The highest risk of psychiatric morbidity is associated with high perceived threat to life, low controllability, lack of predictability, high loss, injury, possibility that the disaster will recur, and exposure to the grotesque [35,52,67–71]. For example, terrorism often can be distinguished from other natural and human-made disasters by the characteristic extensive fear, loss of confidence in institutions, unpredictability and pervasive experience of loss of safety [72]. In a longitudinal national study of reactions to the September 11, 2001 disaster, 64.6% of people outside of New York City reported fears of future terrorism at 2 months and 37.5% at 6 months [73]. In addition, 59.5% reported fear of harm to family at 2 months and 40.6% at 6 months. Terrorism is one of the most powerful and pervasive generators of psychiatric illness, distress and disrupted community and social functioning [35,74].

Vulnerability to psychiatric distress is increased by knowledge that one has been exposed to toxins (e.g., chemicals or radiation) [75,76]. In this case, information itself is the primary stressor. Toxic exposures often have the added stress of being clouded in uncertainty as to whether or not exposure has taken place and what the long-term health consequences may be. Living with the uncertainty can be exceedingly stressful. Typically uncertainty accompanies bioterrorism and is the focus of much concern in the medical community preparing for responses to terrorist attacks using biological, chemical, or nuclear agents [73,77–79].

Symptoms of ASD and PTSD

The diagnostic criteria for ASD closely resemble those of PTSD (see Table 2.3), with the primary difference being time course and the inclusion of dissociative symptoms required for a diagnosis of ASD. The diagnosis of PTSD applies if the symptoms persist longer than 1 month or if the onset of symptoms begins later than 1 month after the traumatic event. Importantly, the severity of symptoms for both ASD and PTSD must be sufficient to cause "clinically significant distress" or impaired functioning (Criterion F) [43]. Symptoms of ASD and PTSD are categorized into three clusters: persistent re-experiencing of the stressor (Criterion B for PTSD and Criterion C for ASD), persistent avoidance of reminders of the event and numbing of general responsiveness (Criterion C for PTSD and Criteria B and D for ASD), and persistent symptoms

TABLE 2.3 Comparison of acute stress disorder (ASD) and post-traumatic stress disorder (PTSD)

	ASD	PTSD
Nature of the trauma/reaction to the trauma		
• Individual experienced, witnessed, or was confronted with an event that involved actual or threatened death or serious injury, or a threat to the physical integrity of self or others	✗	✗
• Individual's response involved intense feelings of fear, horror, or helplessness	✗	✗
Symptom criteria		
• Persistent re-experiencing of the trauma	✗	✗
• Avoidance of reminders of the trauma	✗	✗
• Physical symptoms of hyperarousal	✗	✗
• Symptoms of dissociation during or immediately after the trauma	✗	
• Clinically significant distress or impairment	✗	✗
Time requirements		
• Duration of symptom constellation	2 days–4 weeks	>1 month
• Onset of symptoms in relation to trauma	Within 4 weeks of trauma	Anytime post trauma

of increased arousal (Criterion D). Criterion B for ASD requires that the individual has experienced three or more dissociative symptoms during or following the traumatic event. For ASD, Criterion D requires "marked avoidance of stimuli that arouse recollections of the trauma" [43]. These criteria for ASD overlap with Criterion C for PTSD but are not identical.

The re-experiencing cluster includes symptoms of "recurrent and intrusive recollections" of the event, recurrent distressing trauma-related dreams, acting or feeling as if the event were re-occurring, "intense psychological distress" with exposure to trauma cues, and physiological reactivity to traumatic cues [43]. DSM-IV moved the physiological symptoms related to reminders of the traumatic event from the arousal cluster to the re-experiencing cluster. This change reflects recent advances in understanding the biology of PTSD and its relation to memory [80]. The avoidance/numbing cluster may include purposeful actions as well as unconscious mechanisms, e.g., efforts to avoid trauma-related thoughts, feelings, or conversations; efforts to avoid activities, places, or people reminiscent of the trauma; inability to recall important aspects of the trauma; greatly decreased "interest or participation in previously enjoyed activities"; feeling detached or estranged; restricted range of affect; and a "sense of a foreshortened future" [43]. Increased arousal includes sleep disturbance, "irritability or outbursts of anger", difficulty concentrating, hypervigilance, and exaggerated startle response [43], not precipitated by reminders of the stressor but representing generalized arousal.

PTSD and ASD differ in the numbers of symptoms from each cluster that are required. For a diagnosis of PTSD, there must be at least one re-experiencing symptom, two arousal symptoms and three avoidance/numbing symptoms and it is required that these be temporally related to the stressor. A diagnosis of ASD requires at least one re-experiencing symptom and "marked avoidance of stimuli that arouse recollections of the trauma", and "marked" anxiety or increased arousal as well as three or more dissociative symptoms. The dissociative symptoms can occur during the traumatic event itself or after it. A common early response to traumatic exposure appears to be a disturbance in our sense of time, our internal time clock, resulting in time distortion – time feeling speeded up or slowed down [81]. Along with other ASD dissociative symptoms, time distortion indicates an over four times greater risk for chronic PTSD and may also be an accompaniment of depressive symptoms.

ASD and PTSD also differ in duration of symptoms and temporal relationship to the traumatic stressor. ASD occurs within 4 weeks of the traumatic event and has a duration of 2 days to 4 weeks. For a diagnosis of PTSD, symptoms must be present for more than 1 month. If symptom duration is less than 3 months, acute PTSD is diagnosed. Chronic PTSD is diagnosed when symptoms persist for 3 months or longer. Symptoms of PTSD usually begin within 3 months of exposure.

Delayed onset PTSD (i.e., symptoms that begin 6 months or more after the stressor) is indicated in DSM-IV-TR [43]; however, "true" delayed PTSD (rather than subthreshold that later meets criteria) appears to be much more uncommon than previously reported. Clinically, in cases of late-onset PTSD or reactivation of previously resolved PTSD, current life events should be explored [35]. At symbolically charged times, such as receiving a diagnosis of cancer or retiring from a long military career, emergence of PTSD symptoms may be thought of as the mind's way of expressing metaphorically in the present significant traumatic events in the past that evoked intense feelings. In such cases, exploration of the patient's current situation is generally more productive than focusing on the past.

Other Trauma-Related Disorders

PTSD is not the only trauma-related disorder, nor perhaps the most common [35,66,82] (see Table 2.4). People exposed to trauma and disaster are at increased risk for depression, generalized anxiety disorder, panic

TABLE 2.4   Trauma-related disorders

Psychiatric diagnoses
• Post-traumatic stress disorder
• Acute stress disorder
• Major depression
• Substance use disorders
• Generalized anxiety disorder
• Adjustment disorder
• Organic mental disorders secondary to head injury, toxic exposure, illness, and dehydration
• Somatization
• Psychological factors affecting physical disease (in the injured)

Psychological/behavioral responses
• Grief reactions and other normal responses to an abnormal event
• Change in interpersonal interactions (withdrawal, aggression, violence, family conflict, family violence)
• Change in work functioning (change in ability to do work, concentration, effectiveness on the job; absenteeism, quitting)
• Change in health care utilization
• Change in smoking
• Change in alcohol use

disorder, and increased substance use [1,47,49,83]. 45% of survivors of the Oklahoma City bombing had a post-disaster psychiatric disorder. Of these, 34.3% had PTSD and 22.5% had major depression [35]. After a disaster or terrorist event the contribution of the psychological factors to medical illness can also be pervasive – from heart disease [84] to diabetes [85]. Traumatic bereavement [86], unexplained somatic symptoms [87,88], depression [89], sleep disturbance, increased alcohol, caffeine, and cigarette use [83,90], and family conflict and family violence are not uncommon following traumatic events. Anger, disbelief, sadness, anxiety, fear, and irritability are expected responses following trauma. For example, anxiety and family conflict can accompany the distress and fear of recurrence of a traumatic event, the ongoing threat of terrorism and the economic impact of lost jobs and companies closed or moving as a result of a disaster. The role of exposure to the traumatic event may be easily overlooked by a primary care physician. Medical evaluation, which includes inquiring about family conflict, can provide reassurance as well as begin a discussion for referral, and be a primary preventive intervention for children whose first experience of a disaster or terrorist attack is mediated through their parents.

Major depression, generalized anxiety disorder, substance abuse, and adjustment disorders in disaster victims have been less often studied than

ASD and PTSD, but available data suggest that these disorders also occur at higher than average rates [21,22,29,91]. Major depression, substance abuse, and adjustment disorders (anxiety and depression) may be relatively common in the 6–12 months after a disaster and may reflect survivors' reactions to their injuries, to affects and feelings stimulated by the disaster, and/or to their attributions of the cause of the disaster. The occurrence of these psychiatric disorders may also be mediated by secondary stressors [83,92] (i.e., the problems associated with disaster recovery, such as negotiations with insurance companies for reimbursement, or unemployment secondary to destroyed businesses) following a disaster. Major depression and substance abuse (drugs, alcohol, and tobacco) are frequently comorbid with PTSD and warrant further study [90,93–95]. Grief reactions are common after all disasters. Available studies of grief reactions following trauma do not greatly aid our understanding of who is at risk for persistent depression. One investigation indicated that single parents may be at high risk for developing psychiatric disorders since they often have fewer resources to begin with, and they lose some of their social supports after a disaster [95].

Somatization is common after a disaster and must be managed both in the community and individual patients [96] as well as in disaster and rescue workers [88]. Primary care providers must recognize that somatization is a frequent presentation of anxiety and depression in patients seeking care in medical clinics. Such recognition can help in the appropriate diagnosis and treatment of these psychiatric disorders, thereby minimizing inappropriate medical treatments. In addition, sleep disturbances following trauma are common clinical problems that may require treatment. Sleep difficulties can be due to anxiety related to recurrent disaster events (e.g., aftershocks), the ongoing threat of terrorist attacks, or to underlying psychiatric disease such as depression or PTSD [97]. These disorders must be considered in the differential diagnosis and appropriate treatments initiated as indicated.

Hostility with its accompanying social disruption, feelings of frustration, and perception of chaos, is also common following trauma [98,99]. Although in some cases it is helpful for individuals to recognize that the return of anger can be a sign of a return to normal (i.e., it is again safe to be angry and express one's losses, disappointments, and needs), in others hostility should remind the care provider to assess the risks of family violence and substance abuse.

Co-occurring psychiatric symptoms are frequently seen in injured survivors who may be dealing with the stress of their injury [22, 29,35,67,91,100,101]. Since studies indicate a high rate of psychiatric disorder in the physically injured, a proactive consultation liaison plan is a necessary part of a hospital emergency response plan.

Increasingly, traumatic bereavement is recognized as posing special challenges to survivors [39,86,103,104]. While the death of loved ones is always painful, an unexpected and violent death can be more difficult. Even when not directly witnessing the death, family members may develop intrusive images based on information gleaned from authorities or the media. In children traumatic play, a phenomenon similar to intrusive symptoms in adults, is both a sign of distress and an effort at mastery [105].

COMMUNITY/WORKPLACE RESPONSES TO DISASTER

The degree to which the disaster disrupts the community and workplace influences the development of post-traumatic stress disorders. In the immediate aftermath of a disaster or terrorist attack, individuals and communities may respond in adaptive, effective ways or they may make fear-based decisions, resulting in unhelpful behaviors. Psychiatric disease and psychological function, including the subthreshold distress of individuals, is dependent upon the rapid, effective, and sustained mobilization of health care resources. Knowledge of an individual's and community's resilience and vulnerability before a disaster (or terrorist event), as well as understanding the psychiatric and psychological responses to such an event, enables leaders and medical experts to talk to the public, promoting resilient healthy behaviors, sustaining the social fabric of the community and facilitating recovery [79,106]. The adaptive capacities of individuals and groups within a community are variable and should be understood before a crisis in order to target needs effectively.

The community and workplace serves as a physical and emotional support system. The larger the scale of the disaster, the greater the potential disruption of the community and workplace. It is helpful to examine the generic and unique challenges facing survivors of an airplane crash as well as those confronting victims of disasters such as a tornadoes or earthquakes or victims of terrorist attacks. If family members were not on the same aircraft, the plane crash survivor can return home to family, friends, and co-workers. They will most likely go back to a structurally intact house, to a community unaffected by the accident, to the same job with the same financial security, and so forth. In contrast, a tornado involves additional factors that amplify the trauma. Although the tornado survivor may experience and witness comparably gruesome sights, the recovery environment is markedly different: home and work site may have been destroyed, and relatives, friends, and co-workers may be dead, injured, or displaced. Thus, psychiatric morbidity is affected by the degree a disaster impacts the community [61,107,108].

The economic impact and consequences of disasters (and terrorist attacks) on individuals and communities are substantial. Loss of a job is a major post event predictor of negative psychiatric outcome. These effects can be seen at the macro level, for example, in a dip in consumer confidence during or after the sniper attacks in the Washington area in October 2002. Certain economic behaviors and decisions are affected both by various characteristics of a disaster (or a terrorist attack) and by the psychological and behavioral responses to the disaster. For example, after a terrorist attack, decisions and behaviors related to travel, home purchase, food consumption, and medical care visits are altered directly by changes in availability, but also by changes in perceived safety, optimism about the future and belief in exposure to toxic agents. The fact that threats and hoaxes carry with them economic costs and consequences perhaps best illustrates the importance of psychological and behavioral effects on economic decisions and behaviors and their associated economic costs. The impact on the local or national economy ranges from altered food consumption, savings, insurance and investment, to changes in work attendance and productivity and broader national or industry specific consequences such as altered financial and insurance markets or disrupted transportation, communication and energy networks.

While there are many definitions of disaster, a common feature is that the event overwhelms local resources and threatens the function and safety of the community. With the advent of instantaneous communication and media coverage, word of terrorism or disaster is disseminated quickly, often witnessed in real time around the globe. The disaster community is soon flooded with outsiders: people offering assistance, curiosity seekers and the media. This sudden influx of strangers affects the community in many ways. The presence of large numbers of media representatives can be experienced as intrusive and insensitive. Hotel rooms have no vacancies, restaurants are crowded with unfamiliar faces, and the normal routine of the community is altered. At a time when, traditionally, communities turn inward to grieve and assist affected families, the normal social supports are strained and disrupted by outsiders.

Inevitably, after any major trauma, there are rumors circulated within the community about the circumstances leading up to the traumatic event and the government response. Sometimes there is a heightened state of fear. For example, a study of a school shooting in Illinois noted that a high level of anxiety continued for a week after the event, even after it was known that the perpetrator had committed suicide [44].

Outpourings of sympathy for the injured, the dead, and their friends and families are common and expected. Impromptu memorials of flowers, photographs, and memorabilia are frequently erected. Churches and synagogues play an important role in assisting communities' search for meaning from the tragedy and in assisting in the grief process.

Over time, anger often emerges in the community. Typically, there is a focus on accountability, a search for someone who was responsible for a lack of preparation or inadequate response. Mayors, police and fire chiefs, and other community leaders are often targets of these strong feelings. Scapegoating can be an especially destructive process when leveled at those who already hold themselves responsible, even if, in reality, there was nothing they could have done to prevent adverse outcomes. In addition, nations and communities experience ongoing hypervigilance and a sense of lost safety while trying to establish a new normal in their lives.

There are many milestones of a disaster which both affect the community and may offer opportunities for recovery. There are the normal rituals associated with burying the dead. Later, energy is poured into creating appropriate memorials. Memorialization carries the potential to cause harm as well as to do good. There can be heated disagreement about what the monument should look like and where it should be placed. Special thought must be given to the placement of memorials. If the monument is situated too prominently so that community members cannot avoid encountering it, the memorial may heighten intrusive recollections and interfere with the resolution of grief reactions. Anniversaries of the disaster (one week, one month, one year) often stimulate renewed grief.

GENERAL FEATURES OF PATHOLOGICAL AND NORMAL RESPONSES TO DISASTER

Phases of Psychological Response to Disaster

Although individual patterns of psychological response to trauma and disaster vary, several phases generally emerge over time [96]. Cohen et al. [109] have identified four phases in the response to disaster. The first, immediately following a disaster, generally consists of strong emotions, including feelings of disbelief, numbness, fear, and confusion. People tend to cooperate, and heroic deeds are sometimes seen. These reactions are best understood as "normal responses to an abnormal event". Rescue personnel, family, and neighbors are generally the support systems that are most heavily used.

The second phase usually lasts from a week to several months after the disaster. At this juncture assistance flows in from agencies external to the community, and the cleanup/rebuilding process begins. In this phase of adaptation, denial alternates with intrusive symptoms. The intrusive symptoms generally arise first and consist of unbidden thoughts and feelings accompanied by autonomic arousal (e.g., a heightened startle response, hypervigilance, insomnia, and nightmares). Toward the end of the adaptation phase, denial is more prominent. This is often accompanied by an increase in visits to physicians for complaints of somatic symptoms such as fatigue, dizziness, headaches, and nausea [110]. Anger, irritability, apathy, and social withdrawal are often present.

The third phase lasts up to a year and is marked by disappointment and resentment when expectations of aid and restoration are not met. During this period the strong sense of community may weaken as individuals focus on their personal concerns.

The final phase, reconstruction, may last for years. During this period disaster survivors gradually rebuild their lives, making homes and finding work. Recovery from a disaster involves the resolution of the initial psychological and somatic symptoms [3] through reappraisal of the event, assignment of meaning, and integration into a new concept of self.

Police, paramedics and other first responders who assist the injured and evacuate them to medical care, and hospital personnel who care for the injured, are all groups that need opportunities to process what happened, education on normal responses and information on when to seek further help. Those who are charged with cleaning up the site of the tragedy are also vulnerable to persistent symptoms. Overidentification with the victims (e.g., "It could have been me") and their pain and grief can perpetuate the fear response [111]. This normally health and growth promoting mechanism of identification with victims and heroes can turn against us in this setting like an autoimmune disorder. Inevitably, each disaster situation will also contain individuals who are "silent" victims and often overlooked. By paying close attention to the patterns and types of exposure, these individuals can be identified and receive proper care. For example, traumatically bereaved parents of adult children are a group often forgotten as community programs and neighbors remember the spouse or partner and children of the deceased.

Meaning of Traumatic Events

Clinical studies suggest that the psychiatric consequences following trauma are influenced by the meaning ascribed to the traumatic event by individuals, families, and communities [4,69,112]. Beliefs about the cause of the disaster and the ramifications of these beliefs (such as self-blame, the shattering of assumptions about human nature, and rage at "those responsible" when the event is viewed as preventable) should be assessed in psychiatric evaluation and represent potential areas for intervention. Chronic PTSD may be particularly related to the meaning of the trauma experienced. Therapists can assist patients in modifying distorted attributions (e.g., "It's all my fault; if only I had insisted that we not go away for the weekend, we wouldn't have been caught in the tornado and my wife would still be alive"). Some events are more likely than others to shatter one's faith in a just and safe world [113]. Consider the implications of the following scenarios. An individual has survived an airplane crash in which many people were injured and killed. Various explanations for the crash exist; each would stimulate a different meaning and emotional response. The plane may have crashed because of sudden and unexpected wind shears, because of uncomplicated pilot error, or because of "complicated" pilot error (e.g., the pilot was under the influence of drugs or alcohol). At the far end of this continuum would be a crash caused by an act of terrorism or greed in which the plane was destroyed to further the interests of a group or an individual.

The construction of meaning is an active process that appears to affect the outcome of the traumatic experience and recovery [114,115]. The meaning of a disaster to any one person results from the interaction of his or her past history, present context, and physiological state. The ascribed meaning will then direct individual behaviors of what to do, what to fix, and whom or what to blame. Meaning is dynamic, not static: it changes over time as the individual's psychosocial context changes. Such alterations can aid or inhibit recovery. For example, immediately following the crash of an Air Force C-141 cargo plane, the remaining members of the squadron were convinced that the accident was caused by aircraft failure. However, this belief was modified as the date grew nearer for the squadron members to fly the same type of plane again. By that time, the squadron's belief had changed, and members thought that the crash must have been caused by human error. If it were human error, one could feel safe: "I would never do that."

Resilience

Although the psychiatric consequences of trauma have been associated with debility that can persist for decades, the effects of traumatic events are not exclusively bad. For some people trauma and loss facilitate a move toward health [32,116,117]. A traumatic experience can become the center around which a victim reorganizes a previously disorganized life, reorienting values and goals [3,33]. Traumatic events may function as psychic organizers for memory by linking event-related feelings, thoughts, and behaviors that are later accessed en bloc following symbolic, environmental, or biological stimuli [4]. Many survivors of the 1974 tornado in Xenia, Ohio, experienced psychological distress, but the majority described positive outcomes: they learned that they could handle crises effectively (84%) and believed that they were better off for having met this type of challenge (69%) [118,119]. This "benefited response" is also reported in the combat trauma literature. Sledge *et al.* [120] found that approximately one-third of US Air Force Vietnam-era prisoners of war reported having benefited from their prisoner-of-war experience; they believed that they had developed an important reprioritization of their life goals, placing new emphasis on the importance of family and country. The prisoners reporting these benefits tended to be the ones who had suffered the most traumatic experiences.

CONCLUSIONS

Psychological/behavioral and psychiatric responses to trauma and disasters have a predictable structure and time course. For some, however, the effects of a disaster linger long after its occurrence, rekindled by new experiences that remind the person of the past traumatic event. Even normal life events can cause anxiety and bring to mind a destroyed home or deceased loved ones. The factors influencing resilience and vulnerability to catastrophic events are only now being identified. Although a growing number of studies have investigated psychiatric response to disaster, more empirical research is needed to determine effective treatments for PTSD.

REFERENCES

1. North C.S., Tivis L., McMillen J.C., Pfefferbaum B., Spitznagel E.L., Cox J., et al. (2002) Psychiatric disorders in rescue workers after the Oklahoma City bombing. *Am J Psychiatry*, **159**: 857–859.
2. Foa E.B., Keane T.M., Friedman M.J. (2000) *Effective treatments for PTSD.* Guilford, New York.
3. Ursano R.J. (1987) Commentary. Posttraumatic stress disorder: the stressor criterion. *J Nerv Ment Dis*, **175**: 273–275.
4. Holloway H.C., Ursano R.J. (1984) The Vietnam veteran: memory, social context, and metaphor. *Psychiatry*, **47**: 103–108.
5. Glass A.J. (1966) Army psychiatry before World War II. In R.S. Anderson, A.J. Glass, R.J. Bernucci (Eds.), *Neuropsychiatry in World War II, Zone of the Interior*, Vol. 1, pp. 3–23. Office of the Surgeon General, Department of the Army, Washington, DC.
6. Shephard B. (2000) *A War of Nerves: Soldiers and Psychiatrists in the Twentieth Century.* Harvard University Press, Cambridge, MA.
7. Trimble M.R. (1985) Post-traumatic stress disorder: history of a concept. In C. Figley (Ed.), *Trauma and Its Wake*, pp. 5–14. Brunner/Mazel, New York.
8. Grinker R., Spiegel J. (1945) *Men under Stress.* Blakiston, Philadelphia.
9. Osler W. (1892) *The Principles and Practice of Medicine.* Appleton, New York.

10. American Psychiatric Association (1980) *Diagnostic and Statistical Manual of Mental Disorders*, 3rd edn. American Psychiatric Press, Washington, DC.
11. Chodoff P. (1963) Late effects of the concentration camp syndrome. *Arch Gen Psychiatry*, **8**: 323–333.
12. Eitinger L., Strom A. (1973) *Mortality and Morbidity after Excessive Stress*. Humanities Press, New York.
13. Krystal H. (1968) *Massive Psychic Trauma*. International Universities Press, New York.
14. Matussek P. (1971) *Die Konzentrationslagerhaft und ihre Folgen*. Springer, New York.
15. Lifton R. (1967) *Death in Life – Survivors of Hiroshima*. Random House, New York.
16. Adler A. (1943) Neuropsychiatric complications in victims of Boston's Coconut Grove disaster. *JAMA*, **123**: 1098–1101.
17. Lindemann E. (1994) Symptomatology and management of acute grief. *Am J Psychiatry*, **101**: 141–148.
18. Erikson K.T. (1976) Loss of communality at Buffalo Creek. *Am J Psychiatry*, **133**: 302–306.
19. Gleser G.C., Green B.L., Winget C.N. (1981) *Prolonged Psychosocial Effects of Disaster: a Study of Buffalo Creek*. Academic Press, New York.
20. Titchner J.L., Kapp, F.T. (1976) Family and character change at Buffalo Creek. *Am J Psychiatry*, **140**: 1543–1550.
21. Shore J.H., Tatum E.L., Vollmer W.M. (1986) Psychiatric reactions to disaster: the Mount St. Helens experience. *Am J Psychiatry*, **143**: 590–595.
22. Shore J.H., Vollmer W.M., Tatum E.L. (1989) Community patterns of posttraumatic stress disorders. *J Nerv Ment Dis*, **177**: 681–685.
23. Raphael B., Singh B., Bradbury L., Lambert F. (1983) Who helps the helpers? The effects of a disaster on the rescue workers. *Omega*, **14**: 9–20.
24. Weisaeth L. (1989) Torture of a Norwegian ship's crew. *Acta Psychiatr Scand*, **80**(Suppl.): 63–72.
25. Lima B.R., Pai S., Santacruz H., Lozano J. (1991) Psychiatric disorders among poor victims following a major disaster: Armero, Colombia. *J Nerv Ment Dis*, **179**: 420–427.
26. Ozer E.J., Best S.R., Lipsey T.L., Weiss D.S. (2003) Predictors of posttraumatic stress disorder and symptoms in adults: a meta-analysis. *Psychol Bull*, **129**: 52–73.
27. Wright K.M., Bartone P.T. (1994) Community responses to disaster: the Gander plane crash. In R.J. Ursano, B.G. McCaughey, C.S. Fullerton (Eds.), *Individual and Community Responses to Trauma and Disaster: the Structure of Human Chaos*, pp. 267–284. Cambridge University Press, Cambridge, MA.
28. Helzer J.E., Robins L.N., McEvoy L. (1987) Post-traumatic stress disorder in the general population. *N Engl J Med*, **317**: 1630–1634.
29. Kulka R.A., Schlenger W.E., Fairbank J.A., Jordan B.K., Hough R.L., Marmar C.R., et al. (1990) *Trauma and the Vietnam War Generation*. Brunner/Mazel, New York.
30. Kulka R.A., Schlenger W.E., Fairbank J.A., Jordan B.K., Hough R.L., Marmar, C.R., et al. (1991) Assessment of posttraumatic stress disorder in the community: prospects and pitfalls from recent studies of Vietnam veterans. *Psychol Assess*, **3**: 547–560.
31. Goldberg J., True W.R., Eisen S.A., Henderson W.G. (1990) A twin study of the effects of the Vietnam War on posttraumatic stress disorder. *JAMA*, **263**: 1227–1232.

32. McFarlane A.C. (1989) The aetiology of post-traumatic morbidity: predisposing, precipitating and perpetuating factors. *Br J Psychiatry*, **154**: 221–228.
33. Ursano R.J. (1981) The Vietnam era prisoner of war: precaptivity personality and development of psychiatric illness. *Am J Psychiatry*, **138**: 315–318.
34. Ursano R.J., Boydstun J.A., Wheatley R.D. (1981) Psychiatric illness in US Air Force Vietnam prisoners of war: a five-year follow-up. *Am J Psychiatry*, **138**: 310–314.
35. North C.S., Nixon S.J., Shariat S., Mallonee S., McMillen J.C., Spitznagel E.L., et al. (1999) Psychiatric disorders among survivors of the Oklahoma City bombing. *JAMA*, **282**: 755–762.
36. McFarlane A.C. (1986) Posttraumatic morbidity of a disaster: a study of cases presenting for psychiatric treatment. *J Nerv Ment Dis*, **174**: 4–14.
37. McFarlane A.C. (1988) The longitudinal course of posttraumatic morbidity: the range of outcomes and their predictors. *J Nerv Ment Dis*, **176**: 30–39.
38. McFarlane A.C. (1988) The phenomenology of post-traumatic stress disorders following a natural disaster. *J Nerv Ment Dis*, **176**: 22–29.
39. Fullerton C.S., Ursano R.J., Kao T.C. (1999) Disaster-related bereavement: acute symptoms and subsequent depression. *Aviation, Space, and Environmental Medicine*, **70**: 902–909.
40. Nader K., Pynoos R. (1992) School disaster: planning and initial interventions. *J Soc Behav Personal*, **8**: 1–21.
41. Pynoos R.S., Steinberg A.M., Goenjian A. (1996) Traumatic stress in childhood and adolescence: recent developments and current controversies. In B.A. van der Kolk, A.C. McFarlane, L. Weisaeth (Eds.), *Traumatic Stress: the Effect of Overwhelming Experience on Mind, Body, and Society*, pp. 331–358. Guilford, New York.
42. Shaw J.A. (1996) Twenty-one month follow-up study of school-age children exposed to Hurricane Andrew. *J Am Acad Child Adolesc Psychiatry*, **35**: 359–364.
43. American Psychiatric Association (2000) *Diagnostic and Statistical Manual of Mental Disorders*, 4th edn., text revision. American Psychiatric Association, Washington, DC.
44. Schwarz E.D., Kowalski J.M. (1991) Malignant memories: PTSD in children and adults after a school shooting. *J Am Acad Child Adolesc Psychiatry*, **30**: 936–944.
45. Pynoos R.S., Nader K. (1988) Psychological first aid and treatment approach to children exposed to community violence: research implications. *J Trauma Stress*, **4**: 445–473.
46. Pfefferbaum B., Nixon S.J., Tivis R.D., Doughty D.E., Pynoos R.S., Gurwitch R.H., Foy D.W. (2001) Television exposure in children after a terrorist incident. *Psychiatry*, **64**: 202–211.
47. Kessler R.C., Sonnega A., Bromet E., Hughes M., Nelson C.B. (1995) Posttraumatic stress disorder in the National Comorbidity Survey. *Arch Gen Psychiatry*, **52**: 1048–1060.
48. Resnick H.S., Kilpatrick D.G., Dansky B.S., Saunders B.E., Best C.L. (1993) Prevalence of civilian trauma and posttraumatic stress disorder in a representative national sample of women. *J Consult Clin Psychol*, **61**: 984–991.
49. Breslau N., Davis G.C., Andreski P., Peterson E. (1991) Traumatic events and posttraumatic stress disorder in an urban population of young adults. *Arch Gen Psychiatry*, **48**: 216–222.
50. American Psychiatric Association (1987) *Diagnostic and Statistical Manual of Mental Disorders*, 3rd edn., revised. American Psychiatric Association, Washington, DC.

51. Saigh P.A., Bremner J.D. (Eds.) (1999) *Posttraumatic Stress Disorder: a Comprehensive Text.* Allyn & Bacon, Boston, MA.

52. American Psychiatric Association (1994) *Diagnostic and Statistical Manual of Mental Disorders,* 4th edn. American Psychiatric Press, Washington, DC.

53. Bryant R.A., Harvey A.G. (2000) *Acute Stress Disorder: a Handbook of Theory, Assessment, and Treatment.* American Psychological Association, Washington, DC.

54. Spiegel D., Cardena E. (1991) Disintegrated experience: the dissociative disorders revisited. *J Abnorm Psychol,* 100: 366–378.

55. Solomon Z., Mikulincer M. (1987) Combat stress reactions, posttraumatic stress disorder, and social adjustment: a study of Israeli veterans. *J Nerv Ment Dis,* 175: 277–285.

56. Solomon Z., Mikulincer M., Kotler M. (1987) A two year follow-up of somatic complaints among Israeli combat stress reaction casualties. *J Psychosom Res,* 31: 463–469.

57. Solomon S.D., Smith E.M., Robins L.N., Fischbach R.L. (1987) Social involvement as a mediator of disaster-induced stress. *J Appl Soc Psychol,* 17: 1092–1112.

58. Cardena E., Spiegel D. (1993) Dissociative reactions of the San Francisco Bay area earthquake of 1989. *Am J Psychiatry,* 150: 474–478.

59. Perry S., Difede J., Musngi G., Frances A.J., Jacobsberg L. (1992) Predictors of posttraumatic stress disorder after burn injury. *Am J Psychiatry,* 149: 931–935.

60. Smith E., North C. (1993) Posttraumatic stress disorder in natural disasters and technological accidents. In J.P. Wilson, B. Raphael (Eds.), *International Handbook of Traumatic Stress Syndromes,* pp. 405–419. Plenum, New York.

61. Steinglass P., Gerrity E. (1990) Natural disasters and post-traumatic stress disorder: short-term versus long-term recovery in two disaster-affected communities. *J Appl Soc Psychol,* 20: 1746–1765.

62. Van der Kolk B.A.,Van der Hart O. (1989) Pierre Janet and the breakdown of adaptation in psychological trauma. *Am J Psychiatry,* 146: 1530–1540.

63. Weisaeth L. (1989) A study of behavioral responses to an industrial disaster. *Acta Psychiatr Scand,* 80(Suppl.): 13–24.

64. Weisaeth L. (1989) The stressors and the post-traumatic stress syndrome after an industrial disaster. *Acta Psychiatr Scand,* 80(Suppl.): 25–37.

65. National Institute of Mental Health (2002) *Mental Health and Mass Violence: Evidence-Based Early Psychological Intervention for Victims/Survivors of Mass Violence. A Workshop to Reach Consensus on Best Practices.* US Government Printing Office, Washington, DC.

66. Norris F.H., Friedman M.J., Watson P.J., Byrne C.M., Diaz E., Kaniasty K. (2002) 60,000 disaster victims speak, Part I. An empirical review of the empirical literature: 1981–2001. *Psychiatry,* 65: 207–239.

67. Zatzick D.F., Kang S.M., Hinton L., Kelly R.H., Hilty D.M., Franz C.E., *et al.* (2001) Posttraumatic concerns: a patient-centered approach to outcome assessment after traumatic physical injury. *Med Care,* 39: 327–339.

68. Epstein J.N., Saunders B.E., Kilpatrick D.G. (1997) Predicting PTSD in women with a history of childhood rape. *J Trauma Stress,* 10: 573–588.

69. Green B.L., Wilson J.P., Lindy J.D. (1985) Conceptualizing post-traumatic stress disorder: a psychosocial framework. In C.R. Figley (Ed.), *Trauma and its Wake.* Vol 1. *The Study and Treatment of Post-Traumatic Stress Disorder,* pp. 53–69. Brunner/Mazel, New York.

70. Boudreaux E., Kilpatrick D.G., Resnick H.S., Best C.L., Saunders B.E. (1998) Criminal victimization, posttraumatic stress disorder, and comorbid psychopathology among a community sample of women. *J Trauma Stress*, **11**: 665–678.

71. Schuster M.A., Stein B.D., Jaycox L.H., Collins R.L., Marshall G.N., Elliot M.N., et al. (2001) A national survey of stress reactions after the September 11, 2001 terrorist attack. *N Engl J Med*, **345**: 1507–1512.

72. Fullerton C.S., Ursano R.J., Norwood A.E., Holloway H.C. (2003) Trauma, terrorism, and disaster. In R.J. Ursano, C.S. Fullerton, A.E. Norwood (Eds.), *Terrorism and Disaster. Individual and Community Mental Health Interventions*, pp. 1–20. Cambridge University Press, Cambridge, UK.

73. Silver R.C., Holman E.A., McIntosh D.N., Poulin M., Gil-Rivas V. (2002) Nationwide longitudinal study of psychological responses to September 11. *JAMA*, **288**: 1235–1244.

74. Holloway H.C., Norwood A.E., Fullerton C.S., Engel C.C., Ursano R.J. (1997) The threat of biological weapons: prophylaxis and mitigation of psychological and social consequences. *JAMA*, **278**: 425–427.

75. Baum A., Gatchel R.J., Schaeffer M.A. (1983) Emotional, behavioral, and physiological effects of chronic stress at Three Mile Island. *J Consult Clin Psychol*, **51**: 565–572.

76. Weisaeth L. (1994) Psychological and psychiatric aspects of technological disasters. In R.J. Ursano, B.G. McCaughey, C.S. Fullerton (Eds.), *Individual and Community Responses to Trauma and Disaster: the Structure of Human Chaos*, pp. 72–102. Cambridge University Press, Cambridge, UK.

77. Benedek D.M., Holloway H.C., Becker S.M. (2000) Emergency mental health management in bioterrorism events. *Emergency Medicine Clinics of North America*, **20**: 393–407.

78. DiGiovanni C. Jr. (1999) Domestic terrorism with chemical or biological agents: psychiatric aspects. *Am J Psychiatry*, **156**: 1500–1505.

79. Ursano R.J., Norwood A.E., Fullerton C.S., Holloway H.C., Hall M. (2003) Terrorism with weapons of mass destruction: chemical, biological, nuclear, radiological, and explosive agents. In R.J. Ursano, A.E. Norwood (Eds.), *Trauma and Disaster: Responses and Management*, pp. 125–154. American Psychiatric Press, Arlington.

80. Bremner J.D., Davis M., Southwick S.M., Krystal J.H., Charney D.S. (1993) Neurobiology of posttraumatic stress disorder. In J.M. Oldham, M.B. Riba, A. Tasman (Eds.), *Review of Psychiatry*, Vol. 12, pp. 183–204. American Psychiatric Press, Washington, DC.

81. Ursano R.J., Fullerton C.S. (2000) Posttraumatic stress disorder: cerebellar regulation of psychological, interpersonal and biological responses to trauma? *Psychiatry*, **62**: 325–328.

82. Fullerton C.S., Ursano R.J. (Eds.) (1997) *Posttraumatic Stress Disorder: Acute and Long Term Responses to Trauma and Disaster*. American Psychiatric Press, Washington, DC.

83. Vlahov D., Galea S., Resnick H., Boscarino J.A., Bucuvalas M., Gold J., Kilpatrick D. (2002) Increased use of cigarettes, alcohol, and marijuana among Manhattan, New York, residents after the September 11 terrorist attacks. *Am J Epidemiol*, **155**: 988–996.

84. Leor J., Poole W.K., Kloner R.A. (1996) Sudden cardiac death triggered by an earthquake. *N Engl J Med*, **334**: 413–419.

85. Jacobson A.M. (1996) The psychological care of patients with insulin-dependent diabetes mellitus. *N Engl J Med*, **334**: 1249–1253.

86. Prigerson H.G., Shear M.K., Jacobs S.C., Reynolds C.F., Maciejewski P.K., Davidson J.R., *et al.* (1999) Consensus criteria for traumatic grief: a preliminary empirical test. *Br J Psychiatry*, **174**: 67–73.
87. Ford C.V. (1997) Somatic symptoms, somatization, and traumatic stress: an overview. *Nordic J Psychiatry*, **51**: 5–13.
88. McCarroll J.E., Ursano R.J., Fullerton C.S., Liu X., Lundy A. (2002) Somatic symptoms in Gulf War mortuary workers. *Psychosom Med*, **64**: 29–33.
89. Kessler R.C., Barber C., Birnbaum H.G., Frank R.G., Greenberg P.E., Rose R.M., *et al.* (1999) Depression in the workplace: effects of short-term disability. *Health Affairs*, **18**: 163–171.
90. Shalev A., Bleich A., Ursano R.J. (1990) Posttraumatic stress disorder: somatic comorbidity and effort tolerance. *Psychosomatics*, **31**: 197–203.
91. Smith E.M., North C.S., McCool R.E., Shea J.M. (1989) Acute postdisaster psychiatric disorders: identification of those at risk. *Am J Psychiatry*, **147**: 202–206.
92. Epstein R.S., Fullerton C.S., Ursano R.J. (1998) Posttraumatic stress disorder following an air disaster: a prospective study. *Am J Psychiatry*, **155**: 934–938.
93. Davidson J.R.T., Fairbank J.A. (1992) The epidemiology of posttraumatic stress disorder. In J.R.T. Davidson, E.B. Foa (Eds.), *Posttraumatic Stress Disorder: DSM-IV and Beyond*, pp. 147–169. American Psychiatric Press, Washington, DC.
94. Rundell J.R., Ursano R.J., Holloway H.C., Silberman E.K. (1989) Psychiatric responses to trauma. *Hosp Commun Psychiatry*, **40**: 68–74.
95. Solomon S.D., Smith E.M. (1994) Social support and perceived control as moderators of responses to dioxin and flood exposure. In R.J. Ursano, B.G. McCaughey, C.S. Fullerton (Eds.), *Individual and Community Responses to Trauma and Disaster*, pp. 179–200. Cambridge University Press, Cambridge, UK.
96. Rundell J.R., Ursano R.J. (1996) Psychiatric responses to trauma. In R.J. Ursano, A.E. Norwood (Eds.), *Emotional Aftermath of the Persian Gulf War: Veterans, Communities, and Nations*, pp. 43–81. American Psychiatric Press, Washington, DC.
97. Mellman T.A., Kulick-Bell R., Ashlock L.E., Nolan B. (1995) Sleep events among veterans with combat-related posttraumatic stress disorder. *Am J Psychiatry*, **52**: 110–115.
98. Forster P. (1992) Nature and treatment of acute stress reactions. In L.S. Austin (Ed.), *Responding to Disaster: a Guide for Mental Health Professionals*, pp. 25–51. American Psychiatric Press, Washington, DC.
99. Ursano R.J., Fullerton C.S., Bhartiya V., Kao T.C. (1995) Longitudinal assessment of posttraumatic stress disorder and depression after exposure to traumatic death. *J Nerv Ment Dis*, **183**: 36–42.
100. Brandt G.T., Norwood A.E., Ursano R.J., Wain H., Jaccard J.T., Fullerton C.S., *et al.* (1997) Psychiatric morbidity in medical and surgical patients evacuated from the Persian Gulf War. *Psychiatr Serv*, **48**: 102–104.
101. Goenjian A. (1993) A mental health relief program in Armenia after the 1988 earthquake: implementation and clinical observations. *Br J Psychiatry*, **163**: 230–239.
102. Norris F.H., Murphy A.D., Baker C.K., Perilla J.L., Rodriguez F.G., Rodriguez J. (2003) Epidemiology of trauma and posttraumatic stress disorder in Mexico. *J Abnorm Psychol*, **112**: 646–656.

103. Raphael B. (1977) Preventive intervention with the recently bereaved. *Arch Gen Psychiatry*, **34**: 1450–1454.
104. Shear M.K., Frank E., Foa E., Cherry C., Reynolds C.F., Bander Bilt J., Masters S. (2001) Traumatic grief treatment: a pilot study. *Am J Psychiatry*, **158**: 1506–1508.
105. Terr L.C. (1981) "Forbidden games": post-traumatic child's play. *J Am Acad Child Psychiatry*, **20**: 741–760.
106. IOM (2003) *Preparing for the Psychological Consequences of Terrorism: a Public Health Strategy*. National Academies, Institute of Medicine, Washington, DC.
107. Gerrity E.T., Steinglass P. (1994) Relocation stress following natural disasters. In R.J. Ursano, B.G. McCaughey, C.S. Fullerton (Eds.), *Individual and Community Responses to Trauma and Disaster*, pp. 220–247. Cambridge University Press, Cambridge, UK.
108. Noji E.K (Ed.) (1997) *The Public Health Consequences of Disasters*. Oxford University Press, New York.
109. Cohen R., Culp C., Genser S. (1987) *Human Problems in Major Disasters: A Training Curriculum for Emergency Medical Personnel*. US Government Printing Office, Washington, DC.
110. Green B.L. (1990) Defining trauma: terminology and generic dimension. *J Appl Soc Psychol*, **20**: 1632–1642.
111. Ursano R.J., Fullerton C.S., Vance K., Kao T.C. (1999) Postraumatic stress disorder and identification in disaster workers. *Am J Psychiatry*, **156**: 353–359.
112. Dollinger S.J. (1986) The need for meaning following disaster: attributions and emotional upset. *Pers Soc Psychol Bull*, **12**: 300–310.
113. Holloway H.C., Fullerton C.S. (1994) The psychology of terror and its aftermath. In R.J. Ursano, B.G. McCaughey, C.S. Fullerton (Eds.), *Individual and Community Responses to Trauma and Disaster*, pp. 31–45. Cambridge University Press, Cambridge, UK.
114. Ursano R.J., Fullerton C.S. (1990) Cognitive and behavioral responses to trauma. *J Appl Psychol*, **20**: 1766–1775.
115. Ursano R.J., Kao T.C., Fullerton C.S. (1992) Posttraumatic stress disorder and meaning: structuring human chaos. *J Nerv Ment Dis*, **180**: 756–759.
116. Card J.J. (1983) *Lives after Viet Nam*. Lexington Books, Lexington.
117. Tedeschi R.G., Park C.L., Calhoun L.G. (1998) *Posttraumatic Growth: Positive Changes in the Aftermath of Crisis*. Lawrence Erlbaum, Mahwah, NJ.
118. Quarentelli E.L. (1985) An assessment of conflicting views on mental health: the consequences of traumatic events. In C.R. Figley (Ed.), *Trauma and its Wake*, pp. 173–215. Brunner/Mazel, New York.
119. Taylor V. (1977) Good news about disaster. *Psychol Today*, **11**: 93–94, 124–126.
120. Sledge W.H., Boydstun J.A., Rahe A.J. (1980) Self-concept changes related to war captivity. *Arch Gen Psychiatry*, **37**: 430–443.

Psychiatric Morbidity Following Disasters: Epidemiology, Risk and Protective Factors

Alexander C. McFarlane

University of Adelaide, Queen Elizabeth Hospital, Woodville South, South Australia, Australia

INTRODUCTION

The field of traumatic stress has developed around victims of three types of events: disasters, war and criminal assaults. Disasters are unusual events because they occur randomly and usually involve large numbers of victims in the same window of time. They are events that occur infrequently, in contrast with events such as criminal assaults and motor vehicle accidents that occur daily in large urban communities. These latter events also generally affect single individuals or small groups rather than large populations. Thus, the magnitude of disasters is such that there are particular lessons that can be learned by investigating the collective reactions in the victims, as well as the associated communal processes that mitigate and aggravate the effects of these events.

Disasters, by their nature, are events that capture human attention and concern. However, the public interest in these events tends to be relatively short-lived and their long-term morbidity until recently was often underestimated by welfare and health service providers. Disaster research has highlighted the often very prolonged adverse consequences of such events [1–6]. The first systematic research in the field was conducted by the Swiss psychiatrist E. Stierlin [7,8]. He studied an earthquake that affected Messina in Italy in 1907 and a mining disaster that occurred in 1906. He found that a substantial proportion of the victims developed long-term post-traumatic symptoms. The Messina earthquake was an event of much greater magnitude than usually studied by disaster researchers, having killed

Disasters and Mental Health. Edited by Juan José López-Ibor, George Christodoulou, Mario Maj, Norman Sartorius and Ahmed Okasha.
©2005 John Wiley & Sons Ltd. ISBN 0-470-02123-3.

70,000 of the town's inhabitants. Stierlin found that 25% of the survivors experienced sleep disturbances and nightmares.

History has demonstrated the strange reluctance of psychiatry and the community at large to learn the lessons about the destructiveness of traumatic events to societies and individuals [9,10]. Ever since the last two decades of the nineteenth century, the importance of traumatic events as a cause of psychopathology has been recognised. However, the broader psychiatric community has very slowly grasped the importance of such events as determinants of psychopathology. Equally the social scars and instability that these events bring is all too readily forgotten. This phenomenon of neglect is intriguing, given that the pathological persistence of memory is one of the critical elements of post-traumatic reactions. Yet, societies have an enormous difficulty in holding onto this experience and knowledge about the impact of collective trauma such as disaster and war. The challenge, after any disaster, is to learn from history and to ensure that the knowledge that has been gained is not lost. The research that has been conducted in the last 25 years has done much to ensure that these lessons do not escape from awareness [11,12].

THE ROLE OF DISASTER RESEARCH

Systematic research contributes to the process of challenging this propensity to avoidance and amnesia, allowing the lessons to extend to a much larger community. Ultimately, the challenge for the mental health community is to extend the treatment skills and health delivery systems developed after a disaster to address the needs of other trauma victims who do not come to collective awareness in the same manner that the media coverage ensures for disaster victims. Research also plays a critical role ensuring that there is a systematic review of the experience and lessons that have been learnt. These lessons can then be combined with those from previous disasters to frame the plans for future disaster management. In the interim, the training and health care plans can be further developed to even better manage future situations whilst being flexible enough to be modified in the light of new research.

Large-scale traumatic events impact on social and personal attitudes and have the potential to bring about major, yet sometimes subtle, shifts in societies. Hence, in the aftermath of a disaster, there is a potential for major changes in public and professional attitudes because of the lessons learned by a small group of individuals involved in disaster relief and public administrators. In the longer term, these changes can be instrumental in improving the future management of trauma in the broader community. Research plays a central role in this process by documenting the immediate reactions to the disaster and the long-term outcomes. The lessons learned are also framed in terms of behaviour in the face of threat and how to adapt to the risk of recurrence.

One of the major reasons for the deaths in disasters is the failure of technology and the denial or incorrect appraisal of risk [13]. Perhaps the most iconic symbol of this phenomenon, in Western society, is the sinking of the *Titanic*. The designers claimed that this vessel was constructed so that it was invincible to destruction. As a result, there was insufficient life-saving equipment for all the passengers, owing to the belief that it would never be required. This error of judgement compounded the magnitude of the disaster when the unthinkable happened.

Disaster research as an area of investigation has a number of specific differences from most areas of psychiatric research. The core process of science is the consideration of the previously existing body of knowledge and its further development and refinement through subsequent investigation. The future investigations are driven by the development of hypotheses that emerge with the aim to further refine the existing information that is known about a particular phenomenon. Disaster research has the potential to further the general knowledge about post-traumatic reactions from a phenomenological and aetiological perspective. However, there is a propensity for every disaster to be seen in its own right as a novel event where the questions that have been investigated in previous disasters are re-examined. The instruments available for self-report in interview studies have not varied greatly in the past two decades. Equally, the salient risk factors investigated have not changed substantially during this period time. Therefore the generalisations that come out of this body of literature are contributed to as much by studies conducted in the 1980s as the more recent investigations.

Disaster research has an important social role in highlighting the longer-term effects of these events [14], which in the past tended to be overlooked in disaster recovery plans. This research is therefore part of the social dialectic [15] that is involved in rebuilding a community and also in characterising the less visible aspects of the damage that these events inflict upon communities.

DEFINITION AND TYPOLOGY

The term disaster is rarely defined. The Oxford [16] definition of disaster is: "sudden or great misfortune; calamity; complete failure". Given this breadth of definition, it is an issue of some complexity as to how disasters are clearly separated from other types of traumatic events [17].

The early disaster researchers Kinston and Rosser [18] suggested the term be used to describe "massive collective stress". Norris [19] suggested that these are events in which there are "violent encounters with nature, technology or human kind". Arising out of these definitions, various typologies of disaster have been proposed. These focus on the differentiation of the type of determinants of the destruction. While there is logic to the separation of destructive acts of nature from man-made disasters such as industrial accidents, the differences in terms of the outcomes are not substantial [12]. There has been some interest in separating the effects of man-made acts where there is the potential for malevolence to play a role in contrast to natural disasters. However, these differentiations can be somewhat illusory. For example, arsonists or the careless use of machinery can cause forest fires. Failure to comply with construction codes can lead to the collapse of buildings in earthquakes, with much greater resultant loss of life than would have been the case if the standards were adhered to [20]. Often deaths in natural disasters are due to failures of design or technology. At times these failures involve frank negligence rather than simply failing to foresee a risk, the Bhopal disaster being one such example. These technological disasters have the capacity to divide communities, particularly where one party is seen to represent a sector of privilege and wealth that is exercised with little concern for the welfare of the broader community.

It is on occasions proposed that man-made disasters are more likely to be difficult for individuals to tolerate. Natural disasters possibly can be dismissed as acts of God. At the other end of the extreme are events involving active human design, such as assault, torture and rape. These are premeditated acts that are on occasions purposely planned and implemented. Smith and North [21] articulated the commonly held opinion that technological and human-made disasters are likely to be more traumatic than natural disasters, as they provoke a greater sense of being the deliberate victim of one's fellow human beings. On the other hand, a meta-analysis of the relationship between disasters and trauma related psychopathology [22] came to the opposite conclusion – namely, that natural disasters resulted in greater rates of disorder. This analysis emphasises that any assumptions about typology should be objectively scrutinised.

A classification that has practical implications is the division of disasters according to the intensity and range of their impact (Table 3.1). The first type of disasters are those where there is a clear demarcation of exposure. For example, forest fires and explosions [23] are events where there are clearly defined margins to the disaster. In contrast, events such as an

TABLE 3.1 Classification of disasters

a. Demarcation of exposure
   Clear margins – Fires, explosions
   Graded destruction – Earthquakes, storms

b. Population affected
   Commuter – Impact in local community
   International – Multinational impact

c. Duration
   Warning
   Brief or absent – Earthquakes, terrorist attacks
   Prolonged – Cyclones, floods
   Impact
   Brief – Explosions, accidents
   Prolonged – Fires, floods, hurricanes

earthquake, nuclear accidents and storms have a long gradient of exposure where the precise margins of the disaster are less precise [24]. These disasters pose a risk to all those who live and work in these communities.

Travel accidents and acts of terror are highly concentrated and will strike a group who happen to be congregated by chance. In these events, particularly international flights, very few of the injured or dead may come from the locality of the disaster [25,26]. In some events, there may be significant loss of life and injury for local people as well as for many who come from outside the location of the disaster. These distinctions have major implications for how rescues are mounted and for the provision of services in the aftermath [27]. One such example would be the 2002 Bali bombing, which killed over 200 people. While there were a significant number of Balinese killed, the bombing of a tourist venue meant that people from all around the world were killed and grievously injured.

The impact of these events may be very different for a number of reasons. Firstly, events that are geographically defined are more likely to have a warning phase and the potential for preparatory defence. On the other hand, the community that is destroyed will also be called upon for rescue and recovery, creating a conflict between the role of victim and rescuer for many individuals.

If the aim of a typology is to allow the development of generalisations from research and experience, these distinctions may be of more use than considering the nature of the destructive agent alone.

THE PREVALENCE OF DISASTERS

A report of the Red Cross highlighted the differential impact of disasters in Third World countries. In the period 1967 to 1991, an average of 17,000,000 people living in developing countries were affected by disasters each year, as compared to about 700,000 in developed countries (a striking ratio of 166 to 1) [28]. These communities are particularly at risk in the face of disasters, because they are already under strain and with few resources in reserve to bring to bear at times when rescue and protection are required. Their health systems tend to be rudimentary and to have little mental health capability.

In the last decade, there have been some important investigations of major disasters in non-Western cultures [29]. These initiatives are important to the field, because they provide a test of how culturally specific the earlier findings of disasters in Western cultures are to the broader world community. One of the difficulties is having adequate access to this broader literature that is not readily available through the large electronic databases. Of particular note are the studies conducted into the recent earthquakes that have impacted Kobe in Japan [30,31], China [32], Taiwan [33], India and Turkey [34]. These research projects represent important introductions of the concepts of traumatic stress into these communities and provide valuable data about large-scale events. This volume addresses the consequences of a number of these disasters.

The boundaries between the effects of war and those of disaster are becoming less easy to define, with the onset of more widespread terrorism that targets civilians. For example, the terrorist attacks in Israel, Palestine and Bali and in New York on September 11, 2001 could be considered as acts of war. Another perspective is that these are man-made disasters that are characterised by extreme malevolence. The argument for the latter categorisation is that the victims of these events had no anticipation of the events that unfolded, in contrast to the combatants in a more typical armed conflict.

The threshold of exposure that is required for an individual to be included in a study is one of the issues that are difficult to determine in disaster studies. For instance, the commonsense idea that the trauma due to human negligence or error has a greater capacity to disrupt an individual's psychological assumptions than events such as hurricanes and floods does not appear to be substantiated by the objective evidence. However, this conclusion may be a consequence of differences in the thresholds of inclusion in these studies. Furthermore, the recourse to litigation in man-made disasters will generally result in a degree of financial compensation that is not available to the victims of natural disasters. It may be that adequate financial relief may provide a buffer against some of the negative effects of these events.

The emergence of a more general interest in post-traumatic stress disorder (PTSD) since the publication of DSM-III [35] has led to a dramatic increase in the attention to the impact of disasters. In the past, these events were believed to be outside the range of normal human experience, but systematic examination has now shown that they are more common than previously thought. Norris [19], in a study of 1,000 adults in southern United States, found that 69% of the sample had experienced a traumatic stressor in their lives and this included 21% in the past year alone. In this year, 2.4% of households in the southern United States were subjected to disaster or damage, with a lifetime exposure to disasters of 13%.

Kessler et al. [36], in a stratified population sample in the USA, found that 60.7% of males and 51.2% of females had experienced an event that met the DSM-IV stressor criterion. 18.9% of men and 15.2% of women had been exposed to a natural disaster, with the respective rates of lifetime PTSD being 3.7% and 5.4%. Creamer et al. [37], in a stratified sample of 10,641 Australians, found a similar percentage of lifetime exposure to traumatic experiences, with 19.9% of men and 12.7% of women reporting that they had experienced a disaster. However, of the 158 cases of PTSD in the last 12 months, in only four was a natural disaster nominated as the stressor.

Such studies demonstrate that approximately one in six out of the population has had a lifetime exposure to a natural disaster, but this accounts for a very small component of the post-traumatic morbidity within these communities. When asked to select the most traumatic event in their lives, fewer than 5% nominated their disaster experience. These figures demonstrate the problem of much of research in this area, as they are based on the simple question as to whether the individual has or has not been exposed to a natural disaster, with no definition of threshold given. These definitions about the level of exposure are critical in attempting to make estimates of the risk associated with such events.

TYPES OF DISASTER STUDIES

Disasters have been studied using a range of methodologies:

- Comparison of a representative sample of the exposed population with a control group [38,39].
- Examination of a subgroup of disaster victims, such as those seeking treatment or who are injured. Such studies often provide an opportunity for more in-depth analysis of some of the risk and protective factors [40].
- Investigation of the impact of disaster on particular groups, such as children [41] and emergency service personnel [42,43].

- Longitudinal cohort studies. Typically these studies have followed populations in the aftermath of an event, but there are several studies where a population has been studied for some other reason and then a disaster has impacted on that community [44–48].
- Identifying individuals in a general community sample who have had some disaster exposure and comparing them with people who have been exposed to other traumatic events or have had no traumatic exposure [36,37].

These different types of studies will often come to different conclusions about the same event, because of the issue of the representativeness of the sample [49]. Also the time period that has elapsed between the event and the investigation can have a significant impact on the findings, because of the significant rates of natural remission in the first year.

The majority of the studies that have been published examined the impact of natural disasters (88 = 55%), a further 54 (34%) referred to technological disasters and 18 (11%) documented the impact of massive violence [12]. These events occurred in 29 separate countries, with 57% having occurred in the United States. A further 29% of the events studied had occurred in Europe, Japan and Australia. The developing world – including Eastern Europe, Asia and Africa – accounted for only 14% of the studies.

A range of categories of victim populations has been studied. The vast majority of the survivors investigated were adults, while about 17% were school-aged children and adolescents [50,51]. A few studies have focused on emergency service personnel [52] and family assistance counsellors.

The majority of the studies provide a snapshot of the affected population within a 6 months window. Whilst there have been some substantial longitudinal studies which have followed populations for as long as 32 years [53], approximately half of the reports had their last data point less than one year after the event.

The methods used to measure morbidity varied considerably. Only a minority of studies used structured interviews [54–56], whereas the others used the more easily administered questionnaires [57,58]. A range of instruments has been used to characterise the psychological outcomes, with the most frequent focus being on PTSD [59]. Patterns of non-specific morbidity have been often examined in populations, using instruments such as the General Health Questionnaire (GHQ) [60–63]. Other phenomena, such as disassociation and demoralisation, have also been studied [50,64]. The most comprehensive studies have used structured diagnostic interviews, such as the Composite International Diagnostic Interview (CIDI), allowing the generation of a series of psychiatric diagnoses [43]. Approximately a quarter of the studies have also examined physical health concerns and problems [65–69]. Of particular interest in these studies has been the clinical worsening of physical symptoms and perceived illness burden in disaster-affected communities.

PREVALENCE OF DISORDER

The differential outcomes between disasters are sometimes difficult to determine, because of the previously mentioned variability of the sampling processes that have been used. Equally, the intensity of exposure experienced by the population studied has a major impact on the prevalence of disorders.

Lower rates of impairment have been identified following disasters occurring in the USA in comparison to those occurring in other developed countries [12]. The highest rates have been found in developing countries. This finding may be in part due to the nature of the samples that have been studied, but may also reflect the greater impact of disasters on these communities because of their limited resources to manage the recovery period. Norris et al. [12] identified the Lockerbie [70] and Jupiter cruise ship [71] disasters as those showing the highest rates of impairment.

Conclusions about the type of disaster that is associated with highest rates of impairment are influenced significantly by the amount of research that is done on the different types of events. Hurricane Andrew was a particularly devastating natural disaster and is probably the most researched event [12,48,72,73]. This may affect conclusions about the different impact of natural and man-made technological disasters.

PTSD

The rates of PTSD are very dependent on the sampling used in a study as well as the severity and nature of the event. Therefore, each new disaster should be considered as a novel event and predictions about the rates of morbidity should depend on careful consideration of which group of victims are being considered as well as the time that has elapsed following the disaster.

The Buffalo Creek disaster (dam break), which occurred in 1972, is one of the best studied disasters: a 59% PTSD lifetime rate was found among the victims, with 25% still meeting PTSD criteria some 14 years after the event [17]. One of the highest rates was demonstrated by Goenjian et al. [57] following the Armenian earthquake, with 67% meeting PTSD criteria 18 months after the earthquake. In a study conducted 1 to 4 months after Hurricane Andrew [72], 33% met the criteria for PTSD. However, in some studies of low-exposure groups, the rates of PTSD are sometimes little different from the prevalence in the general population [12]. Shore *et al.* [55] examined the impact of the Mount St. Helens volcanic eruption and compared the exposed population with a control group: the lifetime prevalence of PTSD in the Mount St. Helens group was 3.6% compared to 2.6% in the control.

In a study of an earthquake in Yunnan, China, three villages at increasing distance from the epicentre were evaluated [39]. The rate of PTSD was 23.4% in a village where most houses were destroyed compared with 16.2% where only minor damage occurred.

Gender is also an issue influencing the prevalence, with 20% of men and 36% of women suffering from PTSD one year after a mass shooting [56]. The lasting impact of events on children was demonstrated by the findings of a 33-year follow-up of victims of the Aberfan disaster, where rates of 29% current and 46% lifetime PTSD were found [53].

Other Disorders

Similar issues influence the rates of other disorders following disasters. These disorders may emerge as comorbid conditions with PTSD, in which case they are likely to represent complications of PTSD and an indication of the severity of the underlying traumatic stress response. One review suggests that PTSD occurs four times more frequently in conjunction with comorbid diagnoses than it does alone, even in close proximity to the event [21].

Alcohol usage is often a response to the development of symptoms in disaster-affected populations, an issue which has emerged particularly amongst emergency service workers [12]. On the other hand, there is an increasing body of evidence that depressive and anxiety disorders may emerge following traumatic events in the absence of PTSD [17]. For example, there is an intuitive rationale in the potential role of loss in the onset of depression and of threat and horror as determinants of anxiety disorders [43]. While there have been some explorations of the role that different types of disaster experiences play, in association with risk factors, in the onset of these disorders, this remains an area which needs further investigation [43]. On the other hand, there are studies which have not found an increased prevalence of these non-PTSD disorders, despite high rates of PTSD [53].

One of the problems in defining the prevalence of these disorders is that their assessment requires in-depth structured diagnostic interviews, whose application is time-consuming and sometimes difficult in disaster victims. Furthermore, reported rates of anxiety and depression are often derived from continuous scales, making the clinical and diagnostic interpretation of these data difficult. A further methodological issue is that defining the onset of major depressive disorder or panic disorder is more difficult than for PTSD, which can be tied to a specific event by the content of the intrusive memories. Depressive and anxiety disorders are common in community samples in the absence of disasters, so that the accurate attribution of their onset to a disaster is a difficult task.

The available evidence suggests that depression is the second most common disorder to emerge in the aftermath of a disaster [12]. One important issue is how depression following a disaster relates to pre-existing morbidity in the community. Bravo *et al.* [47] studied the impact of a mud slide and flood in Puerto Rico which killed 800 people. Fortuitously, a year before they had studied this population and were able to re-evaluate 375 of their initial subjects. They found a significant increase in the symptoms of depression and a range of somatic complaints from the pre-disaster levels but failed to demonstrate any increase in panic disorder or alcohol abuse. An increased prevalence of PTSD was identified. Smith *et al.* [74] investigated a series of disaster events in St. Louis involving exposure to dioxin, floods and tornadoes. Exposed individuals had high levels of new PTSD symptoms. However, depressive symptoms increased only in those who had had previous depression.

Following the 1988 Armenian earthquake, a high-impact disaster, major depressive disorder was found in 52% of a stratified sample of 1,785 individuals. Depression was the only disorder in 177 of these individuals and was particularly associated with exposure and loss [75].

In summary, the rates of disorders such as depression are highly variable and affected by the intensity and nature of the disaster. Estimates of the health service needs of a population should take account of the nature of the event and cannot be easily derived from the literature. The question of the rates of anxiety and depressive disorders in the aftermath of disasters is an important issue for further investigation and must consider the interaction with the existing morbidity in the community. The physical presentation of psychiatric disorders also requires better clarification, since the somatic expression of distress in the aftermath of disasters has major practical implications for the post-disaster health services [65,69].

RISK FACTORS

One of the consistent findings emerging from the systematic investigation of disasters is that post-traumatic psychopathology occurs in a minority. This emphasises the need to look at a range of other variables that may be contributing to, as well as protecting against, the onset of symptomatic distress.

Intensity of Exposure

In general, the degree of exposure to a disaster is the critical determinant of who is at risk and the levels of psychological morbidity [76–79]. The total destruction of a family's home and the loss of all possessions have a profoundly disruptive impact on people's sense of identity and social integration. In a world where materialism is often seen from a pejorative perspective, the role of physical possessions in creating a sense of psychological well-being has been given relatively little attention. Multiple bereavements have long been understood as having a particularly detrimental impact on psychological health [75].

The effects of exposure are exemplified by Weisaeth's study of a factory disaster [76,80]. He showed that mortality and injuries were dependent upon the distance from the explosion and this in turn correlated strongly with the later development of PTSD. In the high-exposure group, PTSD prevalence rates were 36% after 7 months, 27% after 2 years, 22% after 3 years and 19% after 4 years. This contrasted to the medium-exposure group, where there was a decrease in the PTSD rate from 17% after 7 months to 2% after 4 years. Thus, the intensity of the stressor not only accounted for the initial prevalence but also for the possible duration of the symptoms. He found that for employees who witnessed the event, even at a close distance, premorbid sensitivity played an important role in the development of symptoms, highlighting the interrelationship between vulnerability factors and exposure.

Several approaches have been used when measuring the severity of exposure. Some investigators have simply used the number of stressful experiences as an index of severity of the trauma [14]. Predictably, the findings suggest that there is a proportional increase in the number of symptoms as the number of stressors experienced increases The alternative approach has been to create ordinal measures of exposure that are based on a series of hypotheses about the relative severity and comparative impact of different components of the disaster [47]. Again, this method has shown that higher rates of exposure can be a good predictor of morbidity. However, over a certain level where extreme threat and horror are ubiquitous, there appears to be a plateau effect.

It is difficult to make any firm recommendations about what is the optimal approach to estimating exposure, because many of the component experiences in a disaster are not independent. For example, the threat to life and rates of injury tend to be highly correlated. Secondly, it is difficult to have a standard measure of exposure that can be applied in all disasters. The nature of the losses and effects that are documented depends upon the nature of the event.

For emergency service workers, measuring exposure is a different challenge [81–84]. To them, the intensity and duration of exposure to the actual disaster site are not the only variables to be taken into account. Other important factors include the extent to which they are involved in body recoveries, or need to deal with the families of the people killed in the event [85].

The interaction between community destruction and individual exposure has seldom been investigated. There is some suggestion that the sense of the collective loss has a modest contribution in addition to that of the individual levels of disaster exposure [86]. Phifer and Norris [87], however, showed that personal loss and community destruction interacted. The individuals who did worst were those who both came from communities with a high level of destruction and had high levels of personal loss.

There are a series of methodological issues involved in developing measures of disaster exposure. Little work has been done examining the validity of such methods of scaling. For example, in a quantitative sense, how does the death of a spouse rank against the death of a child? What is the comparative impact of the loss of property versus death and injury to people? In terms of a numerical rating, it is necessary to make these comparisons, if a score of disaster exposure has to be made.

An example of the problems involved in the development of such measures is given by the study of an earthquake-affected population [88], which surprisingly rated the severity of the impact of major losses as significantly less than comparison populations that were unaffected by the disaster. This finding suggests that traumatised groups have a different perspective on their experience than populations who have not confronted that particular event. This has the potential to create significant errors when investigators are trying to judge the severity of traumatic stresses and to determine what components of disasters are markedly distressing to most people. Furthermore, it suggests that measures of disaster exposure should be scaled on the basis of ratings developed from within communities who have knowledge of the experiences.

This is a complex issue from both a clinical and research perspective. There are many components of disasters whose perception will be influenced by the person's mental state at the time (e.g. the experience of panic or dissociation) and the person's judgement of the risks and capacity to act adaptively. The likelihood of injury and death in part depends on the individual's appraisal and capacity to respond appropriately. The determinants of these behaviours and the degree of exposure may be linked in a way that is not routinely considered. For example, a particular personality attribute may be seen as a risk factor for PTSD in a disaster-exposed individual, while the characteristic in question was actually a determinant of the type of exposure. The estimates people make of the duration of their exposure to a disaster can also be influenced by peritraumatic dissociation [89].

However, there will be objective measures of exposure, such as seeing death and injury or actually being injured. The degree of destruction and loss are also objective issues. Matters that may be equally important in determining the degree of traumatisation include the perceptions that one survived the experience through freak circumstances or was kept safe by chance, and that one had no control over the circumstances for one's behaviour. The DSM-IV [90] recognised the relative importance of these subjective components in determining the nature of the traumatic experience.

Other Risk Factors

Age

The effects of age depend upon the samples examined [91]. The conventional wisdom has been that older persons are at greater risk for morbidity related to disasters [30], as was found in the study of the Newcastle earthquake in Australia [62]. However, Norris et al. [12], in their review of research on disasters, concluded: "In every American sample in which middle-aged adults were differentiated from older adults, the former were almost consistently more affected." The reason for this may be that people in middle age carry many financial burdens and responsibilities for dependants. This life stage is the period in which individuals have least resources in reserve, to cope with the impact of unexpected and threatening demands. Hobfoll's conservation of resources model is a useful theoretical construct in looking at the interaction between a recent major challenge to the individual survival and his/her background attributes that allow him/her to meet further demands [92–94]. The more pronounced impact on older adults had been presumed to arise because their age makes it more difficult for them to physically and financially reconstruct their physical losses. The alternative explanation about the resilience of older people is that their repertoire of life experience has left them with less rigid expectations about the predictability of life.

Intercurrent Adversity

Disasters usually occur at only one time point in the life of a community. Adversity for other reasons will continue to occur [95]. Furthermore, there is often a secondary series of stresses following on from a disaster [96].

These may include legal difficulties in terms of gaining a proper compensation, delays in reconstruction and difficulty in the rehabilitation of physical injuries. Other unanticipated adversities may also hinder the adjustment of the individual. The negative effect of these further events has been demonstrated in a number of studies and has been shown to be an important determinant of the chronicity and severity of post-traumatic symptoms in the aftermath of the disaster [65,97]. In other words, it is important to consider the ongoing impact of the disaster through its secondary effects, modifying the financial stability and relationships of the individual who has survived the event [73,98]. Also, in emergency service personnel, repeated exposures have the potential to sensitise them to subsequent exposure [27].

Gender

It appears that women are at greater risk of psychological distress, measured by a range of outcomes, when exposed to disasters, with the exception of alcohol abuse, where rates are higher in males [17]. These findings are similar to those from general population studies [36] highlighting the relative vulnerability of women when exposed to traumatic events. Although it is difficult to draw conclusions, it appears that women, in general, may be at higher risk of anxiety disorders.

The factors that mediate these differences between men and women are of interest. It appears that when other risk factors exist, such as being a member of an ethnic subculture, the vulnerability of women is magnified. However, the perception of the events by men and women is also different. For example, after the Loma Prieta earthquake, women estimated the duration of the quake as 78 seconds, in contrast to men, who reported the duration was 48 seconds. Similar observations have been made in children, where girls had a greater sense of subjective but not objective threat than boys [99].

Socioeconomic Factors

Ethnic [100] and socioeconomic factors [101] are also important risk factors. Socioeconomic factors have been difficult to examine in some studies, because the affected communities were relatively homogeneous [102]. However, the majority of studies suggest that less education and lower income are risk factors to psychosocial morbidity. A social characteristic that interacts with age is marital status. Solomon [103] found that women with excellent spousal support were more at risk than those with less bonded relationships. The psychological state of mothers appears to be particularly important in terms of the psychological outcome of children [104]. The nature of family interactions is particularly detrimental for the child, if there is overprotection and lack of emotional warmth. These effects are particular likely to follow if the mother is more irritable as a consequence of PTSD. The mothers' distress and anticipation of danger appear to convey a negative sense to the children, that is manifest in their level of observable symptoms and preoccupation with the disaster [105]. However, the impact of maternal bias in reporting children's behaviour needs to be taken into account [106].

Prior Psychological Symptoms

The impact of psychological symptoms prior to the disaster has been extensively studied as a predictor of adjustment in the aftermath. Norris *et al.* [12] concluded that such symptoms are among the best predictors of post-disaster morbidity. However, few studies have considered the fact that, at the time the disaster occurs, a significant minority of the population will be suffering from a psychiatric disorder. Therefore, it is not surprising that prior symptoms are the best predictor of post-disaster symptoms. It is unclear whether these symptoms are exacerbated or whether they are a risk factor for developing PTSD. Most studies have not been able to separate the effects of existing symptoms from the onset of new symptoms and disorders. Since a significant percentage of people suffering from psychological disorders in community samples do not seek treatment, it is difficult to identify this group with any accuracy on the basis of history of previous treatment.

PROTECTIVE FACTORS

The notion of protective factors is of particular appeal because of its implications for prevention and minimisation of morbidity. The problem is that very little research has been done in the area. Most of the protective factors are, in fact, the absence of risk factors such as past psychiatric history or the experience of a negative childhood environment. Attempts to delineate protective factors have proven elusive. One area that has attracted a substantial body of investigation is that of coping. The primary hypothesis that attracted interest was the suggestion that problem-focused coping would have considerable benefits for long-term adjustment with respect to emotion-focused coping. However, several studies [107,108] found that coping behaviour in both problem- and emotion-focused domains was more frequent in those who developed symptoms following a disaster. In other words, individuals who did not develop symptoms after a disaster reported fewer coping behaviours than those who did develop symptoms. Such findings highlight the problems of identifying protective factors in the aftermath of traumatic events, when reporting is contaminated by the presence of symptoms.

Wessely [109] reviewed the literature about the prior screening of troops in World War II and found that many of the characteristics that were thought to be markers of vulnerability had little predictive ability. A study of twin pairs in the US services at the time of the Vietnam war found that there was a genetic vulnerability to PTSD and this was related to personality [110]. The roles that individuals chose in the military were predicted partly by their genetically determined temperamental traits, such as novelty seeking. Individuals with this personality trait were more likely to choose roles that exposed them to high levels of danger in combat. The problem is that such a personality style is likely to characterise those who choose jobs in the emergency services, as those who tend to be harm-avoidant will choose safer careers. Harm-avoidance is a personality trait that is protective but cannot be used as a selection criterion for the emergency services. Such paradoxes highlight the complexity of this domain of interest.

Social Support

Social support is frequently mentioned as a critical factor that protects individuals following exposure to disasters [111]. One of the difficulties that arise in examining this question is the challenge of separating the reality of social support from the perception of its adequacy [112]. The perception of social support is critically determined by the individual's personality. In a prospective study, personality characteristics such as neuroticism were an important determinant of the perception of social support [113].

Perceived social support depends upon the belief about the availability of others to assist rather than the actual receipt of assistance. Solomon *et al.* [114] made the interesting observation that mid-range levels of support availability were associated with the most favourable outcomes for women. In contrast, women with high support availability did poorly. This study also found that women with excellent spouse support had worse outcomes than those with weaker spouse ties. In contrast, men tended to do better if they had a stronger spouse relationship. This suggests that there are important differences between men and women, where the strength of attachment for women may be a burden rather than supportive at times of extreme stress.

Resilience

Vaillant [115] crystallised three models of adaptation (normality, positive psychology and maturity) that provide a context for considering the nature of resilience. Many of the attributes of a well-adjusted life in the circumstances of suburban civility are very different from the skills that would allow an individual to optimally survive some critical life stress. The literature referred to about social support indicates that attachment can be a risk factor in the setting of a disaster, whereas in the absence of such an experience it may have increased the individual's quality of life. Of the three models, maturity is the one that is most likely to characterise resilience in the face of a disaster. Situations of major loss and threat demand the ability to give up previous certainties and to sense the survival of others as bearing major value in contrast to the discomforts and suffering of one's immediate situation, which is essential to embodying a sense of hope.

The real challenge is to develop a framework for investigating resilience. There are a series of time windows when attributes and characteristics can exert their effect. In the pre-disaster period, the willingness to anticipate the risk of predictable disasters can do much to shield an individual and his or her associates through a variety of mitigation and protective steps. A willingness to prepare for a disaster and practice emergence procedures is a measure of personality that predicts survival in a practical and psychological sense [78]. These strategies are about a balance between a realistic appraisal of the future and a capacity for mastery. These attributes contrast with needless risk-taking, on one hand, and phobic avoidance of threat on the other. The latter strategy leaves people with a profound sense of fear and threat with no rehearsal of how to manage adversity, should it arise.

In the face of a rapidly emerging threat, adaptive behaviour depends upon the acceptance of heightened danger and facing rather than bargaining with fate. In the warning phase of disasters, there are often false alarms that must be responded to rather than ignored. In the midst of the disaster, a tolerance of a loss of control and the ability to function in the face of helplessness are attributes that facilitate adaptive behaviour. There is a need to engage in activity that is self-protective rather than exposing the person to needless risks. This reaction depends on an ability to flexibly appraise risk rather than deny one's vulnerability. Only when the risk is not too great can the individual switch from survival behaviour into rescue-directed activities. There are many examples of people's failure to appraise the dangers contributing to their death and injury.

In the post-disaster period, again resilience is characterised by the ability to flexibly use the available assets and resources. The ability to tolerate the new leadership structures and to not indulge in blame but use self-criticism will allow individuals to face and rework the trauma. The individual must be able to move into an active stance when appropriate, rather than presuming that external help will resolve the situation or provide help. At a community and individual level, as the disaster further recedes into the past, an attitude that embodies optimism rather than demoralisation is critical to rebuilding a sense of a future world. Tolerance of distress in oneself and others and the progression beyond post-disaster attachments are likely predictors of a positive outcome.

Age is a factor that may have a range of effects that the earlier discussion has not elucidated. While experience and wisdom are a critical source of resources in the face of extreme threat, the invulnerability of youth and their few material ties mean that youth has cushion against the horror of disasters. On the other hand, the young do not have the support and structure that a career and relationships provide in the face of the threat and disruption created by a disaster. In this regard, it should be emphasised that the ability to survive in the short term may not provide long-term protection.

Hence, there are multiple time windows in which different repertoires of response are likely to be protective. Such behaviours are not static and may only emerge in the face of such adversity. What might be an adaptive behaviour in one setting may not be in another. These characteristics demonstrate why resilience is likely to be very difficult to demonstrate in research studies. While communities are likely to tolerate health impact studies after disasters, they will be less willing to engage in research that has more of a behaviour and purely academic focus. Also, such research requires considerable theoretical development against background knowledge of the literature.

CONCLUSIONS

One contribution of disaster research has been the relevance of the findings to understanding the more general relationship between psychiatric disorder and life events. A major problem that had plagued researchers endeavouring to investigate the relationship between day-to-day adversity and psychiatric disorder has been the question of cause and effect. Longitudinal studies of life events demonstrated that life events were as likely to have been caused by psychiatric disorder, as was the reverse relationship, where the disorder had arisen as a consequence of some adversity.

Disasters by their very nature are beyond individual's control. In other words, they are truly independent life events. Hence, they provide a relatively methodologically sophisticated way of beginning to investigate these causal associations. However, one of the problems, which occur in most disasters, is that pre-existing measures of the adjustment of population do not exist. This is an important issue, because many studies have failed to take account of the existing psychological morbidity in disaster-affected communities. A critical question is the way in which the existing symptoms are modified by traumatic experiences, as well as the nature of the psychopathology which emerges in most people who were otherwise well-adjusted at the time of the traumatic event. Hence, there is a need to differentially investigate PTSD triggered by traumatic events in those with predisposition in contrast to "true PTSD" which emerges in those who are asymptomatic at the time of the event.

Against this background, the epidemiological research into the impact of disasters demonstrates that there are few events that lead to disorder in the majority of people exposed. Hence, it is important to conceptualise the various characteristics of the environment and the individual that may act as relative risk or protective factors. In fact, population studies highlight the variability of the outcome between individuals and these differences are often lost because of the way in which statistical analysis requires the grouping of outcomes. Particularly in situations of relatively low exposure, vulnerability factors such as premorbid personality and previous psychiatric disorder have an important role to play [116].

In summary, vulnerability and protective factors are necessary to explain much of the probability of developing post-disaster morbidity. PTSD and other trauma-related disorders represent the outcome of a complex biopsychosocial matrix of variables. These factors can operate along a variety of axes. The context in which the event occurs in the individual's life is the base from which the disorder emerges. The nature of the stressor and the recovery environment involve a series of interactions modifying the ability of the individual to quench his/her immediate post-traumatic distress. It is in this post-disaster period that these vulnerability factors may play a critical role. On the other hand, it is important to emphasise that PTSD may emerge in previously healthy individuals whose modest vulnerability would otherwise have had little relevance.

REFERENCES

1. Bland S., O'Leary E., Farinaro E., Jossa F., Trevisan M. (1996) Long-term psychological effects of natural disasters. *Psychosom Med*, **58**: 18–24.
2. Bolton D., O'Ryan D., Udwin O., Boyle S., Yule W. (2000) The long-term psychological effects of a disaster experienced in adolescence: II. General psychopathology. *J Child Psychol Psychiatry All Discipl*, **41**: 513–523.
3. Green B., Solomon S. (1995) The mental health impact of natural and technological disasters. In J. Freedy and S. Hobfoll (Eds.), *Traumatic Stress: From Theory to Practice*, pp. 163–180. Plenum, New York.

4. Green B., Grace M., Gleser G. (1985) Identifying survivors at risk: long-term impairment following the Beverly Hills Supper Club fire. *J Consult Clin Psychol*, 53: 672–678.

5. Smith E., North C., Spitznagel E. (1993) Post-traumatic stress in survivors of three disasters. *J Soc Behav Person*, 8: 353–368.

6. Udwin O., Boyle S., Yule W., Bolton D., O'Ryan D. (2000) Risk factors for long-term psychological effects of a disaster experienced in adolescence: predictors of PTSD. *J Child Psychol Psychiatry All Discipl*, 41: 969–979.

7. Stierlin E. (1909) Über psychoneuropathische Folgezustände bei den Überlebenden der Katastrophe von Courrières am 10. Doctoral dissertation, University of Zurich.

8. Stierlin E. (1911) Nervöse und psychische Störungen nach Katastrophen. *Dtsch Med Wochenschr*, 37: 2028–2035.

9. Kardiner A. (1941) *The Traumatic Neuroses of War*. Hober, New York.

10. McFarlane A.C., van der Kolk B.A. (1996) Trauma and its challenge to society. In B. van der Kolk, A.C. McFarlane, L. Weisaeth (Eds.), *Traumatic Stress: The Effects of Overwhelming Experience on Mind, Body and Society*, pp. 24–46. Guilford, New York.

11. Weisaeth L. (1996) PTSD: the stressor response relationship. In E. Giller, L. Weisaeth (Eds.), *Post Traumatic Stress Disorder*. Baillière's Clinical Psychiatry, International Practice and Research, Vol. 2, pp. 191–216.

12. Norris F.H., Friedman M.J., Watson P.J., Byrne C.M., Diaz E., Kaniasty K. (2002) 60,000 disaster victims speak: Part I. An empirical review of the empirical literature, 1981–2001. *Psychiatry*, 65: 207–239.

13. Weisaeth L., Tonnessen A. (2003) Responses of individuals and groups to consequences of technological disasters and radiation exposure. In R.J. Ursano (Ed.), *Terrorism and Disaster: Individual and Community Mental Health Interventions*, pp. 209–235. Cambridge University Press, New York.

14. Briere J., Elliott D. (2000) Prevalence, characteristics and long-term sequelae of natural disaster exposure in the general population. *J Trauma Stress*, 13: 661–679.

15. van der Kolk B.A. (1996) Trauma and memory. In B. van der Kolk, A.C. McFarlane, L. Weisaeth (Eds.), *Traumatic Stress: The Effects of Overwhelming Experience on Mind, Body and Society*, pp. 279–302. Guilford, New York.

16. Sykes J.B. (Ed.) (1987) *The Concise Oxford Dictionary*, 7th edn. Clarendon Press, Oxford.

17. Green B.L. (1996) Traumatic stress and disaster: mental health effects and factors influencing adaptation. In F. Lieh-Mak, C.C. Nadelson (Eds.), *International Review of Psychiatry*, Vol. 2, pp. 177–210. American Psychiatric Press, Washington, DC.

18. Kinston W., Rosser R. (1974) Disaster: effect on medical and physical state. *J Psychosom Res*, 18: 437–456.

19. Norris F. (1992) Epidemiology of trauma: frequency and impact of different potentially traumatic events on different demographic groups. *J Consult Clin Psychol*, 60: 409–418.

20. Pynoos R.S., Goenjian A., Tashjian M., Karakashian M., Manjikian R., Manoukian G., et al. (1993) Post-traumatic stress reactions in children after the 1988 Armenian earthquake. *Br J Psychiatry*, 163: 239–247.

21. Smith E.M., North C.S. (1993) Posttraumatic stress disorder in natural disasters and technological accidents. In J.P. Wilson, B. Raphael (Eds.), *International Handbook of Traumatic Stress Syndromes*, pp. 405–419. Plenum, New York.

22. Rubonis A., Bickman L. (1991) Psychological impairment in the wake of disaster: the disaster–psychopathology relationship. *Psychol Bull*, **109**: 384–399.

23. Tucker P., Dickson W., Pfefferbaum B., McDonald N., Allen G. (1997) Traumatic reactions as predictors of posttraumatic stress six months after the Oklahoma City bombing. *Psychiatr Serv*, **48**: 1191–1194.

24. Dew M., Bromet E. (1993) Predictors of temporal patterns of psychiatric distress during 10 years following the nuclear accident at Three Mile Island. *Soc Psychiatry Psychiatr Epidemiol*, **28**: 49–55.

25. Turner S., Thompson J., Rosser R. (1995) The Kings Cross fire: psychological reactions. *J Trauma Stress*, **8**: 419–427.

26. Selley C., King E., Peveler R., Osola K., Martin N., Thompson C. (1997) Posttraumatic stress disorder symptoms and the Clapham rail accident. *Br J Psychiatry*, **171**: 478–482.

27. Dougall A., Herberman H., Delahanty D., Inslicht S., Baum A. (2000) Similarity of prior trauma exposure as a determinant of chronic stress responding to an airline disaster. *J Consult Clin Psychol*, **68**: 290–295.

28. International Federation of Red Cross and Red Crescent Societies (1993) *World Disaster Report, 1993*. Nijhoff, Dordrecht.

29. Durkin M.S., Khan N., Davidson L., Zaman S., Stein Z. (1993) The effects of a natural disaster on child behavior: evidence for posttraumatic stress. *Am J Publ Health*, **83**: 1549–1553.

30. Kato H., Asukai N., Miyake Y., Minakawa K., Nishiyama A. (1996) Post-traumatic symptoms among younger and elderly evacuees in the early stages following the 1995 Hanshin-Awaji earthquake in Japan. *Acta Psychiatr Scand*, **93**: 477–481.

31. Kitayama S., Okada Y., Takumi T., Takada S., Inagaki Y., Nakamura H. (2000) Psychological and physical reactions of children after the Hanshin-Awaji earthquake disaster. *Kobe J Med Sci*, **46**: 189–200.

32. Wang X., Gao L., Shinfuku N., Zhang H., Zhao C., Shen Y. (2000) Longitudinal study of earthquake-related PTSD in a randomly selected community sample in North China. *Am J Psychiatry*, **157**: 1260–1266.

33. Yang Y.K., Yeh T.L., Chen C.C., Lee C.K., Lee I.H., Lee L.C., Jeffries K.J. (2003) Psychiatric morbidity and posttraumatic symptoms among earthquake victims in primary care clinics. *Gen Hosp Psychiatry*, **25**: 253–261.

34. Salcioglu E., Basoglu M., Livanou M. (2003) Long-term psychological outcome for non-treatment-seeking earthquake survivors in Turkey. *J Nerv Ment Dis*, **191**: 154–160.

35. American Psychiatric Association (1980) *Diagnostic and Statistical Manual of Mental Disorders*, 3rd edn. American Psychiatric Association, Washington, DC.

36. Kessler R.C., Sonnega A., Bromet E. (1995) Posttraumatic stress disorder in the national comorbidity survey. *Arch Gen Psychiatry*, **52**: 1048–1060.

37. Creamer M., Burgess P., McFarlane A. (2001) Posttraumatic stress disorder: findings from the Australian National Survey of Mental Health and Well-Being. *Psychol Med*, **31**: 1237–1247.

38. McFarlane A.C., Clayer J.R., Bookless C.L. (1997) Psychiatric morbidity following a natural disaster: an Australian Bushfire. *Soc Psychiatry Psychiatr Epidemiol*, **32**: 261–268.

39. Cao H., McFarlane A.C., Klimidis S. (2003) Prevalence of psychiatric disorder following the 1988 Yun Nan (China) earthquake. The first 5-month period. *Soc Psychiatry Psychiatr Epidemiol*, **38**: 204–212.

40. Donker G.A., Yzermans C.J., Spreeuwenberg P., van der Zee J. (2002) Symptom attribution after a plane crash: comparison between self-reported symptoms and GP records. *Br J Gen Pract*, **52**: 917–922.
41. Asarnow J., Glynn S., Pynoos R.S., Nahum J., Guthrie D., Cantwell D.P., *et al.* (2000) When the earth stops shaking: earthquake sequelae among children diagnosed for pre-earthquake psychopathology. *J Am Acad Child Adolesc Psychiatry*, **39**: 141–142.
42. Weiss D., Marmar C., Metzler T., Ronfeldt H. (1995) Predicting symptomatic distress in emergency services personnel. *J Consult Clin Psychol*, **63**: 361–368.
43. McFarlane A.C., Papay P. (1992) Multiple diagnoses in posttraumatic stress disorder in the victims of a natural disaster. *J Nerv Ment Dis*, **180**: 498–504.
44. Norris F., Phifer J., Kanisty K. (1994) Individual and community reactions to the Kentucky floods: findings from a longitudinal study of older adults. In R. Ursano, B. McCaughey, C. Fullerton (Eds.), *Individual and Community Responses to Trauma and Disaster: The Structure of Human Chaos*, pp. 378–400. Cambridge University Press, Cambridge, UK.
45. La Greca A., Silverman W., Vernberg E., Prinstein M. (1996) Symptoms of posttraumatic stress in children after Hurricane Andrew: a prospective study. *J Consult Clin Psychol*, **64**: 712–723.
46. Alexander D. (1993) Stress among police body handlers: a long-term follow-up. *Br J Psychiatry*, **163**: 806–808.
47. Bravo M., Rubio-Stipec M., Canino G., Woodbury M., Ribera J. (1990) The psychological sequelae of disaster stress prospectively and retrospectively evaluated. *Am J Commun Psychol*, **18**: 661–680.
48. Warheit G., Zimmerman R., Khoury E., Vega W., Gil A. (1996) Disaster related stresses, depressive signs and symptoms, and suicidal ideation among a multi-racial/ethnic sample of adolescents: a longitudinal analysis. *J Child Psychol Psychiatry All Discipl*, **37**: 435–444.
49. McFarlane A.C., de Girolamo G. (1996) The nature of traumatic stressors and the epidemiology of posttraumatic reactions. In B. van der Kolk, A.C. McFarlane, L. Weisaeth (Eds.), *Traumatic Stress: The Effects of Overwhelming Experience on Mind, Body and Society*, pp. 129–154. Guilford, New York.
50. Laor N., Wolmer L., Kora M., Yucel D., Spirman S., Yazgan Y. (2002) Posttraumatic, dissociative and grief symptoms in Turkish children exposed to the 1999 earthquakes. *J Nerv Ment Dis*, **190**: 824–832.
51. Chemtob C.M., Nakashima J.P., Hamada R.S. (2002) Psychosocial intervention for postdisaster trauma symptoms in elementary schoolchildren: a controlled community field study. *Arch Pediatr Adolesc Med*, **156**: 211–216.
52. Chang C.M., Lee L.C., Connor K.M., Davidson J.R., Jeffries K., Lai T.J. (2003) Posttraumatic distress and coping strategies among rescue workers after an earthquake. *J Nerv Ment Dis*, **191**: 391–398.
53. Morgan L., Scourfield J., Williams D., Jasper A., Lewis G. (2003) The Aberfan disaster: 33-year follow-up of survivors. *Br J Psychiatry*, **182**: 532–536.
54. Yule W., Bolton D., Udwin O., O'Ryan D., Nurrish J. (2000) The long-term psychological effects of a disaster experienced in adolescence: I. The incidence and course of PTSD. *J Child Psychol Psychiatry All Discipl*, **41**: 503–511.
55. Shore J., Tatum E., Vollmer W. (1986) Psychiatric reactions to disaster: the Mount St. Helens experience. *Am J Psychiatry*, **143**: 590–595.
56. North C., Smith E., Spitznagel E. (1997) One-year follow-up of survivors of a mass shooting. *Am J Psychiatry*, **154**: 1696–1702.

57. Goenjian A., Pynoos R., Steinberg A., Najarian L., Asarnow J., Karayan I., *et al.* (1995) Psychiatric co-morbidity in children after the 1988 earthquake in Armenia. *J Am Acad Child Adolesc Psychiatry*, **34**: 1174–1184.

58. Goenjian A., Steinberg A., Steinberg L., Steinberg L., Tashjian M., Pynoos R. (2000) Prospective study of posttraumatic stress, anxiety, and depressive reactions after earthquake and political violence. *Am J Psychiatry*, **15**: 911–916.

59. Asukai N., Kato H., Kawamura N., Kim Y., Yamamoto K., Kishimoto J., *et al.* (2002) Reliability and validity of the Japanese-language version of the Impact of Event Scale-Revised (IES-R-J): four studies of different traumatic events. *J Nerv Ment Dis*, **190**: 175–182.

60. Catapano F., Malafronte R., Lepre F., Cozzolino P., Arnone R., Lorenzo E., *et al.* (2001) Psychological consequences of the 1998 landslide in Sarno, Italy: a community study. *Acta Psychiatr Scand*, **104**: 438–442.

61. Carr V., Lewin T., Webster R., Hazell P., Kenardy J., Carter G. (1995) Psychological sequelae of the 1989 Newcastle earthquake: I. Community disaster experiences and psychological morbidity 6 months post-disaster. *Psychol Med*, **25**: 539–555.

62. Carr V.J., Lewin T.J., Kenardy J.A., Webster R.A., Hazell P.L., Carter G.L., *et al.* (1997) Psychosocial sequelae of the 1989 Newcastle earthquake: III. Role of vulnerability factors in post-disaster morbidity. *Psychol Med*, **27**: 179–190.

63. Carr V., Lewin T., Webster R., Kenardy J., Hazell P., Carter G. (1997) Psychosocial sequelae of the 1989 Newcastle earthquake: II. Exposure and morbidity profiles during the first years post-disaster. *Psychol Med*, **27**: 167–177.

64. Koopman C., Classen C., Spiegel D. (1996) Dissociative responses in the immediate aftermath of the Oakland/Berkeley firestorm. *J Trauma Stress*, **9**: 521–540.

65. McFarlane A.C., Atchison M., Rafalowicz E., Papay P. (1994) Physical symptoms in post-traumatic stress disorder. *J Psychosom Res*, **38**: 715–726.

66. Pfefferbaum B., Doughty D. (2001) Increased alcohol use in a treatment sample of Oklahoma City bombing victims. *Psychiatry*, **64**: 296–303.

67. North C.S., Nixon S.J., Shariat S., Mallonee S., McMillen J.C., Spitznagel E.L., *et al.* (1999) Psychiatric disorders among survivors of the Oklahoma City bombing. *JAMA*, **282**: 755–762.

68. Lutgendorf S., Antoni M., Ironson G., Fletcher M., Penedo F., Baum A., *et al.* (1995) Physical symptoms of chronic fatigue syndrome are exacerbated by the stress of Hurricane Andrew. *Psychosom Med*, **57**: 310–323.

69. Escobar J., Canino G., Rubio-Stipic M., Bravo M. (1992) Somatic symptoms after a natural disaster: a prospective study. *Am J Psychiatry*, **149**: 965–967.

70. Brooks N., McKinlay W. (1992) Mental health consequences of the Lockerbie disaster. *J Trauma Stress*, **5**: 527–543.

71. Yule W., Udwin O., Bolton D. (2002) Mass transportation disasters. In A.M. La Greca, W.K. Silverman, E.M. Vernberg, M.C. Roberts (Eds.), *Helping Children Cope with Disasters and Terrorism*, pp. 223–239. American Psychological Association, Washington, DC.

72. Ironson G., Wynings C., Schneiderman N., Baum A., Rodriguez M., Greenwood D., *et al.* (1997) Posttraumatic stress symptoms, intrusive thoughts, loss, and immune function after Hurricane Andrew. *Psychosom Med*, **59**: 128–141.

73. Maes M., Mylle J., Delmeire L., Janca A. (2001) Pre- and post-disaster negative life events in relation to the incidence and severity of posttraumatic stress disorder. *Psychiatry Res*, **105**: 1–12.

74. Smith E.M., Robins L.N., Pryzbeck T.R. (1986) Psychosocial consequences of a disaster. In J.H. Shaw (Ed.), *Disaster Studies, New Methods and Findings*, pp. 49–76. American Psychiatric Press, Washington, DC.

75. Armenian H.K., Morikawa M., Melkonian A.K., Hovanesian A., Akiskal K., Akiskal H.S. (2002) Risk factors for depression in the survivors of the 1988 earthquake in Armenia. *J Urban Health*, **79**: 373–382.

76. Weisaeth L. (1996) PTSD: vulnerability and protective factors. In E. Giller, L. Weisaeth (Eds.), *Post Traumatic Stress Disorder*. Baillière's Clinical Psychiatry, International Practice and Research, Vol. 2, pp. 217–228.

77. Brewin C.R., Andrews B., Valentine J.D. (2000) Meta-analysis of risk factors for posttraumatic stress disorder in trauma-exposed adults. *J Consult Clin Psychol*, **68**: 748–766.

78. Carlier I., Gersons B. (1997) Stress reactions in disaster victims following the Bijlmermeer plane crash. *J Trauma Stress*, **10**: 329–335.

79. Armenian H.K., Morikawa M., Melkonian A.K., Hovanesian A.P., Haroutunian N., Saigh P.A., *et al.* (2000) Loss as a determinant of PTSD in a cohort of adult survivors of the 1988 earthquake in Armenia: implications for policy. *Acta Psychiatr Scand*, **102**: 58–64.

80. Weisaeth L. (1989) The stressors and the post-traumatic stress syndrome after an industrial disaster. *Acta Psychiatr Scand*, **80**(Suppl. 355): 25–37.

81. Epstein R., Fullerton C., Ursano R. (1998) Posttraumatic stress disorder following an air disaster: a prospective study. *Am J Psychiatry*, **155**: 934–938.

82. Ersland S., Weisaeth L., Sund A. (1989) The stress upon rescuers involved in an oil rig disaster: Alexander L. Kielland 1980. *Acta Psychiatr Scand*, **80**(Suppl. 355): 38–49.

83. Jenkins S. (1997) Coping and social support among emergency dispatchers: Hurricane Andrew. *J Soc Behav Person*, **12**: 201–216.

84. Dyregrov A., Kristofferson J., Gjestad R. (1996) Voluntary and professional disaster-workers: similarities and differences in reactions. *J Trauma Stress*, **9**: 541–555.

85. Jones D. (1985) Secondary disaster victims: the emotional effects of recovering and identifying human remains. *Am J Psychiatry*, **142**: 303–307.

86. McFarlane A.C., Cao H. (1993) The study of a major disaster in the People's Republic of China. The Yunnan Earthquake. In B. Raphael, J. Wilson (Eds.), *The International Handbook of Traumatic Stress Syndromes*, pp. 493-498. Plenum, New York.

87. Phifer J., Norris F. (1989) Psychological symptoms in older subjects following natural disasters: nature, timing and duration in course. *J Gerontol Soc Sci*, **44**: 207–217.

88. Janney J.G, Masuda M., Holmes T.H. (1977) Impact of a natural catastrophe on life events. *J Human Stress*, **3**: 22–34.

89. Anderson K., Manuel G. (1994) Gender differences in reported stress response to the Loma Prieta earthquake. *Sex Roles*, **30**: 725–733.

90. American Psychiatric Association (1994) *Diagnostic and Statistical Manual of Mental Disorders*, 4th edn. American Psychiatric Association, Washington, DC.

91. Knight B., Gatz M., Heller K., Bengston V. (2000) Age and emotional response to the Northridge earthquake: a longitudinal analysis. *Psychol Aging*, **15**: 627.

92. Hobfoll S., Lilly R. (1993) Resource conservation as a strategy for community psychology. *J Commun Psychol*, **21**: 128–148.

93. Arata C.M., Picou J.S., Johnson G.D., McNally T.S. (2000) Coping with technological disaster: an application of the conservation of resources model to the Exxon Valdez oil spill. *J Trauma Stress*, **13**: 23–39.

94. Benight C.C., Ironson G., Klebe K., Carver C., Wynings C., Greenwood D., *et al.* (1999) Conservation of resources and coping self-efficacy predicting distress following a natural disaster: a causal model analysis where the environment meets the mind. *Anxiety, Stress, and Coping*, **12**: 107–126.

95. McFarlane A.C. (1989) The aetiology of post-traumatic morbidity: predisposing, precipitating and perpetuating factors. *Br J Psychiatry*, **154**: 221–228.

96. Burnett K., Ironson G., Benight C., Wynings C., Greenwood D., Carver C., *et al.* (1997) Measurement of perceived disruption during rebuilding following Hurricane Andrew. *J Trauma Stress*, **10**: 673–681.

97. Kwon Y., Maruyama S., Morimoto K. (2001) Life events and posttraumatic stress in Hanshin-Awaji earthquake victims. *Environ Health Prevent Med*, **6**: 97–103.

98. Havenaar J.M., Rumyantzeva G.M., van den Brink W., Poelijoe N.W., van den Bout J., van Engeland H., *et al.* (1997) Long-term mental health effects of the Chernobyl disaster: an epidemiologic survey in two former Soviet regions. *Am J Psychiatry*, **154**: 1605–1607.

99. Goenjian A.K., Molina L., Steinberg A.M., Fairbanks L.A., Alvarez M.L., Goenjian H.A., *et al.* (2001) Posttraumatic stress and depressive reactions among Nicaraguan adolescents after Hurricane Mitch. *Am J Psychiatry*, **158**: 788–794.

100. Jones R., Frary R., Cunningham P., Weddle J., Kaiser L. (2001) The psychological effects of Hurricane Andrew on ethnic minority and Caucasian children and adolescents: a case study. *Cultural Diversity and Ethnic Minority Psychology*, **7**: 103–108.

101. Lima B., Pai S., Santacruz H., Lozano J. (1991) Psychiatric disorders among poor victims following a major disaster: Armero, Colombia. *J Nerv Ment Dis*, **179**: 420–427.

102. McFarlane A.C. (1986) Long-term psychiatric morbidity of a natural disaster: the implications for disaster planners and emergency services. *Med J Australia*, **145**: 561–563.

103. Solomon S. (2002) Gender differences in response to disaster. In G. Weidner, S. Kopp, M. Kristenson (Eds.), *Heart Disease: Environment, Stress, and Gender*, NATO Science Series I: Life and Behavioural Sciences, 327, pp. 267–274. IOS Press, Amsterdam.

104. Green B.L, Korol M., Grace M.C., Vary M.G., Leonard A.C., Gleser G.C., *et al.* (1991) Children and disaster: age, gender, and parental effects on PTSD symptoms. *J Am Acad Child Adolesc Psychiatry*, **30**: 945–951.

105. McFarlane A.C., Policansky S.K., Irwin C.P. (1987) A longitudinal study of the psychological morbidity in children due to a natural disaster. *Psychol Med*, **17**: 727–738.

106. Bromet E.J., Goldgaber D., Carlson G., Panina N., Golovakha E., Gluzman S.F., *et al.* (2000) Children's well-being 11 years after the Chernobyl catastrophe. *Arch Gen Psychiatry*, **57**: 563–571.

107. Spurrell M., McFarlane A.C. (1993) Posttraumatic stress disorder and coping after a natural disaster. *Soc Psychiatry Psychiatr Epidemiol*, **28**: 194–200.

108. Chung M., Easthope Y., Chung C., Clark-Carter D. (2001) Traumatic stress and coping strategies of sesternary victims following an aircraft disaster in Coventry. *Stress and Health*, **17**: 67–75.

109. Wessely S. (2003) The role of screening in the prevention of psychological disorders arising from major trauma: pros and cons. In R.J. Ursano, C.S. Fullerton, A.E. Norwood (Eds.), *Terrorism and Disaster: Individual and Community Mental Health Interventions*, pp. 121–145. Cambridge University Press, Cambridge, UK.
110. True W., Lyons M. (1999) Genetic factors for PTSD: a twin study. In R. Yehuda (Ed.), *Risk Factors for Posttraumatic Stress Disorder*, pp. 61–78. American Psychiatric Association Press, Washington, DC.
111. Norris F., Kaniasty K. (1996) Received and perceived social support in times of stress: a test of the social support deterioration deterrence model. *J Person Soc Psychol*, **71**: 498–511.
112. Kaniasty K., Norris F., Murrell S. (1990) Perceived and received social support following natural disaster. *J Appl Soc Psychol*, **20**: 85–114.
113. Henderson S., Byrne G., Duncan-Jones P., Scott R., Adcock S. (1980) Social relationships, adversity and neurosis: a study of associations in a general population sample. *Br J Psychiatry*, **136**: 574–583.
114. Solomon Z., Mikulincer M., Hobfoll S.E. (1987) Objective versus subjective measurement of stress and social support: combat-related reactions. *J Consult Clin Psychol*, **55**: 577–583.
115. Vaillant G.E. (2003) Mental health. *Am J Psychiatry*, **160**: 1373–1384.
116. Maj M., Starace F., Crepet P., Lobrace S., Veltro F., De Marco F., *et al.* (1989) Prevalence of psychiatric disorders among subjects exposed to a natural disaster. *Acta Psychiatr Scand*, **79**: 544–549.

4

Re-evaluating the Link between Disasters and Psychopathology

Rachel Yehuda and Linda M. Bierer

Bronx Veterans Affairs Medical Center, New York, USA

INTRODUCTION

Some individuals are vulnerable to the development of psychopathology following exposure to events that elicit feelings of helplessness and terror, but the majority of persons show only transient symptoms that, for the most part, resolve within weeks or months. Attempting to delineate what makes a response pathological is difficult, because it is not clear whether and to what extent the presence of psychological symptoms following trauma exposure should be defined as a function of time, that is, using a "recovery" model, or, alternatively, whether a pathological response following trauma exposure represents an alternative trajectory to the normative response. In the first model, psychopathology is defined by the persistence of symptoms that within some specified period of time immediately following the event would otherwise be considered normal. The second model posits that pathology is defined by the presence of a fundamentally different initial response to stress, leading to a cascade of events that results in persistent symptoms of intrusive recollections of the trauma, avoidance of reminders, and hyperarousal.

Attempting to delineate which of an individual's responses following a traumatic experience should be considered to represent or predict psychopathology is similarly difficult, because the distinction between "pathologic" and "normal" implies a dichotomy that may not exist clinically. It has never been completely clear whether to consider long-lasting symptoms following trauma on the basis of a spectrum with respect to level of functioning, or whether those who develop mental illness following trauma exposure constitute, in essence, a different population. The latter would support the idea of thinking about responses to trauma

Disasters and Mental Health. Edited by Juan José López-Ibor, George Christodoulou, Mario Maj, Norman Sartorius and Ahmed Okasha.
©2005 John Wiley & Sons Ltd. ISBN 0-470-02123-3.

dichotomously, for example, as either normal or pathological, but the former is more consistent with most traditional conceptions of post-traumatic stress responses, as well as with current clinical practices.

There are many different kinds of responses to an event perceived as potentially life-threatening, which reflect the trauma-associated experiences of loss, threat, or injury, and how they are viewed in consideration of the individual's past history and current life circumstances. To date, however, it has been difficult to predict long-term responses to trauma based on the acute response to a traumatic event – particularly for any given individual. Examining the question of whether the development of either short-term or long-term psychological symptoms following trauma exposure is a reflection of *risk factors* or the presence of *resilience factors*, may assist in discriminating which responses are likely to represent pathology. If we assert that recovery is the normal response to trauma, then risk factors become important in understanding how psychopathology develops. If we assert that trauma exposure in and of itself is a potent enough toxin to elicit long-lasting pathology, risk factors will become less important to under-standing such responses, and the focus might then shift to the impact of dose of trauma, and/or of failing to marshal resources post-trauma, such as social support, that, under normal circumstances, buffer individuals from the natural course of symptom development (i.e., factors that contribute to resiliency).

HOW DO WE KNOW WHETHER A RESPONSE TO TRAUMA IS PATHOLOGICAL IN ITS IMMEDIATE AFTERMATH?

In the immediate aftermath of a traumatic event, most people will exhibit symptoms such as difficulties in sleeping and concentrating, irritability, nightmares, having recurrent thoughts about the trauma, or experiencing distress at being reminded of the event, but these symptoms will not last for a long time. The question becomes whether having even an abundance of such symptoms at a time when it is reasonable to have them constitutes pathology. The question of how to think about such symptoms is important from a public health perspective, since it raises the even greater issue of whether or not the presence of early symptoms requires intervention.

It is clear that most people recover from early post-traumatic symptoms. This phenomenon can be illustrated by results of several prospective, longitudinal studies, as well as recent surveys conducted by the New York Academy of Medicine following the attacks of September 11, 2001 in New

York City. Five to eight weeks after the attacks, a prevalence rate of 7.5% of randomly sampled subjects living south of 110th Street had reportedly developed symptoms of post-traumatic stress disorder (PTSD) [1], with those having the most severe exposure or personal loss at higher risk than others. When another randomly sampled group taken from the same cohort was studied 6 months after the attacks, only 1.7% demonstrated PTSD [2]. Certainly one can conclude from these findings that there was recovery of the New York community as a whole from the initial effects of the September 11 attacks. Two important questions are raised by these findings. First, did the clinical symptoms contributing to the initial estimates of PTSD constitute a real clinical syndrome requiring treatment, or simply reflect temporary distress rather than mental illness? Second, would the smaller group with persistent symptoms be identifiable immediately post-trauma?

WHAT KIND OF RESPONSES TO TRAUMA SHOULD MENTAL HEALTH PRACTITIONERS BE CONCERNED ABOUT?

In most discussions of long-term pathologic responses following a traumatic event, there is an implicit assumption that the critical outcome being referred to is PTSD. Yet, PTSD is but one among several possible outcomes following trauma exposure. Trauma survivors, compared to persons who have not experienced trauma, are at increased risk for the development of other mental disorders, such as major depression, panic disorder, generalized anxiety disorder, and substance abuse, as well as persistent anxiety symptoms and distress that do not meet criteria for a specific psychological disorder [3]. Furthermore, they are at risk for developing somatic symptoms and physical illnesses, particularly hypertension, asthma, chronic pain syndromes and other psychosomatic illnesses. Interestingly, the focus of most investigations in the wake of disasters that affect large numbers of persons, whether they be natural or man-made events, has been related to PTSD, even though this disorder is neither an inevitable outcome nor a prototypic one (e.g., 5). Because of this, a lack of understanding of the associations between trauma exposure and other potentially detrimental consequences constitutes a major gap in our knowledge. Future studies must utilize a more broadly based evaluation of trauma survivors, both in the acute and chronic aftermath, so as to ensure that the full spectrum and time-course of mental health consequences has been captured.

DOES THE PTSD DIAGNOSIS EFFECTIVELY CLASSIFY SYMPTOMATIC PERSONS POST-TRAUMA?

When PTSD was established as a diagnosis in 1980, it was not conceptualized as a pathologic response, but rather as a normative response to the abnormal circumstance of extreme trauma. PTSD was considered to represent "psychopathology" only in so far as this "normative response" resulted in a maladaptive complex of symptoms. The idea behind PTSD was that victims should not need to justify the existence of symptoms or poor social, occupational or interpersonal functioning, because exposure alone explained symptom formation. The framers of the PTSD diagnosis were concerned that, in the absence of this diagnosis, stress-related symptoms had been viewed as transient, and not requiring intensive treatment (reviewed in 6). Thus, the extent to which the diagnosis of chronic PTSD has become an indication of a psychopathologic response to trauma represents a major paradigmatic shift from the original intention of the diagnosis.

The PTSD diagnosis was initially proposed in the absence of prospective, longitudinal data describing the natural course of symptoms. Rather, it was based on the clinical presentation of chronically symptomatic and often disabled patients. Further, no attempt was made to differentiate the symptoms of trauma survivors who appeared less disabled and showed greater overall functioning. It is now clear that trauma survivors who may not meet full diagnostic criteria for PTSD, and who appear to be functioning well (for example, they do not report high levels of subjective distress and largely maintain pre-exposure levels of occupational and interpersonal functioning) may still endorse experiencing distress at reminders of the traumatic event, and active avoidance symptoms such as forgetting aspects of the trauma, and avoiding reminders of the event. Can these symptoms be considered pathological if they are associated with only moderate or manageable subjective distress, and occur in the absence of functional impairment? Do more specific criteria reflecting functional disability, such as absenteeism from work or family obligations, reduced productivity, loss of employment, and increased utilization of health care systems, need to be included in assessing whether long-term responses are pathological? Moreover, are there some symptoms whose persistence is associated with greater functional impairment than others? Without a critical examination of these issues, it is difficult to consider the trajectory from the acute response to psychopathology.

CORE PREDICTORS OF CHRONIC DYSFUNCTION IN THE ACUTE PHASE

Generally speaking, researchers have failed to demonstrate that the severity of intrusive, avoidance and hyperarousal symptoms within several days following a traumatic event is associated with the later development of PTSD. However, greater symptom severity from 1 to 2 weeks post-trauma and onwards has been positively associated with subsequent symptom severity [7]. On the other hand, it is fairly certain that persons with low symptom levels in the immediate aftermath of a traumatic event are not at risk for the development of subsequent PTSD. These findings are consistent with the idea that PTSD as a psychopathologic process reflects a failure of recovery.

Numerous studies have found a relationship between peri-traumatic dissociation and the subsequent development of PTSD (e.g., 5,8–10). One recent meta-analysis reported that peri-traumatic dissociation was the single best predictor ($r = 0.35$) of subsequent PTSD development among trauma-exposed individuals [11]. However, this association has not been a consistent finding [12–15] and, when present, has often been attributed to the effects of covariate interactions [16,17]. Prospective studies have also failed to identify peri-traumatic dissociation as a reliable predictor of chronic PTSD (e.g., 15–18). One important methodologic consideration is the distinction between true peri-traumatic dissociation, that is dissociative symptoms occurring during or immediately following the trauma, and the subsequent experience of depersonalization or derealization, occurring in the first weeks after exposure. The latter are required for a diagnosis of acute stress disorder (ASD), but have not been shown to predict PTSD any more than does the emergence of PTSD symptoms in the acute aftermath of trauma, i.e., re-experiencing, avoidance and arousal symptoms. Further, studies of dissociation in the aftermath of trauma have generally not accounted for compromised intellectual function, which in itself is a risk factor for PTSD, and is linked with dissociation [19]. Indeed, McNally [19] recently concluded that it remains undetermined whether dissociation in the aftermath of trauma predicts chronic PTSD over and above the development of other acute PTSD symptoms.

Closely related to dissociation is the potentially important role of panic during and after trauma exposure. There is evidence that panic attacks occur in 53–90% of trauma survivors during the traumatic experience [20]. Further, the majority of people with ASD report peri-traumatic and post-traumatic panic attacks [21]. Galea et al. [1] found peri-traumatic panic to be the best predictor of PTSD in the post September 11 survey of 1,008 residents living south of 110th Street in Manhattan. This observation is consistent with the results of a study of 747 police officers in which panic reactions during exposure were highly predictive of post-September 11 symptom development [22].

In attempting to formulate a psychological explanation as to why symptoms such as peri-traumatic dissociation or panic might be particularly predictive of PTSD, McNally [19] suggested that such symptoms can promote catastrophic interpretations of the trauma, and/or constitute a somatic experience that gives rise to the erroneous idea that the symptoms are harbingers of more serious problems. Indeed, some investigators have demonstrated the power of negatively appraising any aspect of the event in the peri-traumatic period to predict long-term pathology. For example, having a negative perception of other people's responses (e.g., "I feel that other people are ashamed of me now"), is associated with the development of PTSD above that predicted by initial symptom levels [23]. Similarly, catastrophic attributions of responsibility for the trauma in the acute post-trauma phase have been shown to predict PTSD [24,25].

BIOLOGICAL CORRELATES OF ACUTE POST-TRAUMA PREDICTORS OF CHRONIC SYMPTOM DEVELOPMENT

It is not clear whether or to what extent these cognitive processes are related to or mediated by stress hormones. An increased catecholaminergic response to trauma could underlie or be the proximal cause of intense panic, and persons in a more intense biologic state of fear are likely to interpret bodily cues to indicate greater danger. Alternatively, anticipatory fears, or other predisposing cognitive factors, might mediate an exaggerated catecholaminergic response to the event, leading to panic. Thus, pre-existing cognitive factors, in turn, may or may not be the cause, result, or correlate of pre-existing biological alterations, either or both setting the stage for an extreme response to the trauma.

Basic science research on memory consolidation and fear conditioning during states of heightened arousal (i.e., adrenergic activation) is consistent with the idea that peri-traumatic panic, or even intense distress during and immediately after a traumatic event, might contribute to the production of intrusive recollections. However, clarifying the precise nature and biological correlates of symptoms that appear in the immediate aftermath of a trauma, and/or that predict the continued presence of long-term symptoms, will no doubt assist in developing models for potential prophylactic interventions and early treatments. For example, to the extent that panic reactions are associated with increased catecholamine responses at the time of trauma, early and aggressive intervention with adrenergic blocking agents [26], or cognitive-behavioral stress management techniques emphasizing relaxation, may be the most appropriate interventions for persons who panic in the hours immediately following trauma exposure.

For persons who are not in a position to receive intervention within several hours or days post-trauma, it will be necessary to determine the relative importance of specific behaviors and other factors, such as the availability of social support, on the longitudinal course of post-traumatic responses and on the development of persistent psychopathology. Such data could be used, for instance, to inform families and loved ones of the importance of their availability, of simply providing comfort, reassurance, and of not encouraging the survivor to recount (i.e., relive) the trauma unless, and only to the extent that, he or she wishes.

PRE-TRAUMA RISK FOR THE DEVELOPMENT OF POST-TRAUMATIC MENTAL HEALTH PROBLEMS

Although being able to predict potential long-term pathologies from the acute response, such as peri-traumatic panic, is important, understanding the development of psychiatric disorders post-trauma will ultimately involve an appreciation of risk factors for those early responses. The finding that only a proportion of those exposed to trauma develop short and long-term symptoms justifies an exploration of the factors that increase the risk for, as well as those that might serve to protect individuals from, developing symptoms following trauma exposure. While the concept of risk can be used to describe characteristics of a trauma that make an event more or less likely to result in symptoms, or to describe the specific nature of the response to a trauma that may predict persistent symptomatology, as in the preceding discussion, it is equally used to describe characteristics of the persons who undergo a traumatic experience that make them more likely to develop post-traumatic psychopathology. We will limit the remaining discussion to pre-trauma risk for PTSD, for which a variety of factors, ranging from situational or environmental, to familial and even genetic risk factors have now been identified (e.g., 27).

It appears, on the basis of retrospective studies, that those at greatest risk for developing PTSD following trauma are persons with a family history of psychopathology [28], childhood abuse [29], prior trauma exposure [30,31], cognitive factors such as lower IQ [32], female gender in some circumstances [31], and poor social support [29,33]. To a large extent, prospective studies have supported these findings, in that persons showing less recovery following traumatic exposure tended to have more of these risk factors than those who did not. However, when such risk factors have been entered into discriminant function analyses for the prediction of subsequent PTSD in prospective studies, no single variable emerged as a significant predictor. Biological risk factors, including genetic susceptibility, have not been firmly established, but constitute a possible avenue of exploration, given the increased concordance for PTSD in monozygotic compared with dizygotic twins [34]. Furthermore, adult children of Holocaust survivors with PTSD show a greater prevalence of PTSD in response to their own traumatic events compared to adult children of Holocaust survivors without PTSD [35]. To establish a genetic basis would require the identification of a gene or genes involved in stress vulnerability. In the absence of such data, it is difficult to know to what extent the increased vulnerability to PTSD in family members of trauma survivors is related to biological or genetically transmitted phenomena, as opposed to experiential ones, because of the large degree of shared environmental influences in families.

THE ROLE OF BIOLOGICAL STUDIES IN HELPING TO IDENTIFY PATHOLOGICAL RESPONSES

Biological findings in PTSD have become increasingly relevant to the issue of the identification of psychopathology. Initially, the biology of stress and the stress response was adopted as a relevant model for the study of PTSD. This assumption provided the intellectual justification for interpreting PTSD as one manifestation along a continuum of "normal" responses to adversity. Although a comprehensive review of the neurobiology of PTSD is beyond the scope of this chapter, the results of neurobiological studies of PTSD pertain directly to the issue of the identification of PTSD as a pathological or non-normative response to trauma. Most relevant to this discussion are the repeated observations and nature of a distinct set of biological alterations associated with PTSD symptoms (see 36). At least some of the biological alterations that have been observed reflect changes in stress-responsive systems (e.g., the hypothalamic–pituitary–adrenal axis) that are quite different from what would be predicted based on the stress literature. Furthermore, the alterations in individuals with PTSD have been found to be distinct from those of similarly exposed individuals without PTSD, and also different from those found in other psychiatric disorders, such as mood and other anxiety disorders. Together, these findings suggest that the biology of PTSD is not simply a reflection of a normative stress response, but rather, a pathologic one [6].

GENERAL MECHANISMS WHEREBY BIOLOGICAL FINDINGS IN PTSD MIGHT REFLECT A PATHOPHYSIOLOGY OF THE DISORDER

In tandem with observations of the phenomenology and psychology of PTSD, neurobiological examinations of trauma survivors have supported the possibility that the development of PTSD is facilitated by a failure to contain the normal stress response at the time of the trauma, resulting in a cascade of biological alterations that, eventually, underlie the enhanced recall, distress at reminders, avoidance, and hyperarousal symptoms that characterize PTSD. In contrast to the normal fear response, which is characterized by a series of biological reactions that help the body modulate, and gradually recover from stress (e.g., high cortisol levels), prospective biologic studies have shown that individuals who develop PTSD or PTSD-related symptoms appear to have more attenuated cortisol increases in the acute aftermath of a trauma than those who do not develop the disorder [37,38]. Moreover, persons who develop PTSD show elevated heart rates in the emergency room, and at one week post-trauma, compared to those who ultimately recover [39], suggesting, if not a greater degree of sympathetic nervous system activation, one that is prolonged and "abnormally" persistent. These findings indicate that unrestrained noradrenergic activation in association with trauma exposure predicts the development of subsequent PTSD psychopathology.

Thus, even subtle alterations in the degree of physiological activation that an individual experiences at the time of trauma exposure and in its immediate aftermath may have considerable consequences with respect to symptomatic and functional outcome. Some aspects of the physiological responses of persons who develop PTSD are typical, or consistent with the "normative" stress response, while others are not. Further, a number of observations suggest that at least some of the biological alterations associated with PTSD (e.g., enhanced dexamethasone-induced suppression; decreased hippocampal volumes) may represent risk factors for the development of the disorder, rather than either a consequence of trauma exposure or a reflection of the pathophysiology of the disorder [40,41].

SPECIFIC MECHANISMS POTENTIALLY CONTRIBUTING TO THE PATHOPHYSIOLOGY OF PTSD

While the precise mechanisms whereby even well-established biological risk factors may influence a person's acute response to trauma have not yet been fully elaborated, it is important to consider the possibilities. With respect to the neuroendocrine alterations, for example, since cortisol inhibits its own release through negative feedback at the level of the pituitary and the hypothalamus, lower circulating cortisol levels may disrupt (or delay) the process of physiological stress recovery by failing to inhibit the activation of the hypothalamus/pituitary. This failure of inhibition will result in increased corticotropin releasing factor (CRF) stimulation, in synergy with other neuropeptides, such as arginine vasopressin, resulting in a higher magnitude adrenocorticotropin hormone (ACTH) response, which in turn might further stimulate the sympathetic nervous system through a direct effect [42]. Moreover, since glucocorticoids inhibit norepinephrine release from sympathetic nerve terminals, relatively lower cortisol levels may be expected to prolong norepinephrine availability at synapses, both in the periphery and in the brain [43]. Importantly, enhanced negative feedback inhibition may be present at the time of the trauma (i.e., may be a pre-trauma risk factor), and may contribute to the premature suppression of ACTH and cortisol among individuals at increased risk for the development of PTSD in response to trauma [44].

There may be consequences of increased catecholamine levels in the acute aftermath of a trauma in promoting the consolidation of the traumatic memory. Indeed, adrenergic activation in the presence of low cortisol has been shown to facilitate "learning" in animals [45]. If this was the neurohumoral state of an individual during and in the immediate aftermath of a traumatic exposure, the event would not only be strongly encoded in memory, but associated with extreme subjective distress. This level of distress, in turn, would set the stage for the occurrence of perceptual and cognitive distortions in the acute aftermath of the event, particularly regarding the estimation of danger and subjective assessment of ability to respond effectively to the threat. Such altered beliefs would serve to further inhibit recovery by leading to a failure to quell fearful recollections. The repeated experience of the trauma memory with its associated fear response, as may occur at the time of an intrusive recollection or in response to a traumatic reminder, serves to enhance, rather than reduce, the association of trauma-related and distorted cognitions with the fear response, further increasing the likelihood of spontaneous re-emergence of the memory. In this way, re-experiencing symptoms becomes a form of re-traumatization, that not only perpetuates, but can intensify the intrusive and arousal symptoms of PTSD, and provide further provocation for avoidance behaviors. This cascade can produce a series of secondary biological changes. Indeed, the exaggerated startle response in PTSD is not observed until one month following trauma, and not earlier, reflecting the developmental progression of at least some aspects of the pathophysiology of PTSD [44].

BIOLOGICAL RISK FACTORS CONTRIBUTING TO PTSD

If there is a predisposing biology of PTSD, it appears to comprise a set of conditions that impede an individual's ability to contain the stress response. According to the cascade described above, trauma exposure will further the development of these conditions and consequences, resulting in a progressive sensitization to subsequent trauma exposures. It is conceivable that any one of a number of biological conditions could have the effect of stimulating or sustaining heightened levels of physiological arousal, and consequently distress, at the time of the traumatic experience, and thereby, of facilitating a biological sensitization to subsequent traumatic events.

PTSD has been associated with numerous other biological alterations, including, for example, those affecting immune function [46], catecholaminergic regulation [47], psychophysiologic responsivity [48], and changes in sleep architecture [49], each of which could be studied prospectively and in high-risk samples. Furthermore, both structural and functional neuro-imaging studies have revealed changes in brain volume and/or activation in response to traumatic reminders in brain regions associated with the experience of fear and recognition of danger, e.g., the amygdala and hippocampus [50]. The future identification of genetic factors may provide a context for interpreting the relative contributions of pre-, peri-, and post-traumatic factors to the emergence of various pathophysiologic responses to trauma.

Thus, biological studies in PTSD have begun to provide a framework for understanding how similar events could result in biologically hetero-geneous outcomes, and for identifying specific mediators related to the presence and severity of PTSD symptomatology. The concept of biological risk, as it may be elaborated in future studies, will help to characterize and to predict individual differences in vulnerability to develop PTSD, versus other potential post-traumatic outcomes, and may eventually suggest a rationale for selecting subgroups of exposed individuals with a high likelihood of developing psychopathology, even before the expression of functional impairment.

IMPLICATIONS OF BIOLOGICAL FINDINGS IN PTSD FOR STRATEGIES OF PHARMACOLOGICAL PROPHYLAXIS

The biological conditions that appear to promote the development of PTSD suggest two promising strategies for pharmacological prophylaxis. The first is to develop interventions aimed at diminishing adrenergic hyperactivity. Two trials have been initiated to date using propranolol for this purpose. Pitman et al. [26] performed double-blind treatment with placebo ($n = 23$)

and propranolol ($n = 18$) at doses sufficient to effect beta-adrenergic blockade (40 mg qid) in patients within 6 hours of a psychologically traumatic event. Treatment continued for 10 days and Clinician Administered PTSD Scales (CAPS) were administered to 11 propranolol- and 20 placebo-completers after 1 month. Whereas total CAPS scores did not differ significantly between the treatment groups, the propranolol-treated subjects were significantly less physiologically reactive to traumatic reminders, suggesting that this or a related approach might provide an effective preventative strategy. Vaiva et al. [51] initiated a similar study in which 11 subjects were treated, immediately following a traumatic experience, for only 7 days and at somewhat lower doses of propranolol (40 mg tid), followed by a slow propranolol taper over the following 8–12 days. Propranolol-treated subjects were compared to eight patients who refused propranolol treatment. At 2 months following the trauma, both the occurrence of PTSD and the severity of PTSD symptoms were significantly reduced by propranolol treatment. Although based on few subjects, these results suggest that the pharmacologic modulation of adrenergic neuro-transmission in the immediate aftermath of traumatic exposure may interrupt the pathophysiologic cascade initiated by heightened adrenergic responsivity.

Alternatively, the model considered in this chapter would suggest that increasing the level of glucocorticoids would be an effective method of suppressing adrenergic outflow, and in fact, posits that this is an endogenous mechanism by which threat-associated elevations in adrenergic transmission are dampened. While even short-term administration of glucocorticoids has not yet been proposed as a viable prophylactic strategy, recent observations by Schelling et al. [52,53] in the setting of a medical intensive care unit (ICU) have provided proof-of-concept data to indicate that this is not only a theoretical but in fact an effective strategy for the prevention of ICU-related PTSD and PTSD symptoms.

Survivors of long-term treatment in the ICU for critical medical illness report the vivid recall of traumatic memories, i.e., aspects of their ICU stay associated with anxiety, respiratory distress, nightmares, etc. Higher doses and more prolonged administration of adrenergic agents (usually administered as pressors to critically ill patients) were not only associated with increased recollection of trauma memories (e.g., enhanced encoding) but also with the post-discharge development of PTSD. The additional administration of corticosteroids, however, protected against the emergence of PTSD. This was interpreted as an effect of steroids to inhibit memory retrieval, and thereby to diminish the contribution of reliving symptoms to the generation of PTSD. However, the effect might additionally reflect the action of glucocorticoids to modulate the experiential and pharmacologic effects of functional adrenergic hyperactivity.

CONCLUSIONS

In recent years most research has focused on a linear relationship between acute psychological variables (e.g., panic, dissociation, appraisals of threat, perceived ability to cope) and the subsequent occurrence of disorder. Yet, in the future, it will be necessary to adopt a more sophisticated approach that allows for multivariate consideration of the many factors involved in predicting short- and long-term responses to trauma, and the relationship between these responses, functional disability, and the need and/or response to treatment.

REFERENCES

1. Galea S., Ahern J., Resnick H., Kilpatrick D., Bucuvalas M., Gold J., et al. (2002) Psychological sequelae of the September 11 terrorist attacks. N Engl J Med, 346: 982–987.
2. Galea S., Boscarino J., Resnik H., Vlahov D. (in press) Mental health in New York City after the September 11 terrorist attacks: results from two population surveys. In R.W. Manderscheid, M.J. Henderson (Eds.), Mental Health, United States, 2002. US Government Print Office, Washington, DC.
3. Kessler R.C., Sonnega A., Bromet E., Hughes M., Nelson C.B. (1995) Posttraumatic stress disorder in the National Comorbidity Survey. Arch Gen Psychiatry, 52: 1048–1060.
4. Boscarino J.A. (1996) Posttraumatic stress disorder, exposure to combat, and lower plasma cortisol among Vietnam veterans: findings and clinical implications. J Consult Clin Psychol, 64: 191–201.
5. Shalev A.Y., Freedman S., Peri T., Brandes D., Sahar T., Orr S.P., Pitman R.K. (1998) Prospective study of posttraumatic stress disorder and depression following trauma. Am J Psychiatry, 155: 630–637.
6. Yehuda R., McFarlane A.C. (1995) Conflict between current knowledge about posttraumatic stress disorder and its original conceptual basis. Am J Psychiatry 152: 1705–1713.
7. Harvey A.G., Bryant R.A. (1998) The relationship between acute stress disorder and posttraumatic stress disorder: a prospective evaluation of motor vehicle accident survivors. J Consult Clin Psychol, 66: 507–512.
8. Ehlers A., Mayou R.A., Bryant B. (1998) Psychological predictors of chronic PTSD after motor vehicle accidents. J Abnorm Psychol, 107: 508–519.
9. Koopman C., Classen C., Spiegel D. (1994) Predictors of posttraumatic stress symptoms among survivors of the Oakland/Berkeley, Calif., firestorm. Am J Psychiatry, 151: 888–894.
10. Murray J., Ehlers A., Mayou R.A. (2002) Dissociation and post-traumatic stress disorder: two prospective studies of road traffic accident survivors. Br J Psychiatry, 180: 363–368.
11. Ozer E.J., Best S.R., Lipsey T.L., Weiss D.S. (2003) Predictors of posttraumatic stress disorder and symptoms in adults: a meta-analysis. Psychol Bull, 129: 52–73.

12. Simeon D., Greenberg J., Knutelska M., Schmeidler J., Hollander E. (2003) Peritraumatic reactions associated with the World Trade Center disaster. *Am J Psychiatry*, **160**: 1702–1705.
13. Panasetis P., Bryant R.A. (2003) Peritraumatic versus persistent dissociation in acute stress disorder. *J Trauma Stress*, **16**: 563–566.
14. Gershuny B.S., Cloitre M., Otto M.W. (2003) Peritraumatic dissociation and PTSD severity: do event-related fears about death and control mediate their relation? *Behav Res Ther*, **41**: 157–166.
15. Marshall G.N., Schell T.L. (2002) Reappraising the link between peritraumatic dissociation and PTSD symptom severity: evidence from a longitudinal study of community violence survivors. *J Abnorm Psychol*, **111**: 626–636.
16. Ladwig K.H., Marten-Mittag B., Deisenhofer I., Hofmann B., Schapperer J., Weyerbrock S., *et al.* (2002) Psychophysiological correlates of peritraumatic dissociative responses in survivors of life-threatening cardiac events. *Psychopathology*, **35**: 241–248.
17. Engelhard I.M., van den Hout M.A., Kindt M., Arntz A., Schouten E. (2003) Peritraumatic dissociation and posttraumatic stress after pregnancy loss: a prospective study. *Behav Res Ther*, **41**: 67–78.
18. Dancu C.V., Riggs D.S., Hearst-Ikeda D., Shoyer B.G., Foa E.B. (1996) Dissociative experiences and posttraumatic stress disorder among female victims of criminal assault and rape. *J Trauma Stress*, **9**: 253–267.
19. McNally R.J. (2003) Psychological mechanisms in acute response to trauma. *Biol Psychiatry*, **53**: 779–788.
20. Bryant R.A., Panasetis P. (2001) Panic symptoms during trauma and acute stress disorder. *Behav Res Ther*, **39**: 961–966.
21. Nixon R., Bryant R.A. (2003) Peritraumatic and persistent panic attacks in acute stress disorder. *Behav Res Ther*, **41**: 1237–1242.
22. Marmar C., Best S., Metzler T., Chemtob C., Gloria R., Killeen A., *et al.* Impact of the World Trade Center attacks on New York City police officers: a prospective study. Unpublished study.
23. Dunmore E., Clark D.M., Ehlers A. (2001) A prospective investigation of the role of cognitive factors in persistent PTSD after physical and sexual assault. *Behav Res Ther*, **39**: 1063–1084.
24. Andrews B., Brewin C.R., Rose S., Kirk M. (2000) Predicting PTSD in victims of violent crime: the role of shame, anger and blame. *J Abnorm Psychol*, **109**: 69–73.
25. Delahanty D.L., Herberman H.B., Craig K.J., Hayward M.C., Fullerton C.S., Ursano R.J., *et al.* (1997) Acute and chronic distress and posttraumatic stress disorder as a function of responsibility for serious motor vehicle accidents. *J Consult Clin Psychol*, **65**: 560–567.
26. Pitman R.K., Sanders K.M., Zusman R.M., Healy A.R., Cheema F., Lasko N.B., *et al.* (2002) Pilot study of secondary prevention of posttraumatic stress disorder with propranolol. *Biol Psychiatry*, **51**: 189–192.
27. Yehuda R. (Ed.) (1999) *Risk Factors for Posttraumatic Stress Disorder*. American Psychiatric Association, Washington, DC.
28. Breslau N., Davis G.C., Andreski P., Peterson E. (1991) Traumatic events and posttraumatic stress disorder in an urban population of young adults. *Arch Gen Psychiatry*, **48**: 216–222.
29. Brewin C.R, Andrews B., Valentine J.D. (2000) Meta-analysis of risk factors for posttraumatic stress disorder in trauma-exposed adults. *J Consult Clin Psychol*, **68**: 748–766.

30. Nishith P., Mechanic M.B., Resick P.A. (2000) Prior interpersonal trauma: the contribution to current PTSD symptoms in female rape victims. *J Abnorm Psychol*, **109**: 20–25.
31. Breslau N., Chilcoat H.D., Kessler R.C., Davis G. (1999) Previous exposure to trauma and PTSD effects of subsequent trauma: results from the Detroit Area Survey of Trauma. *Am J Psychiatry*, **156**: 902–907.
32. Silva R.R., Alpert M., Munoz D.M., Singh S., Matzner F., Dummitt S. (2000) Stress and vulnerability to posttraumatic stress disorder in children and adolescents. *Am J Psychiatry*, **157**: 1229–1235.
33. Coker A.L., Smith P.H., Thompson M.P., McKeown R.E., Bethea L., Davis K.E. (2002) Social support protects against the negative effects of partner violence on mental health. *J Women's Health Gend Based Med*, **11**: 465–476.
34. True W.R., Rice J., Eisen S.A., Heath A.C., Goldberg J., Lyons M.J., et al. (1993) A twin study of genetic and environmental contributions to liability for posttraumatic stress disorder. *Arch Gen Psychiatry*, **50**: 257–264.
35. Yehuda R., Schmeidler J., Wainberg M., Binder-Brynes K., Duvdevani T. (1998) Vulnerability to posttraumatic stress disorder in adult offspring of Holocaust survivors. *Am J Psychiatry*, **155**: 1163–1171.
36. Yehuda R. (2004) Risk and resilience in posttraumatic stress disorder. *J Clin Psychiatry*, **65**(Suppl. 1): 29–36.
37. Resnick H.S., Yehuda R., Foy D.W., Pitman R. (1995) Effect of prior trauma on acute hormonal response to rape. *Am J Psychiatry*, **15**: 1675–1677.
38. Delahanty D.L., Riamonde A.J., Spoonster E. (2000) Initial posttraumatic urinary cortisol levels predict subsequent PTSD symptoms in motor vehicle accident victims. *Biol Psychiatry*, **48**: 940–947.
39. Bryant R.A., Harvey A.G., Guthrie R., Moulds M. (2000) A prospective study of acute psychophysiological arousal, acute stress disorder, and posttraumatic stress disorder. *J Abnorm Psychol*, **109**: 341–344.
40. Yehuda R., Bierer L.M., Schmeidler J., Aferiat D.H., Breslau I., Dolan S. (2000) Low cortisol and risk for PTSD in adult offspring of holocaust survivors. *Am J Psychiatry*, **157**: 1252–1259.
41. Gilbertson M.W., Shenton M.E., Ciszewski A., Kasai K., Lasko N.B., Orr S.P., et al. (2002) Smaller hippocampal volume predicts pathologic vulnerability to psychological trauma. *Nature Neurosci*, **5**: 1242–1247.
42. Holsboer F. (2001) The corticosteroid receptor hypothesis of depression. *Neuropsychopharmacology*, **23**: 477–501.
43. Pacak K., Palkovitz M., Kopin I.J., Goldstein D.S. (1995) Stress-induced norepinephrine release in the hypothalamic paraventricular nucleus and pituitary-adrenocortical and sympathoadrenal activity: in vivo microdialysis studies. *Frontiers in Neuroendocrinology*, **16**: 89–150.
44. Yehuda R. (2002) Posttraumatic stress disorder. *N Engl J Med*, **346**: 108–114.
45. Cahill L., Prins B., Weber M., McGaugh J.L. (1994) Adrenergic activation and memory for emotional events. *Nature*, **371**: 702–704.
46. Maes M., Lin A.H., Delmeire L., Van Gastel A., Kenis G., De Jongh R., et al. (1999) Elevated serum interleukin-6 (IL-6) and IL-6 receptor concentrations in posttraumatic stress disorder following accidental man-made traumatic events. *Biol Psychiatry*, **45**: 833–839.
47. Southwick S.M., Krystal J.H., Morgan C.A., Johnson D., Nagy L.M., Nicolaou A., et al. (1993) Abnormal noradrenergic function in posttraumatic stress disorder. *Arch Gen Psychiatry*, **50**: 266–274.

48. Orr S. (1997) Psychophysiologic reactivity to trauma-related imagery in PTSD: diagnostic and theoretical implications of recent findings. In R. Yehuda, A.C. McFarlane (Eds.), *Psychobiology of Posttraumatic Stress Disorder*, pp. 114–124. New York Academy of Sciences, 821.

49. Neylan T.C., Lenoci M., Maglione M.L., Rosenlicht N.Z., Metzler T.J., Otte C., *et al.* (2003) Delta sleep response to metyrapone in post-traumatic stress disorder. *Neuropsychopharmacology*, **28**: 1666–1676.

50. Rausch L.S., Shin L.M., Pitman R.K. (1997) Evaluating the effects of psychological trauma using neuroimaging techniques. *Annual Review of Psychiatry*, **17**: 67–96.

51. Vaiva G., Ducrocq F., Jezequel K., Averland B., Lestavel P., Brunet A., *et al.* (2003) Immediate treatment with propranolol decreases posttraumatic stress disorder two months after trauma. *Biol Psychiatry*, **54**: 947–949.

52. Schelling G. (2002) Effects of stress hormones on traumatic memory formation and the development of posttraumatic stress disorder in critically ill patients. *Neurobiol Learn Mem*, **78**: 596–609.

53. Schelling G., Briegel J., Roozendaal B., Stoll C., Rothenhausler H.B., Kapfhammer H.P. (2001) The effect of stress doses of hydrocortisone during septic shock on posttraumatic stress disorder in survivors. *Biol Psychiatry*, **50**: 978–985.

5

Psychological Interventions for People Exposed to Disasters

Mordechai (Moty) Benyakar[1] and Carlos R. Collazo[2]

[1]University of Buenos Aires, Buenos Aires, Argentina
[2]University of El Salvador, Buenos Aires, Argentina

INTRODUCTION

Disasters confront us with the complex interweaving of different dimensions of human life. Therefore, in order to deal with the psychological consequences of disasters, we need to integrate various disciplines. In this chapter we address the specific field of mental health care. Our experience as psychiatrists with people exposed to several wars, terrorist attacks, massive accidents and "natural" disasters made us aware of some paradoxes, which are presented below. Subsequently, the reader will find what one of us called the "10 Ws", i.e., 10 key concepts on which to base psychological assistance during disasters. We will then analyze the various psychological approaches to people exposed to disasters.

Disasters are external events that harm both people and their habitat. They affect populations as well as individuals. Most of them irrupt unexpectedly, a fact that gives them a high psycho-pathogenic potential [1–3]. They are usually referred to as traumatic, but we prefer to call them "disruptive", leaving the words "trauma" and "stress" to name certain subjective reactions. This terminology allows us to consider disruptive situations as not unavoidably pathogenic for the affected individuals [4–6].

PARADOXES IN PSYCHOLOGICAL ASSISTANCE IN DISASTERS

(1) The pathogenic character of a disruptive situation lies in the situation itself, external to the individual, more than in his/her biological or psychological condition.

Disasters and Mental Health. Edited by Juan José López-Ibor, George Christodoulou, Mario Maj, Norman Sartorius and Ahmed Okasha.
©2005 John Wiley & Sons Ltd. ISBN 0-470-02123-3.

(2) As assisting and assisted persons are under the same threats, it is especially difficult for the therapists to establish a proper therapeutic distance.

(3) Highly trained teams have to be prepared to act in situations whose character, time and place of occurrence they cannot anticipate.

(4) Almost everyone undergoing a disruptive event is a "damaged person", but not necessarily a patient. The presence of hidden psychological injuries needs to be checked.

(5) In helping "damaged" people, we must avoid their victimization. From a psychosocial point of view, a "victim" is a person whose subjectivity becomes and remains trapped by a given situation. "Victims" are usually produced by "harmed" groups who need them in order to guarantee the memory of the "harming event". This production is the result of an unconscious process. As assisting professionals, we must help "damaged" people to recover their subjectivity by getting rid of the role of "victims". Victimization is a major obstacle to rehabilitation [7,8].

(6) Post-traumatic stress disorder (PTSD) is the main diagnostic category we have for psychic injuries due to disasters. Yet, at present, it is an unspecific syndrome, placing stress and trauma under the same diagnostic heading, thus failing to acknowledge the variety of psychic consequences of disasters [9,10]. We prefer to use the expression "disorders by disruption", a category encompassing various psychological manifestations such as stress, depression, different types of anxiety disorders, etc. This diagnostic construct specifies some features included in PTSD more precisely and highlights others not considered in that diagnosis [7,11].

(7) Although for each individual who is physically injured during a disaster there are more than 200 psychologically damaged people, the ratio between the personnel who assist the former and the latter is 20 to 1 [12–14].

(8) The disorganizing impact of disasters also affects those who assist. They tend to create small groups which not rarely compete with each other, as if they were unconsciously acting out the environment's disorganizing effects.

These paradoxes lead to the following key concepts (10 Ws), on which to base psychological assistance methods during disasters.

THE 10 Ws

1. Warding (Warding Psychological Stability)

Despite the unpredictability of disasters, populations can be prepared psychologically in advance to meet their impact [15,16]. People living under constant threat (especially that of terrorism) show a tendency to develop mechanisms like denial, which leads to the belief that the menace will never be effective or will not affect them directly. Based on this evidence, on the principles of somatic immunity and on the conviction that strong psychological and physical preparation helps people to accept reality, we developed the concept of "mental immunity", emphasizing the development of defenses so that attacks can be thought of as possible [7]. Mental immunity means that the individual can: (a) recognize the menace and its characteristics; (b) use psychological capacities to cope with threatening situations; (c) take preventive and objective measures in case threat becomes a fact.

2. Why (Why Are Mental Health Professionals Necessary during a Disaster?)

They are needed because disruptive situations have the potential to cause various mental disorders. Therefore, one function of these professionals is to serve as a bridge between the disruptive external world and the inner world of each person. As the outer world is perceived as harmful, therapists must present themselves as part of that same world, but with a protective attitude. In this way they will prevent a permanent damage in the individual's relation with the outer world. Another function is to screen the main pathological reactions. A third one is to decide what kind of interventions should be carried out. A final one is to adapt interventions to actual needs, time and place [17,18].

3. What (What Is Our Objective While Assisting during Disasters?)

In a collapsing environment, endangered or actually harmed psychological processing abilities are the core of our interventions [19,20]. There are two concepts to be stressed: (a) the recovery of the individual's subjectivity; (b) the maintenance of the ability to elaborate the inner–outer world relation. Therapists should be finely tuned with the timing, place and manner of the intervention and highly sensitive to cultural characteristics.

4. Who (Who Must Intervene to Ensure People's Psychological Stability?)

As the ratio between available practitioners and people in need of mental health care is so inadequate, the population as a whole must become a resource. Mental health professionals play an important role in acknowledging people's ability to assume responsibility (this applies especially to prominent members of the community, such as religious leaders, educators, etc.), building a network including them as health agents, and coordinating it [21,22].

5. Whom (Whom Are We Going to Assist?)

During disasters, mental health care is usually given to those showing their needs in the most evident way. Yet, we need to be sensitive in order to identify those who remain silent, apart or make-believe that "nothing happened to them". Some groups are special targets: children, the elderly, pregnant women, disabled people, and those at risk due to psychological weakness and lesser capacity to deal with threats [23,24].

6. Whose (Whose Responsibility Is at Stake?)

This question concerns individuals and social institutions in two different aspects: (a) the mere presence makes human beings subjectively responsible; even though we may have no relation at all with the occurrence of external facts, we still are inevitably responsible for our reactions to them; (b) communities must have institutions which are accountable socially and legally for disasters. That is, not only who is "guilty" but who is in charge of administering assistance [25].

7. When (When Do We Have to Intervene?)

Intervention during disasters involves four different stages: (a) the pre-impact phase, in which actions are directed towards building "mental immunity" in all members of the community so that they will become capable of recognizing the nature and importance of the menace, organizing available resources and acting properly and according to the circumstances [26]; (b) the impact phase, in which actions are directed to evaluate the impact of the event on the population and to respond to urgent and acute needs; (c) the phase immediately after the occurrence of the event, in which actions are directed to evaluate individual responses, to prevent the development of pathogenic mechanisms and to respond to emerging pathologies [27]; (d) the long-term phase, in which actions are directed to provide treatment to people that need long-term assistance or cases of late appearance of mental disturbances, and in which strategies for building "mental immunity" should be reinforced as a preventive measure for the future [28,29].

8. Where (Where Do We Have to Intervene?)

Mental health professionals will often need to be flexible and create adequate therapeutic milieus even in completely inadequate environments. Any place can become a suitable one for therapy if it is signified as such; for example, in the open by underlining the sheltering character of a tree. We have called this process "from the couch to the stones" [30].

9. Ways (In Which Ways Are We Going to Intervene?)

Treatment can consist of individual, family or group interventions. Professionals must stick to the core of their theoretical frameworks while adapting techniques to the circumstances. During disasters people are not aware of the psychic damage they may be suffering. Therefore, they do not demand treatment. This is why we postulate the concept of "intervention by presence" instead of "by demand", which means to be present offering direct care in different places and moments.

10. Wholeness

Wholeness means an integrative approach based on the previous nine Ws and on a consistent vision of the problem, the ways to intervene and the organization of assistance. The complexity of disasters requires not only the integration of psychiatric and psychological aspects, but also knowledge about social, political, economic and cultural processes. This does not mean that we will take care of all aspects of the problem. On the contrary, we must restrict our interventions to our specific role, preserving the ethical values of our profession [31,32].

PSYCHOLOGICAL DEBRIEFING

Over the last 20 years, it has become customary and then almost mandatory to apply early intervention after disasters and other traumatic events, in the hope of accelerating the resolution of trauma-associated symptoms. Early interventions are intuitively appealing and appear to be a response to a perceived need, but whether or not they are useful remains unclear.

The procedure of choice has become psychological debriefing, in which the subject is encouraged to talk about the trauma in narrative detail, recounting the facts and elaborating on his or her thoughts and feelings during the event. Debriefing is typically provided in a single session, within 72 hours of the trauma, in an individual or group setting. This is based on the assumption that the earlier the intervention occurs the less opportunity there is for maladaptive and disruptive cognitive and behavioral patterns to become established.

The concept of group debriefing grew out of the work of Marshall during World War II. He noticed that when a person could describe what happened to him during a very stressful experience this served not only an abreactive purpose but allowed colleagues to correct misperceptions and render social support. This appeared to reduce the likelihood of combat stress reactions and to restore the readiness to combat [33].

Debriefing has become increasingly popular as a treatment for victims of a wide range of traumatic events, from violent crime to natural disasters. In some circumstances and in certain occupations it has become mandatory. Organizations which routinely send their employees into potentially traumatizing situations are compelled to use it in order to protect the health of employees and minimize the impact of litigation seeking compensation.

Psychological debriefing is a formal type of post-traumatic care, for which several models have been developed in the past two decades. Among them, the Critical Incident Stress Debriefing (CISD), also known as the Mitchell model, is the most popular. This is a preventive method proposed by Jeffrey Mitchell to minimize adverse effects of the normal stress response [34,35]. It is one of the most widely practiced forms of early intervention in disruptive situations, promoting emotional processing, ventilation, normalization of reactions and preparation for possible future experiences. It aims to reduce pathological patterns, by focusing on the "here and now", during the 48–72 hours after the disruptive event, in a group meeting that lasts approximately 2 or 3 hours, led by one or two debriefers. Groups of participants are led in an active process of abreaction, sharing, and normalizing of stress reactions while participants are told that they are not "patients".

Mitchell describes several stages in the process of debriefing: (a) the introductory phase (introduction of the team, purpose of the meeting, confidentiality, ground rules, etc.); (b) the fact phase (reconstruction of the event in detail, in chronological order, viewed from all sides and perspectives, and by each group member); (c) the thought phase (sights, smells, other sensory impressions and thoughts about what happened; participants are asked to share what "thoughts" they had at key moments); (d) the reaction phase (to identify and ventilate feelings regarding self, victims or colleagues and raised by the event); (e) the symptom phase (review of symptoms and signs of distress; description of the normal stress response legitimizing participants' physical symptoms and behavioral reactions; challenging inappropriate feelings of guilt and responsibility); (f) the teaching phase (emphasizing that the feelings and stress symptoms are normal reactions to abnormal situations and that they are expected to resolve normally; teaching coping strategies to deal with possible psychological symptoms, with family, friends and work; explaining when, where and under what circumstances to get further help if necessary); (g) the reentry phase (summarize, discuss selected issues, complete and close the debriefing).

Perren-Klingler [36] identifies seven stages for debriefing: (a) introducing the procedure; (b) processing the thread connecting different aspects of the event; (c) transition to the next stage by elaborating emotions and feelings related to the event; (d) going over impressions and sensations; (e) information and normalizing of reactions; (f) separation rituals; (g) recovering contact with reality and daily routine. Herman [37] proposes a "three-phase model": the first aims to re-establish a sense of safety and self-control, as well as control over the environment, and to learn how to handle symptoms that put the subject at risk; the second is that for remembrance and mourning, that is, when the patient reconstructs the traumatic event through a narration where fragments of memory and emotional and physical sensations become integrated; the third is for reconnection (the patient is again connected with his/her present and future and with significant relationships and activities).

The timing of debriefing is considered of vital importance. Defenses start to work almost immediately and the individuals begin to deny and project anger. Therefore, it is commonly maintained that many groups should be debriefed as soon as possible to avoid the crystallization of such maladaptive defenses.

How effective is psychological debriefing? Is psychological debriefing a waste of time [38]? We can find numerous anecdotal reports suggesting that providing debriefing for everyone involved in a disruptive experience reduces subsequent psychopathological morbidity [39–41]. We became accustomed to using psychological debriefing with no research available as to whether it was helpful or not. Despite its popularity, this technique had been studied only sporadically over the years, and it is only in the last decade that high-quality research (i.e., high-quality clinical trials in which traumatized people were randomly assigned to be debriefed or not) has been published.

In recent years, studies have, in fact, shown that the procedure has no positive effect on post-traumatic stress symptoms. One study found no difference between victims of motor vehicle accidents who received debriefing and those who did not, 3 months after they experienced the trauma [42]. Moreover, longer-term studies have suggested that debriefing may impede the natural process of recovery: in a study of burn victims, there was no difference between those who did and did not receive the intervention 3 months later, but, at 13 months, those who had had debriefing did worse: 15% met criteria for PTSD, compared with none [43].

A Cochrane review [44] of eight randomized trials found no evidence that debriefing has any impact on psychological morbidity (in particular, no strong evidence that debriefing reduces a person's odds of developing PTSD, depression and anxiety; is safe and effective for children; or can be an effective form of group therapy). Furthermore, there is no information about debriefing for those who had psychiatric disorders prior to the trauma, because such people have been excluded from all studies. The most troubling finding came from the controlled trials with the longest follow-up (one tracked participants for 13 years), which provided evidence that some people are worse off after debriefing. The reviewers concluded that, for some people, "debriefing may actually cause the post-traumatic stress it is intended to prevent. This may be because talking about and reliving the trauma is a further traumatic event in itself" [44]. The reviewers also found that people most likely to develop PTSD are unlikely to be helped by a single debriefing session, and "indeed such an intervention may be harmful" [44]. These findings were so alarming that the reviewers recommended to stop the practice of compulsory post-trauma debriefing in people with certain occupations.

In the above review, it was hypothesized that the relatively recent changes in awareness of the psychological effects of traumas could render debriefing obsolete. Due to this awareness, "everybody experiences a 'bit of debriefing' anyway, thus reducing the possibility of showing any effects from a formal intervention" [44]. Concerning the apparent harmful effect of the intervention, it was postulated that debriefing may "medicalize" normal distress, thus increasing "the expectancy of developing psychological symptoms in those who would otherwise not have done so" [44].

Evidence about the ineffectiveness of debriefing has come from randomized trials which used broad definitions of the intervention. Therefore, it might be that these findings were obtained because an inappropriate form of debriefing was used. In particular, if a specific model like CISD had been used, the outcome could have been different. However, there have been no published, randomized controlled trials using such specific models. There has also been no randomized controlled trial comparing the different types of debriefing. Therefore, there is no evidence supporting the use of one type of debriefing instead of another.

Debriefing is a very popular intervention among many health and allied practitioners. Many organizations are likely to continue using it, since there is no comparable broadly acceptable early intervention with a similar low cost.

Everly and Mitchell [45] pointed out several methodological problems in research carried out up to now on debriefing. Some studies pooled the results of interventions offered by practitioners with varied levels of skills and training, and possibly using different debriefing models. Other studies involved an improper application of debriefing, using it as a freestanding intervention rather than as one component of a complete critical incident stress management (CISM) program. Apparently, similar difficulties commonly arise whenever researchers attempt to study the efficacy of psychotherapy using randomized experimental designs. The only way to get an accurate picture of the effectiveness of these interventions may be to allow a broader research approach, including the use of non-randomized designs and survey research [45].

A National Institute of Mental Health (NIMH) workshop on mass violence concluded that early intervention in the form of ventilation of events and emotions evoked by a traumatic event does not consistently reduce risk for later PTSD or related adjustment difficulties [46]. However, the same workshop concluded that early, brief, and focused psychotherapeutic intervention can reduce stress in bereaved spouses, parents, and children and that selected cognitive-behavioral approaches may help reduce incidence, duration, and severity of acute stress disorder (ASD), PTSD and depression in survivors.

CISD was never designed to be a stand-alone intervention, but, instead, a component of a broader, multi-component CISM-type intervention, that included training in being prepared for a crisis, follow-up, and referral. Therefore, debriefing should be used carefully and always as part of a broader crisis intervention program including ongoing education, social support and, when necessary, psychotherapy.

COGNITIVE-BEHAVIORAL INTERVENTIONS

Cognitive-behavioral interventions are rooted in learning theories, especially classical conditioning and operant avoidance. Early studies focused exclusively on fear and anxiety reactions. The first treatment approach to be proposed for treating trauma-related symptoms was Stress Inoculation Training (SIT) [47]. The main goal of SIT is to help the patients to understand and manage their trauma-related fear reactions and, as a result, decrease avoidance behavior.

SIT can be conducted in either group or individual format and the classic protocol consists of three steps: education, skills-building and application. During the education phase, the patients receive an explanation for their symptoms and are taught to identify their different "channels" of response (emotions, behaviors, thoughts and sensorimotor level). During the second step, the patients are taught coping skills for each of the channels. Coping skills include relaxing, relaxing imagery, recognition of "stress deposit" areas in the body, identification of cues that trigger fear reactions, thought stopping, redirection of thinking, covert rehearsal, etc. During the third step (application), the patient learns how to apply these coping skills in daily situations that provoke anxiety.

Exposure techniques have also been applied to persons suffering from post-traumatic disorders. They use careful, repeated, detailed imagining of the trauma (exposure) in a safe, controlled context to help the survivor face and gain control of the anxiety, fear and distress that was overwhelming during the disrupting event. In some cases memories or reminders can be confronted all at once ("flooding"). For other individuals, it is preferable to work up to the most severe symptoms gradually by using relaxation techniques and by starting with less upsetting life stresses, or by taking the trauma one piece at a time ("desensitization").

Systematic desensitization involves the pairing of relaxation with either stimuli reminiscent of the traumatic event ("in vivo" desensitization) or images of the disrupting event (imaginal desensitization). In vivo exposure to traumatic cues would include a return to the scene of a disruptive event and a gradual approach to the cues that are most evocative of the emotions associated with the event together with the practice of cued relaxation responses such as deep breathing and relaxing imagery. Previously, a graduated hierarchy of anxiety-inducing cues is built by the therapist together with the patient and this enables the therapist to control the extent to which the patient is successfully coping with the anxiety and thus determine whether the patient is ready to face the next step in the hierarchy.

Following the same fundamental principles used in "in vivo" desensitization, imaginal desensitization uses memories, images or other cognitive representations of the disruptive event. The patient is trained in using relaxation skills, and is then confronted with fear cues in imagination, along a graded hierarchy, while in a relaxed state. During each session the exposures are brief, repetitive and focused on one fear cue alone. There is input and feedback from the patient along the sessions, which allows him/her to develop a sense of control in the process.

In the flooding technique, the patient undergoes an extended exposure to moderate or strong fear-producing cues in the safety of the therapeutic relationship. The fear sequences are repeated as many times as necessary until the event or cues progressively become less aversive.

Along with exposure, cognitive behavioral interventions for trauma include: (a) learning skills for coping with anxiety (such as breathing retraining or biofeedback) and negative thoughts ("cognitive restructuring");

(b) managing anger; (c) preparing for stress reactions ("stress inoculation"); (d) handling future symptoms related to disruptive events; (e) addressing urges to use alcohol or drugs when trauma symptoms occur; (f) communicating and relating effectively with people (social skills or marital therapy).

A large number of studies have examined the effectiveness of cognitive-behavioral interventions in preventing or treating PTSD or ASD.

Foa et al. [48] reported on the preliminary findings of a therapeutic intervention intended to prevent the development of PTSD in female rape and assault victims. The intervention consisted of four 2-hour sessions. During the first meeting, the therapist introduced the program and gathered information about the subject's symptoms and distorted beliefs related to the disruptive experience they suffered. Also, a list of avoided people and/or situations was generated. In the second session, this list was organized into a hierarchy based on the level of anxiety each item produced. The person was trained in relaxation and deep breathing and then asked to recall the experience (imaginal exposure). The therapist led the person to examine the accuracy of his/her beliefs through oriented questions (cognitive restructuring). This dialogue was audiotaped and the person was instructed to listen to it several times during the week. Also he/she was encouraged to confront daily some of the anxiety-releasing detected situations. The third meeting began with a review of the "homework" followed by a new session of imaginal exposure and cognitive restructuring. Again, the person was instructed to listen to the audiotape every day, to confront feared situations, to update a daily diary to record cognitive distortions and negative feelings and thoughts. During the fourth session, imaginal exposure was repeated, followed by cognitive restructuring using the daily diary records. Finally, both the therapist and the person reviewed the new skills the person had obtained. The results were very positive: 2 months after the trauma, 10% of the group of persons who received the program met criteria for PTSD, compared to 70% of the control group.

Bryant et al. [49], treating motor vehicle and industrial accident victims who met criteria for ASD, compared five sessions of non-directive supportive counseling (providing support and education and teaching problem solving skills) with brief cognitive-behavioral treatment (trauma education, progressive muscle relaxation, imaginal exposure, cognitive restructuring, and graded in vivo exposure to avoided situations). At the conclusion of treatment, 8% of the participants in the cognitive-behavioral treatment group and 83% of those in the supportive counseling group met criteria for PTSD. Six months after the trauma, these criteria were met by 17% in the former group and 67% in the latter. There was also a significant reduction in depressive symptoms in the former group compared to the latter.

The magnitude of treatment effects appears greater with cognitive-behavioral interventions than with any other treatment. The questions for the clinician, then, are with what patients is exposure therapy most effective, for what kind of symptoms and at what time. When utilized within a comprehensive treatment program that addresses the psychological, social and physiological elements of the disorder, exposure therapies offer innovative methods to deal with this type of human suffering. The creativity and flexibility of the therapist are essential when focusing on the key symptoms of the affected persons in order to promote the optimal exposure.

EYE MOVEMENT DESENSITIZATION AND REPROCESSING

Eye movement desensitization and reprocessing (EMDR) is a technique developed by Shapiro [50] on the basis of the observation that lateral eye movements facilitate cognitive processing of traumatic material. It is a form of exposure (desensitization) with evident cognitive components accompanied by rhythmic eye movements. Designed originally as a treatment for traumatic memories, it was called eye movement desensitization (EMD). Its essence was as follows. After identifying a traumatic target memory, the therapist asked the patient to articulate a self-referent negative cognition associated with the memory and a positive cognition to replace the negative one. The therapist then moved his/her fingers back and forth in front of the patient's eyes, instructing the patient to track his/her fingers visually while concentrating on the distressing memory. After each set of 10–12 eye movements, the therapist asked the client to provide ratings of distress and strength of belief in the positive cognition. The therapist repeated this procedure until distress subsided and belief in the positive cognition increased.

According to Shapiro [50], a single 50-minute session of EMD was 100% successful in abolishing distress associated with a traumatic memory in survivors of combat, rape, and childhood sexual or emotional abuse. To explain these impressive results, she hypothesized that the crucial component of the EMD procedure is the repeated eye-movements while the memory is maintained in awareness. Shortly thereafter, Shapiro reconceptualized EMD in terms of accelerated information processing and renamed it eye movement desensitization and reprocessing (EMDR). The shift from EMD to EMDR appears, however, more conceptual than procedural.

Vaughan et al. [51] found no difference among the effects of EMDR, applied relaxation, and "image habituation training" in cases of civilian PTSD, although all treatments were better than a wait-list.

EMDR has been controversial for a number of reasons, especially the lack of theoretical foundation for the therapeutic impact of eye movements and the lack of empirical data obtained with reliable methodology. Researchers have compared EMDR to the relationship between therapist and patient used in EMDR technique without eye movements and in most of the studies they did not find differences in the effects [52]. Therefore any efficacy demonstrated by EMDR may be more attributable to the facilitation of information processing than to eye movements. According to one view, what is effective in EMDR (imaginal exposure) is not new, and what is new (eye movements) is not effective [53]. Consistent with this interpretation, a meta-analysis revealed that EMDR produced effects similar to those produced by conventional behavioral and cognitive-behavior therapy treatments for PTSD [54].

SOMATIC AWARENESS APPROACHES

Persons who suffer a disruptive situation usually show an altered relationship among cognitive, emotional and sensory-motor (body) levels of information processing. The sensory-motor (body) processing level must be integrated with cognitive and emotional processing in the treatment of the patient. By using the body (rather than cognition or emotion) as a primary entry point in processing trauma, sensory-motor psychotherapy aims to directly treat the effect of trauma on the body, which in turn should facilitate emotional and cognitive processing [55].

The essentials of sensory-motor psychotherapy are (a) regulating affective and sensory-motor states through the therapeutic relationship, and (b) teaching the patient to self-regulate by mindfully contacting, tracking and articulating sensory-motor processes independently. This approach aims to allow the patient to increase his/her awareness of inner body sensations, facilitating the processing of unassimilated body reactions to trauma and their disturbing effects on cognition and emotion. At present, there is no systematic study confirming the efficacy of this approach.

PSYCHOANALYTICALLY ORIENTED PSYCHOTHERAPY

Lindy used brief psychoanalytic psychotherapy techniques to treat PTSD [56]. His therapy has three main elements: (a) therapeutic alliance; (b) disclosure and interpretation of transference; (c) detection and therapeutic use of counter-transference. According to Lindy, the disruptive event damages the patient's perceptive capacity negatively, affecting his/her reality judgment. The analyst must bring the patient's attention to those aspects of everyday reality associated with trauma that can be elaborated. Later on the patient, after internalizing the psychoanalyst's discriminative capacity, will recover his reality judgment. At present, there is no systematic study confirming the efficacy of this approach.

CONCLUSIONS

Several psychological interventions are currently applied in people exposed to disasters. However, research evidence concerning the efficacy of most of them is currently insufficient. For psychological debriefing, the most frequently used technique, the available evidence is even predominantly negative. However, several methodological problems should be taken into account in this respect, and innovative research designs are probably needed.

A common objective of the various interventions is to elaborate the articulation between the disruptive event which took place and the patient's psychic experience. Counter-transference needs to be adequately managed: the risk of "compassion fatigue" has to be taken into account. Some flexibility is needed to adapt therapeutic models to the circumstances in which therapists have to work.

Therapists must differentiate between bizarre but normal reactions and the pathological consequences of a disaster, in order to avoid "over-treating" people. They must bear in mind that they do not treat "traumas" or "stress", but people who assume a disruptive event as trauma or stress. The difference may seem subtle, even artificial, but it is very important in terms of the therapeutic process.

The core of mental health interventions in disasters is to deal with the suffering of the damaged person avoiding fixing him/her in the role of victim.

REFERENCES

1. Crocq L. (1997) The emotional consequences of war 50 years on. A psychiatric perspective. In L. Hunt, M. Marshall, C. Rowlings (Eds.), *Past Trauma in Late Life*, pp. 39–48. Kingsley, London.
2. Cohen R. (2002) Mental health services for victims of disasters. *World Psychiatry*, 1: 149–152.
3. López-Ibor J.J. (2002) The psycho(patho)logy of disasters. Presented at the 12th World Congress of Psychiatry, Yokohama, August 24–29.
4. Benyakar M., Kutz I., Dasberg H., Stern M. (1989) The collapse of a structure: a structural approach to trauma. *J Trauma Stress*, 2: 431–449.

5. Benyakar M. (in press) Five wars. In *Living with Terror, Working with Trauma: A Clinician's Handbook*. Aronson, New York.
6. Benyakar M., Knafo D. (in press) Disruption: individual and collective threats. In *Living with Terror, Working with Trauma: A Clinician's Handbook*. Aronson, New York.
7. Benyakar M. (2003) *Disruption: Collective and Individual Threats*. Biblos, Buenos Aires.
8. López-Ibor J.J. (2003) Foreword. In M. Benyakar (Ed.), *Disruption: Collective and Individual Threats*, pp. 11–13. Biblos, Buenos Aires.
9. Crocq L. (1996) Critique du concept d'état de stress post-traumatique. *Perspectives Psychologiques*, December.
10. Shalev A.Y. (2000) Post-traumatic stress disorder: diagnosis, history and life course. In D. Nutt, J. Davison, J. Zohar (Eds.), *Post-traumatic Stress Disorder. Diagnosis, Management and Treatment*, pp. 1–12. Dunitz, London.
11. Benyakar M., Collazo C., de Rosa E. (2002) Anxiety by disruption. http://psiquiatria.com.
12. McFarlane A.C. (1989) The treatment of post-traumatic stress disorder. *Br J Med Psychol*, **18**: 354–358.
13. Ursano R.J., Fullerton C., McCaughey B.G. (2000) *Trauma and Disaster*. Cambridge University Press, Cambridge, UK.
14. Susser E.S., Susser M. (2002) The aftermath of September 11: what's an epidemiologist to do? *Int J Epidemiol*, **31**: 719–721.
15. Cohen R. (1999) *Mental Health for Victims of Disasters. Instructors Guide*. Pan-American Health Organization, Washington, DC.
16. Cohen R. (1999) *Mental Health for Victims of Disasters. Workers Manual*. Pan-American Health Organization, Washington, DC.
17. López-Ibor J.J., Soria J., Cañas F., Rodriguez-Gamazo M. (1985) Psychopathological aspects of the toxic oil syndrome catastrophe. *Br J Psychiatry*, **147**: 352–365.
18. López-Ibor J.J. (1987) Social reinsertion after catastrophes. The toxic oil syndrome experience. *Eur J Psychiatry*, **1**: 12–19.
19. Mark B.S., Layton A., Chesworth M. (1997) *I'll Know What To Do: A Kid's Guide to Natural Disasters*. American Psychological Association, Washington, DC.
20. Murthy S. (2002) *Riots. Psychosocial Care by Community Level Helpers for Survivors*. Books for Change, Bangalore.
21. Kretsch R., Benyakar M., Baruch E., Roth M. (1997) A shared reality of therapists and survivors in a national crisis as illustrated by the gulf war. *Israel J Psychiatry*, **34**: 28–33.
22. Benyakar M. (2002) Frame in social disasters, war and terrorism. In J. Raphael-Left (Ed.), *Between Sessions and Beyond the Couch*, pp. 126–129. University of Essex, Colchester.
23. Tyano S. (1996) Seven year follow-up of child survivors of a bus–train collision. Personal communication.
24. Benyakar M. (2000) *Aggression of Life and Violence of Death. The Infant and His Environment*. http://w.w.w.winnicott.net/patron_esp.htm.
25. Collazo C. (1985) Psychiatric casualties in Malvinas war: a provisional report. In P. Pichot, P. Berner, R. Wolf, K. Thau (Eds.), *Psychiatry: The State of the Art*, Vol. 6, pp. 499–503. Plenum Press, New York.
26. Lebigot F. (1998) The advantages of immediate and postimmediate care following psychic trauma. Presented at the 5th World Congress of the International Association for Emergency Psychiatry, Brussels, 15–17 October.

27. Crocq L., Doutheau C., Louville P., Cremniter D. (1998) Psychiatrie de catastrophe. Réactions immédiates et différées, troubles séquellaires. Paniques et psychopathologie collective. In *Encyclopédie Médico-Chirurgicale, Psychiatrie*, 37-113-D-10. Elsevier, Paris.

28. Solomon Z., Laor N., Weiler D., Muller U., Hadar O., Waysman M., *et al.* (1991) The psychological impact of the Gulf War: a study of acute stress in Israeli evacuees. *Arch Gen Psychiatry*, 50: 320–321.

29. Solomon Z. (1993) Immediate and long-term effects of traumatic combat stress among Israeli veterans of the Lebanon War. In J.P. Wilson, B. Raphael (Eds.), *International Handbook of Traumatic Stress Syndromes*, pp. 321–332. Plenum, New York.

30. Benyakar M. (1994) Trauma and post traumatic neurosis: from the psychological experience to theoretical consideration. *Actualidad Psicológica*, 211: 26–32.

31. Okasha A., Arboleda-Florez J., Sartorius N. (2000) *Ethics, Culture and Psychiatry: International Perspectives*. American Psychiatric Press, Washington, DC.

32. Fariña J., Benyakar M., Arboleda Flórez J. (2003) International bioethical information system: multimedia on ethics in catastrophes. Presented at the Interamerican Congress of Psychology, Lima, July 13–18.

33. Marshall C. (1979) *Bringing up the Rear: A Memoir*. Presidio Press, San Rafael.

34. Mitchell J.T. (1983) When disaster strikes: the critical incident stress debriefing process. *J Emergency Med Serv*, 8: 35–39.

35. Dyregov A. (1997) The process of psychological debriefings. *J Trauma Stress*, 10: 589–605.

36. Perren-Klingler G. (2003) *Debriefing. Models and Applications. From the Traumatic History to the Integrated Story*. Psychotrauma Institute, Switzerland.

37. Herman J. (1997) *Trauma and Recovery. The Aftermath of Violence. From Domestic Abuse to Political Terror*. Basic Books, New York.

38. Wessely S., Deahl M. (2003) Psychological debriefing is a waste of time. *Br J Psychiatry*, 183: 12–14.

39. Armstrong K., O'Callahan W., Marmar C.R. (1991) Debriefing Red Cross disaster personnel: the multiple stressor debriefing model. *J Trauma Stress*, 4: 581–593.

40. Dyregov A. (1989) Caring for helpers in disaster situations: psychological debriefing. *Disaster Management*, 2: 25–30.

41. Chemtob C., Toma S., Law W., Cremniter D. (1997) Post-disaster psychological interventions: a field study of the impact of debriefing on psychological distress. *Am J Psychiatry*, 154, 415–417.

42. Hobbs M., Mayou R., Harrison B., Worlock P. (1996) A randomised controlled trial of psychological debriefing for victims of road traffic accidents. *Br Med J*, 313: 1438–1439.

43. Bisson J.I., Jenkins P.L., Alexander J., Bannister C. (1997) Randomised controlled trial of psychological debriefing for victims of acute burn trauma. *Br J Psychiatry*, 171: 78–81.

44. Rose S., Bisson J., Wessely S. (2002) Psychological debriefing for preventing post-traumatic stress disorder. *Cochrane Library*, issue 2. Update Software, Oxford.

45. Everly G.S. Jr., Mitchell J.T. (1999) The debriefing "controversy" and crisis intervention: a review of lexical and substantive issues. *Int J Emergency Mental Health*, 2: 211–225.

46. National Institute of Mental Health (2002) *Mental Health and Mass Violence: Evidence-Based Early Psychological Intervention for Victims/Survivors of Mass Violence. A Workshop to Reach Consensus Based on Practices.* US Government Printing Office, Washington, DC.

47. Kilpatrick D.G., Veronen L.J., Resick P.A. (1982) Psychological sequelae to rape: assessment and treatment strategies. In D.M. Dolays, R.L. Meredith, A.R. Ciminero (Eds.), *Behavioral Medicine: Assessment and Treatment Strategies*, pp. 473–497. Plenum Press, New York.

48. Foa E.B., Hearst-Ikeda E., Perry K.J. (1995) Evaluation of a brief cognitive behavioral program for the prevention of chronic PTSD in recent assault victims. *J Consult Clin Psychol*, **152**: 116–120.

49. Bryant R.A., Sackville T., Dang S.T., Moulds M., Guthrie R. (1999) Treating acute stress disorder: an evaluation of cognitive behavior therapy and supportive counseling techniques. *Am J Psychiatry*, **156**: 1780–1786.

50. Shapiro F. (1989) Eye movement desensitization: a new treatment for post traumatic stress disorder. *J Behav Ther Exper Psychiatry*, **20**, 211–217.

51. Vaughan K., Armstrong M.S., Gold R., O'Connor N., Jenneke W., Tarrier N. (1994) A trial of eye movement desensitization compared to image habituation training, and applied muscle relaxation in posttraumatic stress disorder. *J Behav Ther Exper Psychiatry*, **25**: 237–248.

52. Devilly G.J., Spence S.H., Rapee R.M. (1998) Statistical and reliable change with eye movement desensitization and reprocessing: treating trauma within a veteran population. *Behav Ther*, **29**: 435–455.

53. McNally R.J. (in press) On eye movements and animal magnetism: a reply to Greenwald's defense of EMDR. *J Anxiety Disord.*

54. Van Etten M.L., Taylor S. (1998) Comparative efficacy of treatments for posttraumatic stress disorder: a meta-analysis. *Clin Psychol Psychother*, **5**: 126–145.

55. Ogden P., Minton K. (2000) Sensorimotor psychotherapy: one method for processing traumatic memory. *Traumatology*, **6**.

56. Lindy J.D. (1993) Focal psychoanalytic psychotherapy of posttraumatic stress disorder. In J.P. Wilson and B. Raphael (Eds.), *International Handbook of Traumatic Stress Syndromes*, pp. 803–810. Plenum, New York.

6

Organization of Mental Health Services for Disaster Victims

Louis Crocq[1], Marc-Antoine Crocq[2], Alain Chiapello[3] and Carole Damiani[4]

[1]Necker Hospital, Paris, France
[2]Rouffach Hospital, Rouffach, France
[3]French Red Cross Society, Paris, France
[4]INAVEM (Institut National d'Aide aux Victimes), Paris, France

INTRODUCTION

In the past, the care of disaster victims was limited to rescuing them, tending their wounds, offering shelter and material assistance, helping them to relocate and resume their previous occupation. In the last three decades, increasing attention has also been given to the victims' psychological suffering, and to the psychosocial and moral burden of the individual and the community. Thus, programs for medical, psychological, and psychosocial intervention have been devised in various countries. They are implemented at different stages of the disaster and its aftermath. The guiding principles are: (a) to take into account psychological distress; (b) to manage the psychosocial impact on the individual and society; and (c) to prevent the development of late sequelae that would handicap individual or group functioning. Various initiatives have been proposed by governments, non-governmental organizations (NGOs), international associations, and private groups. Some of these initiatives have been quite successful. However, there is a need to integrate these various initiatives into a coherent whole. At a certain level, rescue and rehabilitation need to be coordinated by government authorities.

Disasters and Mental Health. Edited by Juan José López-Ibor, George Christodoulou, Mario Maj, Norman Sartorius and Ahmed Okasha.
©2005 John Wiley & Sons Ltd. ISBN 0-470-02123-3.

THE IMPACT OF DISASTERS ON INDIVIDUAL AND COLLECTIVE MENTAL HEALTH

In 1988, the World Health Organization estimated that natural disasters had afflicted 26 million persons between 1900 and 1988. In that number, 10 million had been made homeless. A 1992 report by the International Federation of the Red Cross and Red Crescent Societies identified 7,766 disasters that had occurred in the world between 1967 and 1991, killing 7 million and affecting 3 trillion individuals [1]. Natural disasters predominantly afflict poor populations – 68 out of 109 natural disasters that occurred in the world between 1960 and 1987 concerned developing countries, and only 41 affluent countries. Furthermore, the casualty rate is higher when disasters happen in poor countries, as compared with richer countries, because of factors such as overcrowding in areas that are prone to natural (e.g., floodland) or industrial disasters (e.g., chemical plants).

Regardless of the degree of material destruction, disasters are first and foremost characterized by the intensity of human trauma. The psychosocial aspect of disasters is underlined in our definition of a disaster by a combination of five criteria: (a) the occurrence of a negative event that brings distress to the people and the community (a revolution that frees a country from a tyrant is not considered a disaster, even when it causes thousands of casualties); (b) the causation of material destruction that significantly alters human environment (an avalanche in an uninhabited mountain valley is not a disaster, contrary to an avalanche in a populated valley); (c) a great number of victims, dead, injured, homeless, who suffer significant somatic injuries and psychological suffering; (d) the overwhelming disruption of local means of rescue and protection; and (e) the interruption of services that are normally offered by society (i.e., sheltering; producing, distributing, and consuming energy, water, food; health services; transportation; communication; public order; and even... burying the dead). It should be remembered that victims have been threatened not only in their individual ego, but also in their collective ego, or sense of belonging to a community. Their individual misfortune is also a collective misfortune. Gerrity and Steinglass [2] developed similar hypotheses about the familial group, on the basis of Reiss's "family paradigm" [3]. The family elaborates a set of beliefs about the environment. Its response to a disaster will be determined by its cognitive and emotional perception of the traumatic event and its relationship with the family's history.

The term "victim" is somewhat unclear. In the broadest meaning of the term, a victim is anyone who has been affected by the disaster in his/her physical or mental health, properties, or social life. Victims are usually classified into five groups on the basis of their distance to the disaster [4]:

(a) primary victims (dead, wounded, uninjured survivors), who have been directly exposed to the disaster; (b) secondary victims, who have not been directly affected, but who mourn a close relative who is part of the primary victims; (c) third-level victims, such as rescuers, health personnel, who intervened on the scene and have often witnessed traumatizing events; (d) fourth-level victims, such as government or media workers, who may have suffered emotionally when taking decisions or witnessing scenes; (e) fifth-level victims, in the general public, who were not physically present at the scene but suffered by proxy when exposed to the media coverage.

MENTAL CONDITION AND HEALTH CARE NEEDS OF DISASTER VICTIMS

The mental state of victims should be considered at the three different stages of disaster and aftermath: (a) the immediate reaction (usually, from a few hours to less than a day); (b) the post-immediate phase, that begins on the second day and lasts from a couple of days to a couple of months; (c) the delayed and long-lasting sequelae, that may be transitory (from 2 to 6 months) or become chronic (longer than 6 months).

Immediate Phase

About 75% of victims show no mental disorder, but only short-lived neuro-vegetative and psychological symptoms that are transitory (a few hours) and are part of the normal adaptive stress reaction. A short period of physical and psychological exhaustion may follow, because stress depletes energy. From a psychological viewpoint, this adaptive stress reaction is characterized by an adaptive focusing of attention on the danger situation, by the recruitment of mental capacities, and by the facilitation of action. Adaptive stress leads to decision-taking, acting on a decision, and adaptive fight-or-flight reactions. However, adaptive stress is an exceptional response that has a high cost in energy and discomfort. Therefore, individuals who exhibited this adaptive response may still need psycho-logical help afterwards.

A smaller proportion (25%) of victims may present with abnormal and maladaptive stress reactions, which may follow one of four patterns [5,6]: stupor, agitation, panic flight, automatic reaction. These maladaptive stress reactions always comprise elements of peri-traumatic dissociation [7], including confusion, derealization, fright, impression of absence of relief, and abulia. In ICD-10, such reactions are termed "acute stress reaction". DSM-IV proposes no diagnosis for this acute stress reaction, since the criteria of "acute stress disorder" require that the disturbance lasts for a minimum of 2 days, which exceeds the duration of the immediate stress reaction. Individuals who responded with maladaptive stress should be viewed as "psychological casualties"; they have lost their capacity for autonomy and should be given psychological help.

Post-immediate Period

Either the mental state returns to normal in a few days (neuro-vegetative and psychological symptoms subside, the individual is no longer entirely preoccupied by the event and can resume his previous activities), or a psychotraumatic syndrome appears, characterized by the re-experience of the event, avoidance of stimuli reminiscent of the trauma, hyperreactivity, and constant preoccupation with the trauma. Psychotraumatic symptoms may appear only after weeks, or months. This is the so-called "latency period", which had been identified in traumatic neurosis by Charcot and Janet, and called period of incubation, contemplation, meditation or rumination. The duration of this period is variable: each individual needs a different amount of time to organize new defense mechanisms. Furthermore, if the individual is still hospitalized, he may wait till he recovers his autonomy to start coping with the trauma. ICD-10 and DSM-IV propose the diagnostic term "post-traumatic stress disorder" (PTSD) (acute type, since the duration is short) for this syndrome. In addition, DSM-IV offers the category "acute stress disorder" for the cases with dissociative symptoms (appearing in the immediate phase) and psychotraumatic symptoms such as re-experiencing (appearing within 4 weeks of the trauma). Individuals who presented with a maladaptive acute stress reaction are more at risk to present with acute PTSD afterwards. However, this course is not unavoidable, and there are cases of maladaptive stress reaction that recover without consequences, whereas individuals who initially responded adaptively to the trauma may later develop severe PTSD.

Delayed and Chronic Period

Cases of acute stress and post-traumatic stress that occur during the post-immediate phase may resolve – spontaneously, or with treatment – fairly rapidly (in less than 3 months). However, they may also persist, and even become chronic. The typical clinical picture of PTSD may then become manifest during the delayed and chronic period, with its key features of: (a) exposition to a traumatic event, evoking a response of intense fear or helplessness; (b) persistent re-experience of the traumatic event (in intrusive recollections, dreams, flashback episodes, etc.); (c) avoidance of stimuli associated with the trauma and numbing of general responsiveness; and (d) symptoms of increased arousal.

It is worth noting that the above criteria (c) and (d) together reproduce the personality changes that were described in the former European diagnostic category termed "traumatic neurosis". According to Fenichel, this personality change was characterized by the blocking of such functions of the ego as: (a) filtering of the environment; (b) presence; (c) relationship with others. Briefly, the victim no longer has the same relationship with others and the world since the traumatic event. He has developed a new way of perceiving, thinking, loving, wanting, and acting. In addition to PTSD, ICD-10 provides another diagnostic category entitled "enduring personality change after catastrophic experience" (F62.0), defined by criteria such as a mistrustful attitude toward the world, social withdrawal, feelings of emptiness or of being threatened, and estrangement.

Traumatic neurosis, as it was described in Europe, associated several non-specific symptoms, such as physical, psychological, and sexual asthenia; anxiety; hysterical, phobic, or obsessive overlay symptoms; somatic complaints (notably in children); psychosomatic complaints; conduct disorders, addiction, suicide attempts. Many patients still present with these symptoms, which are considered "comorbid" in DSM-IV and ICD-10, like the pseudo-depression that is linked to psychological numbing. These non-specific symptoms may be prominent in the clinical picture, and lead to errors in diagnosis and treatment. In clinical practice, many patients do not meet all the DSM criteria for PTSD, or the ICD criteria for "enduring personality change after catastrophic experience". There are many atypical cases of varying onset, duration and severity, with a diverse degree of handicap. All disaster victims who still present with symptoms at this stage should be offered psychological or psychiatric care until recovery.

Numerous surveys have shown that a substantial proportion of disaster victims still present with PTSD symptoms several years after the traumatic event. Green and Lindy [8] observed a PTSD prevalence of 44% two years after the 1972 Buffalo Creek flood disaster, and of 14% after 14 years. Bromet and Dew [9] mention a 22% rate of psychological sequelae (including 11% PTSD) after a hurricane in Honduras. In a survey of 43 terrorist attack victims, Bouthillon-Heitzmann et al. [10] reported a 79% PTSD rate 3 years after the event; one-third of subjects showed clear psychosomatic disorders.

MENTAL STATE OF THE AFFLICTED COMMUNITY

A disaster strikes a whole community, causing types of collective behavior which cannot be reduced to the mere sum of instances of individual behavior. Collective behavior is influenced by a community's psychology, by the crowd's state of mind, and is characterized by its own specific features. After a disaster, collective behavior may be either adaptive or maladaptive.

Adaptive collective behavior is often rehearsed and expected. Instances of adaptive collective behavior during the immediate phase are remaining at one's post, orderly evacuation, helping others. Adaptive collective behavior is characterized by three features: (a) group structure is preserved; (b) leadership is maintained or reestablished; (c) mutual help is organized. During the post-immediate and long-term phases, adaptive collective behavior is manifested by normal mourning, regaining autonomy, reconstruction and resuming normal professional and social activities.

Maladaptive collective behavior during the immediate phase may show as: (a) collective stupor (the population remains reactionless or evacuates the impact zone in a long centrifugal exodus); (b) collective panic (headlong flight, scrambling for safety); or (c) exodus. These three types of collective behavior are characterized by: (a) the loosening of group structure; (b) the collapse of leadership; and (c) the lack of solidarity. Additionally, it is possible to observe, during the post-immediate period, the spread of rumors, and violence outbursts (riots, hooliganism, and search for scapegoats). The delayed and chronic phase may give rise to a paranoid collective mentality (hostility toward the world and demanding redress), and a dependent mentality, with feelings of being entitled to assistance, and the inability to recover autonomy.

The leaders who are responsible for organizing rescue operations must be aware of these behavior patterns, and their predisposing factors. Raphael et al. [11] identified some pathogenic factors in the social context of disaster: (a) the extent of material destruction, (b) the disturbance of the normal channels of psychosocial support, (c) a history of previous collective trauma, (d) the pre-existing state of the community (e.g., migration), and (e) the separation of families. Additional negative factors are the composition of the population (proportion of elderly, children, women), its lack of structure and preparedness, its mental state on the eve of the disaster (the "expectant attention", described by Le Bon, facilitates panic), rumors fostering feelings of panic or abandonment, and the presence of specific individuals who overtly spread alarmist views and will "contaminate" others. After a disaster, individual interventions should be complemented by collective measures aimed at restoring collective psychological health.

HISTORY OF MENTAL HEALTH INTERVENTIONS AFTER DISASTERS

The detection and treatment of mental disorders caused by disasters began in the USA, thanks to the advent of the PTSD diagnostic category in the aftermath of the Vietnam War, and the subsequent application of this diagnosis to civilian situations. A literature survey [12] revealed that a great variety of treatment methods have been proposed at different times. Treatment has been offered to victims [13,14], relatives and other community members [15,16], or rescuers [17,18]. The usefulness of treatment was accepted only gradually in the community, and Lindy [19] mentions that the main difficulty was gaining access to victims.

As early as 1983, Mitchell [20] defined debriefing procedures, on the basis of cognitive techniques. His method aimed at treating police officers or firemen who had been exposed to a critical event. Mitchell's method can be applied during the post-immediate period (first week); it follows a seven-step procedure (introduction; facts; thoughts; reactions; symptoms; education; conclusion). Mitchell's approach is mainly cognitive (it helps the patients to gain an exact knowledge of the event); it aims at prevention (lack of knowledge might lead to PTSD) and restoring operational capability. It is not meant to treat and to be applied to victims. Mitchell's debriefing techniques were modified by several authors: some established a distinction between didactic, psychological, and therapeutic debriefing; others placed debriefing in a "continuum of care", and emphasized the importance of coping mechanisms and cognitive structuring. After the San Francisco earthquake in 1989, Armstrong et al. [21] developed a "multiple stressor debriefing model", taking into account all stressors and comprising four steps: disclosure of the event and all stressors; feelings and reactions; coping strategies; and conclusion and return to the familial group. In 1992, Dyregrov [22] developed a collective debriefing method, which made use of the group's capacity to provide mutual help. In France and Belgium, debriefing has been based on the verbal expression of the experience, both cognitive and emotional, and considered to be an early therapeutic intervention, which could be followed by longer-term management.

It is only in the 1990s that American authors started proposing more comprehensive management programs [23] that included reducing symptoms (intrusive re-experience and avoidance), restoring emotional control, incorporating the personal significance of the event, and social reinsertion. Similar initiatives happened in Europe at the same time. In the United Kingdom, the police used to take care of the initial psychological needs of the victims, before medical and social services intervened. In 1995, Turner et al. [24] surveyed, 7 years after the event, the mental health of the survivors of King's Cross underground station fire in London (18 November 1987), which killed 31 people. The authors remarked that physical wounds were adequately treated, whereas psychological wounds and long-term consequences were neglected. After the *Herald of Free Enterprise* car ferry capsized (1987), a special group – the Herald Assistance Unit – was created by the Kent Social Services to coordinate social and psychological help over a 15-month period. The group produced a newsletter and operated a 24-hour telephone hotline; further treatment was given in London. Similar initiatives were launched in Belgium, the Netherlands, Germany, Sweden, Finland, and Norway.

In Norway, the military is in charge of first aid, including psychological and psychiatric assistance (it intervened as early as 1985 at a factory fire, and at an avalanche site). In Sweden, psychologists and psychiatrists practicing in civilian hospitals will also evaluate and treat victims, as was the case, for instance, after the rail collision at Lerum, on the Stockholm to Göteborg line, which caused 9 dead and 100 wounded, on 16 November 1987 [25].

In France, initiatives to treat disaster victims were taken as early as 1987. A specialized consultation was created at Saint Antoine Hospital in Paris in 1988 by Crocq, Alby and Puech, first for victims of terrorist acts, and later for victims of different kinds of psychological traumata. Special interventions were made to assist survivors of the collapse of a spectator stand at a soccer game in Bastia, Corsica, on 5 May 1992; relatives of passengers of the DC-10 of the French airline UTA destroyed by a midair explosion over the Tenere desert of Niger in 1989; and passengers of an airliner hijacked between Algiers and Paris on 24 December 1994.

However, it was a terrorist attack in the Paris subway that triggered a decision by the President of the Republic to create a network of cells for medical and psychological emergencies (Cellules d'Urgence Médico-Psychologiques – CUMP). The CUMP network is present with a cell in each one of the French *départements* (i.e., counties); each cell comprises psychiatrists, psychologists, and nurses, who are trained in disaster psychiatry. The CUMP is guided by a proactive philosophy, which is to assist disaster victims as early as possible, anticipating the subject's request [26].

In Israel, Shalev *et al.* [27] intervene early, as soon as the victims of terrorist attacks are admitted into the hospital. They described how the mental state can vary, according to external factors and time (first hours, first week, etc.). They favored a flexible therapeutic approach, taking into account the victim's needs and the course.

The example of the severe earthquake in the Sea of Marmara region in Turkey on August 17, 1999 shows how the notion of mental help after disasters has become accepted by national and international organizations. The earthquake, reaching 7.4 on the Richter scale, damaged several villages in an area of 20 million inhabitants; 18,000 died, 50,000 were wounded, and thousands were left homeless. The Turkish government and the international community reacted immediately. Gökalp [28] described a 6-month post-immediate period, when survivors expressed confusion, grief, regressive demands, and lack of initiative. In the area of Adazpar, where 39% had lost a relative, 60% of the sample were diagnosed with PTSD after 12 months, with comorbidity in 40%. In the areas of Yenikoy, Otosan, and Mehmetcik [29], 47% of subjects had PTSD and 33% depression. Gökalp stressed the importance of preparing for disaster.

The recent earthquake that damaged the whole region east of Algiers (May 2003) exemplifies how mental health has become a priority. On the first day of the disaster, the psychiatrists and psychologists of the region were called to assist victims; later, they were relieved in 10-day shifts by their colleagues from neighboring areas. In addition, 30 psychologists intervened in refugee camps. Three months after the earthquake, these personnel were debriefed to prevent burnout; they expressed a wish for additional training on trauma.

In Latin America, the Pan American Health Organization (PAHO) has been actively engaged for the last 20 years in efforts to assist disaster victims, in particular after hurricanes in the Caribbean [30]. The first strategy consisted in sending teams to the afflicted community. However, sending teams from outside did not help the countries to prepare for future disasters. Thus, a new strategy was adopted to elaborate national rescue plans in several stages: (a) creation of an agency to evaluate needs and priorities; (b) training of first-level personnel (first-aid teams, social workers, cadres) to identify serious casualties; (c) training of medical and psychiatric services; (d) creation of teams that can train first- and second-level rescuers; (e) systems to educate the population. Such plans can be successful only if they are supported by competent teams at the ministry of health.

In Asian countries, the recent earthquake in Kobe, Japan, on 17 January 1995, showed that installing a mental health service in a disaster area is fraught with difficulties. The Hanshin-Awaji earthquake left 5,500 dead and 350,000 homeless in that conurbation of 1.5 million. Local authorities were overwhelmed and could not respond immediately in an adapted manner. One and a half million volunteers came from all over Japan, mostly students and relatives of victims. They helped victims salvage their belongings and find shelter, water, and food. Often, they listened to the victims' stories. However, this spontaneous rescue action was not coordinated; rescuers were too few in some isolated areas, and too numerous in more accessible centers. A few psychiatrists organized mental health rescue centers; however, survivors were more interested in salvaging their belongings and satisfying material needs. Psychiatrists prepared booklets containing guidelines for volunteer rescuers. Shinfuku [31] reported that mental symptoms followed three successive stages: (a) a first immediate phase of stupor and derealization; (b) a second phase, during a few weeks, of anxiety, fear of a recurrence, and psychosomatic symptoms (hypertension, gastric ulcer); (c) a third phase, after a few weeks, characterized by depression and mourning of human and material losses. After a year, problems were more of a social nature than purely mental (loss of drive, alcohol abuse, etc.). The prevalence of PTSD was not reported. However, the publicity around PTSD in the media helped reduce the social stigma attached to mental problems. Kobe University inaugurated a Research Center for Urban Health, with a department of disaster medicine. Five years after the earthquake, the population of Kobe was reduced by 100,000, but it seemed to have returned back to its usual life.

Recently, McFarlane [32] gave more indications about the management of psychiatric morbidity in disasters. It is important to reduce the impression of chaos and to inventory needs by rapidly drawing a map of the situation, assessing the number of casualties, and the extent of destructions. Public health plans, prepared beforehand, should be enacted. However, types of disaster are so varied that it necessary to show flexibility rather than strict adherence to plans. Often, disaster victims will initially cope with the situation, and present with symptoms only weeks or months later. The attack on the World Trade Center on September 11, 2001 showed that rescuers can, in turn, become primary victims. The popularity of mental help intervention in the public led to an increase in requests for assistance, but also to an influx of poorly trained volunteers who have little experience in psychological help and team work. Such volunteers may embark on the treatment of a victim, whom they will abandon after a short while when they realize the task's difficulty. The intervention of outside experts, even if they are highly competent, may thwart the efforts of the local services. Often, victims prefer to be taken care of by their own local teams, with whom they can relate better.

In 2002, Raquel Cohen wrote a survey of mental health intervention with disaster victims [4]. She stressed that mental health intervention should be integrated within the larger frame of the public organization of rescue operations, and establish links with other partners. She suggested that the psychological intervention plan should be refined in several modules according to the type of victims (primary, secondary) and the stage of the disaster (immediate, aftermath). One of the key tasks is to give emotional support to the survivors, to help them understand the stress they experienced, and to help them put their thoughts in order. The operational concept is based on the "individual–situation–configuration" model. Post-crisis intervention aims at giving back to the individual the capacity to adjust to the new stressful situations. The three objectives are: (a) helping victims to recover their capacities; (b) helping them organize their new environment; (c) assist victims in their interactions with the bureaucracy in charge of rehabilitation. The methods to achieve these objectives are a function of the different schools of thought, but flexibility and creativity must always complement a classical clinical approach. It will be necessary to take care of mourning families, in particular after they have been called to identify the corpses of deceased relatives. Population groups housed in camps and temporary shelters have to endure poverty and promiscuity and may be prompt to react with depression, anger, violence, alcohol or other drugs. It will be necessary to assist these refugees, help them organize their new life and recover their ability to take care of themselves, and also to help them express their emotions. Treatment can rely on a wide variety of methods: medications, cognitive therapies, individual or group psychotherapy, family therapy. It will also be necessary to consider prevention, as well as social and professional rehabilitation, for instance the children's schooling. Finally, it will be necessary to identify patients who evolve towards chronicity and need particular treatment. It may be useful to include collaborators from the private sector, from allied health professions (nurses, etc.), and also members of the clergy if they are trained and correspond to the cultural and religious needs of the victims. The relationship with the media is of crucial importance. The media are fond of interviews with psychiatrists, and it is important to use them to convey information to the population about mental health services.

ORGANIZATION OF MENTAL HEALTH SERVICES FOR DISASTER VICTIMS

The organization of mental health services for disaster victims should be able to answer the following questions: (a) What type of disaster? (b) Which victims? (c) What types of mental disturbances (they vary according to the victims and the stage of the disaster)? (d) What type of mission? (e) Which personnel? (f) What is the administrative frame?

What Type of Disaster?

The nature and severity of the disaster will influence the mental symptoms presented by the victims, and government or local authority approach.

Natural disasters, such as earthquakes, can concern many people, cover a wide area, and last a significant length of time. An erupting volcano may affect only a few hamlets, or completely destroy a large city, as was the case with the Nevado del Ruiz eruption in Colombia that obliterated the city of Armero with its 20,000 inhabitants. A collapsed dam may damage only one city (e.g., in Malpasset, France, 1959; or Buffalo Creek, USA, 1972), whereas heavy rain and floods may cover whole provinces (the Gard *département* in France, July 2001) or even whole countries (Bangladesh in 1987), disorganizing health structures. The effects of an earthquake may be limited to one city (e.g., Kobe, Japan, 1995), or afflict a whole region (Sea of Marmara, Turkey, 1999).

Technological and industrial disasters (train or plane crashes, sinking boats, explosions or fires in factories) are usually limited in space, which simplifies the organization of rescue operations. However, the Chernobyl radioactive cloud, in April 1986, threatened most of Europe. Disasters that are deliberately provoked by man (terrorist attacks, war bombings) are also usually limited in time and space, but the threat of recurrence may leave insecurity feelings in the population. Also, bombings of cities like Dresden, Tokyo, Hiroshima, and Nagasaki in World War II erased entire cities. Finally, society disasters, such as the panics in stadiums (Brussels, 29 April 1985; Sheffield, 15 April 1989) or at other places (the tunnel at Mecca, 1991) are generally limited in time and space. Whereas natural disasters can be attributed only to fate, destiny or the gods, man-made disasters involve questions of fault, cruelty, responsibility, which will complicate the psychological reaction to the disaster.

Which Victims?

Mental health teams will first have to take care of the primary victims of the disaster, i.e., with those who have been in direct contact with the disaster. Also, a few witnesses and rescuers who have been shocked by the sight of death and destruction may have to be taken care of fairly early. Later on, it will be necessary to assist the secondary victims, such as mourning relatives or evacuated populations. Thirdly, rescuers and health personnel will have to be assisted to cope with the stressors experienced at different stages of the disaster: (a) when arriving on the site, because of the sudden confrontation with corpses, etc.; (b) during the phase of maximum activity, because of various stressors (working rapidly in dangerous conditions, lack of sleep, the guilt induced by triage and the impossibility of spending enough time with individual patients); (c) during the final post-disaster evaluation (impression that the task was not completed, or of having failed). It is now generally accepted that rescuers may have to be taken care of during the mission because some of them will not be able to continue functioning adequately, and after the mission to free them from intrusive recollections before they go back to their families. Fourthly, officials and media representatives may also be exposed to various stressors and may benefit from psychological help, although many of them would be reluctant to admit it for fear of appearing soft or weak. Fifthly, one may wonder whether the population at large should be helped, at a time when the disaster can be experienced "live" through the realistic images broadcast by television. These "fifth level" victims are not traumatized in the same way as direct victims and rescuers, because they did not face death directly and were not threatened in their life or physical integrity; however, their psychological sense of security and illusion of immortality have been shattered because they realized how fragile human life is. The attack on the World Trade Center on September 11, 2001 showed how the collective ego and morale of a whole nation can be afflicted [33,34].

What Types of Mental Disturbances?

The types of disorders occurring during and after disasters have been reviewed above. Briefly, the immediate phase may be associated with distressing symptoms accompanying adaptive stress; symptoms of mal-adaptive stress, such as confusion, agitation, panic flight, automatic behavior; and, exceptionally, neurotic or psychotic reactions; the post-immediate phase may be characterized by a return to normal health, or by the insidious onset of a post-traumatic syndrome (PTSD or PTSD-like); the chronic phase may present with the persistence of PTSD, or personality changes.

In addition to individual symptoms, it may be possible to observe collective symptoms, such as collective inhibition, collective panic flight, fleeing, rumors, and post-disaster abnormal behavior (e.g., riots, pogroms, etc.). Although mental health specialists may help prevent such abnormal collective behaviors, it is the responsibility of public authorities to control them and restore public order. Psychiatrists, psychologists, and sociologists may act as advisers.

What Type of Mission?

Organization, Coordination, Planning

In many countries, organizing the initial rescue operations is the responsibility of the government, or its agencies at various levels (federal, provincial, and town) according to the severity of the disaster. In France, for instance, the prefect (French: *préfet*), who heads the *département*, is responsible for organizing the rescue operations. He commands public sector personnel, as well as the personnel from the private sector and NGOs (Red Cross, Médecins sans Frontières, etc.). In matters of health, the prefect delegates his authority to an intensive care physician, who will be in charge of the medical aspects of rescue operations and supervise other physicians, nurses, and psychologists. In other countries, where the public sector is less developed, it may happen that private personnel and NGO members perform the bulk of relief operations.

The most important factor is the presence of a clear organization, preventing anarchy. Tasks, timetables, places, and actors should be clearly defined. It has been too often the case that NGO members behaved with excessive independence, infringing on tasks that had been assigned to others and reporting only to their own headquarters. Also, there have been instances where some refugee camps, located near major roads, were abundantly cared for, whereas other camps, isolated in remote areas, were neglected. Therefore, it is important that government authorities organize the rescue operations. Often, there is no time for improvisation and rescue plans have to be drafted, tested and rehearsed in advance for the different types of disaster that can be anticipated.

Evaluation of Mental Health Needs

A second key mission is evaluation. Among the mental health personnel at the scene, one psychiatrist must assume this task, even if it means that his treatment mission will be taken over by one of his colleagues. On the basis of information contributed by colleagues and first aid staff, this psychiatrist has to evaluate the number of "psychiatric" casualties, and the types of disorders that are present or will occur soon (stupor, agitation, panic). Assessment of needs may point to the need for requesting reinforcement from the rear. Evaluating accurately is sometimes complex. For instance, after the Concorde crash at Roissy airport (Paris) on July 25, 1999, different needs had to be anticipated at different times. Just after the crash, there were no survivors among plane passengers and crew, but survivors from the houses on which the aircraft had crashed who required immediate attention. There were also witnesses who had been shocked (air-traffic controllers, airport personnel), as well as the inhabitants of neighboring villages who realized that they were living under a sword of Damocles. It was anticipated that victims' relatives would be arriving from Germany on the following day. It was then necessary to arrange for the presence of German-speaking psychiatrists and psychologists for a few days. Further, it was necessary to anticipate that the Air France personnel, who would accompany the grieving relatives, would themselves have to be helped. Also, provision had to be made for the church memorial service that gathered 9,000 persons at the airport 3 days after the crash. In the longer term, it was necessary to debrief the personnel (firemen, police, etc.) who had to recover and examine human remains at the crash site. This example shows the complexity of evaluation, when taking into account both the immediate and post-immediate phases of the disaster [35].

Whenever possible, it is advisable to try to evaluate the possible long-term symptoms and sequels, in order to have an idea of the needs for long-term treatment and of the related costs.

Triage of Psychiatric Casualties

In many disasters, advanced rescue stations on the scene are flooded by a sudden influx of casualties, to the point that they risk being clogged and paralyzed. Thus, triage is essential. Triage means establishing a diagnosis, even if provisional. The diagnosis, along with the main symptoms, should be indicated on the records and the documents that accompany the patient when he is evacuated to the rear. Thus, the continuity of care can be preserved.

Medical and Psychological Care

Although the psychological assistance to victims may sound simple and straightforward, it is in fact a complex task. It may be preferable to call this kind of care "medical and psychological" rather than "psychiatric", because many individuals present with psychological and neuro-vegetative symptoms that reflect adaptive stress; also, individuals with symptoms of maladaptive stress cannot, and do not want to, be viewed as psychiatric patients. Only a few clearly abnormal symptoms (delirium, delusions, and acute anxiety) can be qualified as psychiatric. Victims presenting with mental symptoms can be treated only by medical teams. However, other victims, without mental symptoms, can be taken care of by "psychosocial" workers (rescuers, social workers, etc.).

It has often been mentioned that the material and physical help given by the first rescue team on the site also has a beneficial psychological effect on the victims. The arrival of the first rescue team on the site dissipates the victims' feelings of isolation. The close physical contact restores the "psychic envelope". Satisfying primordial needs (hunger, thirst, and warmth) brings about a sense of psychological well-being. However, this effect is due to non-specific factors, and not to a true psychological intervention. It is advisable that rescuers be trained in recognizing the symptoms of stress, in the victims and in themselves.

The psychological and psychiatric methods employed are left to the judgment of the mental health teams (anxiolytic, antidepressant, or hypnotic drugs; brief psychological support; verbalization of emotions). In some cases, psychological support can be given in small groups (defusing), which will save time. It is good to keep in mind that individuals with physical symptoms always present to some degree with psychological symptoms; in other words, physical casualties are also psychological casualties. This shows the need for collaboration between psychiatrists and other medical specialists.

If necessary, psychological treatment should be continued during the post-immediate phase. As was already mentioned, symptoms will sometimes appear only after a latency period of weeks or months. Therefore, it is important to give the victims some information on the possible appearance of symptoms, and on places to contact for outpatient treatment. This information can be given in the form of a leaflet that is distributed to survivors. Subsequent psychiatric treatment can be given by the individual's general practitioner or by a psychiatrist. However, it should be kept in mind that some physicians are not adequately trained to identify trauma-related symptoms and may misdiagnose the problems as mere cases of "depression", "anxiety", or "insomnia", deserving only non-specific and superficial treatment.

The post-immediate period is the ideal time for debriefing sessions. The meaning of the term debriefing may be ambiguous. First, it may refer to a preventive and educational intervention in a group of non-symptomatic subjects who have experienced a critical incident (e.g., firemen, police officers, etc.). Second, it may be understood as a treatment method in a group of individuals presenting with post-traumatic symptoms. In the latter case, one debriefing session may be insufficient to eliminate the symptoms and cure the patients; however, the patient may be motivated to start a longer therapeutic process.

The symptoms (initial stress reaction or symptoms of later onset) will disappear quickly in some patients. In others, symptoms may persist longer or tend toward chronicity. In these cases, the question of long-term treatment is raised, along with the question of choice of therapist and treatment method (cognitive and behavioral methods, drugs, hypnosis, eye movement desensitization and reprocessing (EMDR), psychotherapy, catharsis, or even psychoanalysis).

Prevention and Education

Prevention can be envisaged at three stages: primary, secondary, and tertiary. Primary prevention is information and education before the event. Secondary prevention means intervening as soon as possible after the event to prevent the onset or persistence of psychotraumatic symptoms. Tertiary prevention means treating the late-onset or persisting symptoms, and helping subjects recovering their health and social capacities.

Primary prevention starts at school, and continues at work and at home. It consists of four complementary actions [36,37]: (a) educating the population, and stressing the moral obligation of helping one's neighbor; (b) informing about possible risks and their consequences; (c) teaching the reactions and behavior to adopt in case of danger; (d) rehearsing the likely scenarios. Primary prevention has to be decided and enforced by government authorities. The methods can include television, pamphlets and brochures, lectures given by experts (fire department, Red Cross/Red Crescent). Experience has shown that theory is not sufficient, and that regular practical exercises will be the most efficient way to rehearse adaptive reactions ("the memory in arms and legs"). Japan is a good example. In that country, authorities stage collective exercises every year on September 1 (the anniversary day of the Tokyo earthquake of September 1, 1923, which caused 200,000 deaths): on that day, schools and factories are evacuated and relief exercises are practiced on the street. A specialized information and training center has been created in Tokyo, and replicas of apartments have been mounted on hydraulic jacks to simulate the shaking produced by an earthquake.

Secondary prevention implies that the mental health worker is able to identify subjects at risk after a disaster. A first objective is to make sure that immediate abnormal stress symptoms, notably dissociation, have been treated. Certain clinicians [38] have reported that the presence of dissociative symptoms during the post-immediate period predicted the evolution toward PTSD. Others [39] have shown that the experience of loss and mourning can lead to depression. Ursano et al. [40] have reported a rate of probable PTSD of 11% at 1 month and 2% at 13 months in volunteers who had handled bodies after the USS Iowa gun turret explosion. Secondary prevention can be performed either in personal interviews, or in collective debriefing sessions (often based on Mitchell's method).

Certain authors [41] think that secondary prevention can be achieved by developing the resilience capacity of the victims. There have also been reports of individuals who managed to use the experience of trauma and loss to reorganize their defense mechanisms, change their values, and reorganize their shattered lives. As part of their education, survivors may be given an information leaflet. Robertson et al. [42] reported a high degree of satisfaction with a two-page leaflet, entitled "Surviving Trauma", consisting of six parts: (a) description of the authors; (b) immediate symptoms; (c) impact of trauma on the environment; (d) evolution of symptoms during the first months; (e) how to help oneself; (f) places where help can be found.

Tertiary prevention is part of long-term therapy. It aims at curing or alleviating protracted disorders, such as PTSD. This disorder may be incomplete, or atypical, or dominated by comorbid symptoms. The ultimate objective is not only the disappearance of symptoms. Obviously, the patient cannot forget the trauma, but he must integrate it into the dynamics of his life. The patient must be delivered from his regressive relationship to others and his fascination by his trauma.

Which Personnel?

Generally, mental health is the province of specialized personnel: psychiatrists, psychologists, psychiatric nurses. Further, the support of administrative and paramedical (e.g., Red Cross) personnel is required.

During the immediate phase, rescuing the wounded is usually the task of volunteer or professional first-aid teams, who will carry the victims on stretchers to the first-aid station. These paramedical personnel are often the victims' first contact. Therefore, they should be given some psychological training about the needs of the victims and how to approach them. It is important that the victim be given some information on the situation and what happened. Once he has arrived at the first-aid station, the victim will be taken care of by emergency medicine specialists who will practice life-saving measures and triage. These specialists will perform well-rehearsed technical actions; however, they should keep in mind that the psychological condition of a patient may aggravate his physical health. The emergency medicine physician should be able to diagnose maladaptive stress symptoms, and to call a psychiatrist or psychologist if necessary. When possible, the patient should be reassured and given information such as the name of the person treating him, or his destination of evacuation.

During the immediate phase, we recommend [43] installing a medical/psychological station (MPS) near the advanced medical station of the emergency medicine teams. The MPS should be operated by as many mental health practitioners (psychiatrists, psychologists, psychiatric nurses) as required (hence, the importance of the initial evaluation of needs). Individuals presenting with manifest psychiatric symptoms (delusions, stupor, agitation) or adaptive or maladaptive stress reactions will be directed toward the MPS. A first triage of psychiatric cases can be performed at that level. The attitude toward patients should be more interventionist and directive than the traditional psychoanalyst's neutrality. It is important to offer sympathetic listening, and also to encourage the person to verbalize his/her experience. At that early stage, this type of defusing may be able to prevent the constitution of a psychotraumatic process.

The post-immediate phase is crucial and follow-up of the survivors is necessary. Either the acute stress symptoms abate, or a PTSD appears. Many victims, still in the euphoria of having survived, do not notice the onset of the first psychotraumatic symptoms. Because the survivors may not be aware of their initial psychotraumatic symptoms, it is important that mental health professionals other physicians, and paramedical personnel try to detect their onset before they are reported by the patients.

The post-immediate period is the best time to carry out debriefing sessions. The debriefing of rescuers, which has a preventive purpose, can be performed either by mental health professionals or, as suggested by certain authors [44], by trained peers. The debriefing of victims, which pursues both therapeutic and preventive objectives, can be carried out only by trained psychiatrist or psychologists [45–47].

At the chronic stage, patients with protracted symptoms are best treated by mental health professionals with a good training in psychotraumatology. However, these patients are often treated by their general practitioners, who may limit themselves to prescribing drugs for the most obvious symptoms, such as insomnia or anxiety, without approaching the question of trauma. Since these patients are reluctant to discuss their traumatic history, it may require clinical acumen to detect the traumatic etiology of the disorder.

What is the Administrative Frame?

Mental health is usually under the control of the government, notably the ministry of health. Therefore, it is understandable that mental health in time of disaster should also be controlled by government authorities, even though NGOs, the Red Cross, private practitioners, volunteers, etc. may take part in relief operations. Specifically, the emergency plans are prepared by government administrations, with the advice of experts. When disaster strikes, intervention on the site must be ultimately coordinated by government authorities. This applies of course to the logistics. It also applies to medical relief. Physicians and other health and paramedical personnel on the site have to be integrated into a hierarchical structure, in the frame of pre-existing emergency plans. This prevents anarchy, and also ensures that central headquarters have valid information about the situation and can direct relief towards areas that might otherwise be neglected.

During the post-immediate and long-term phases, government control can no longer be so strict. However, government offices have to make sure that structures do exist to take care of the long-term treatment of victims. It is also essential to make sure that the victims are adequately informed about possible abnormal psychotraumatic symptoms and places to turn to for treatment. Finally, government offices must be able to evaluate the level of long-term morbidity caused by a disaster.

Different solutions have been applied in different countries. In some countries, government agencies will be in charge of all mental health interventions in disasters; in others, non-governmental initiatives are integrated into the structure; finally, there are countries where most of the tasks have been delegated to private agencies.

THREE EXAMPLES OF SYSTEMS OF MENTAL HEALTH INTERVENTION

The French System for Medical and Psychological Emergencies

The impetus for forming a French system for medical and psychological emergencies started in 1995. In French, this system is abbreviated as CUMP (Cellules d'Urgence Médico-Psychologiques). One significant event was a terrorist attack at the Paris subway station "Saint-Michel" on July 26, 1995. The image of French president Jacques Chirac visiting the wounded in hospital was widely broadcast by the media. A directive from the Ministry of Health officially created the system on May 28, 1997. The creation of the system was supervised by Louis Crocq, a French Army psychiatrist with a long experience in stress and traumatic neuroses.

This system comprises about 100 "cells", i.e., one cell in each French *département* (or county). In each *département*, a government-employed, hospital-based psychiatrist volunteered to coordinate a group of voluntary psychiatrists, psychologists, and psychiatric nurses. Their mission is to intervene as soon as possible on the site in the case of disaster, terrorist attacks, etc. These cells are meant to intervene when there are a large number of casualties, in a collective disaster. However, at times, they may also intervene in situations with one or a few casualties that produced much awe and distress among witnesses. Examples are suicides or accidental deaths in schools.

During disasters, in the immediate phase, the intervention of the psychological cells is supervised by the SAMU (Service d'Aide Médicale Urgente), the French system of emergency medicine.

European Red Cross Societies Network for Psychological Support (ENPS)

In his text that stimulated the creation of the Red Cross (1862), Henri Dunant mentioned the psychological distress of the wounded on the battlefield. Generally, Red Cross workers take care not only of physical wounds, but also of mental distress. Red Cross workers often arrive on disaster sites before mental health specialists; they are also confronted with psychological suffering in refugee camps.

The European Red Cross/Red Crescent Societies Network for Psychological Support (ENPS) was established in 2000. The ENPS is driven by a steering committee which consists of the Belgian, French, Hungarian, Dutch and Swiss Red Cross Societies. The secretariat is held by the French Red Cross. Conferences on psychological support were held in Copenhagen (1995) and in Lyon (1998) where the advantages of creating a network were pointed out.

The objectives of the ENSP include: (a) taking an inventory and share experiences and practices in psychological support in the national European societies (this includes action and team training programs adapted to cultural sensitivities); (b) establishing and developing the specificities of psychological support in the Red Cross movement at the European level; (c) setting up a cooperation between the national societies, the authorities and the European institutions; (d) working in contact with the international Red Cross reference center for psychological support based in Danish Red Cross.

In order to set up and share the inventory of structures and resource persons in the European Red Cross societies, a questionnaire has been sent to each national society. A workshop on "First Aid and Psychological Support" was held at the 6th European Red Cross and Red Crescent Regional Conference in Berlin, 14–19 April 2002.

Interface between Judicial Protection and Mental Health

Disaster victims have suffered loss, damage, or injury, to their person or property. Sometimes, this may have occurred through the omission, negligence, or unlawful acts of others. Therefore, they may be entitled to a pecuniary compensation or indemnity. Besides the purely judicial aspects, the fact that damages are awarded and a responsibility is established by a law court can help the healing process. Conversely, the judicial process, the experience of testifying, recounting one's experience, establishing proof, may reactivate symptoms such as intrusive recollections or distressing dreams of the event. In several countries, systems have been set up to help victims exert their rights. Often, such systems require the interaction of social workers, lawyers, and psychologists. In France, the INAVEM (Institut National d'Aide aux Victimes – National Institute for the Help to Victims) was created in 1986. INAVEM is partially funded by the French Ministry of Justice [48].

CONCLUSIONS

The objectives of the mental health care of disaster victims are to alleviate psychological distress, to manage the psychosocial impact on individuals and the community, and to prevent the development of late psychical sequelae. The organization of mental health care must be planned in advance, taking into account that disasters differ in type and severity. Mental health intervention must be initiated as soon as possible, on the site, in the immediate phase (first hours), but it should also cover the post-immediate (second day until two months) and chronic phases (after two months); further, it must be adapted to the specific disorders occurring in each of these three phases. Treatment must be given to the primary victims (who have come in direct contact with the disaster), secondary victims (relatives of victims), tertiary victims (shocked and exhausted rescuers and caregivers), fourth-level victims (leaders and media who have witnessed traumatizing scenes), and even fifth-level victims (population shocked through the media).

Only government officials can supervise, organize and coordinate relief operations, including mental health care. In the immediate phase, evaluation and triage of mental casualties are essential. During the post-immediate phase, it becomes necessary to survey the mental status of victims – even if they are not asking spontaneously – because it is the phase where PTSD can appear. In the chronic phase, treatment must include not only symptomatic techniques, but also true treatment of the trauma, with the objective of helping the victim to give a meaning to his experience and place it in the continuum of his life story.

Even though the intervention of the paramedical personnel (who are the victims' first contact after the disaster) has a good psychological effect (especially if this personnel has received a basic training in disaster psychology), mental health care must be given by psychiatrists and clinical psychologists with a special training in psychotraumatology and disaster psychiatry. Techniques such as defusing and psychiatric debriefing of victims must be viewed as specific therapeutic methods, or as the beginning of a longer therapeutic process. They differ from mere critical incident stress debriefing, which is a preventive measure for teams who have been exposed to a potentially traumatic event, but who do not present with abnormal symptoms.

REFERENCES

1. Joseph S., Williams R., Yule W. (1997) *Understanding Post-traumatic Stress. A Psychosocial Perspective on PTSD and Treatment.* Wiley, Chichester.

2. Gerrity E.T., Steinglass P. (1994) Relocating stress following natural disasters. In R.J. Ursano, B.G. MacCaughey, C.S. Fullerton (Eds.), *Individual and Community Responses to Trauma and Disaster. The Structure of Human Chaos*, pp. 220–247. Cambridge University Press, Cambridge, UK.

3. Reiss D. (1982) The working family: a researcher's view of health in the household. *Am J Psychiatry*, **139**: 1412–1420.

4. Cohen R. (2002) Mental health services for victims of disasters. *World Psychiatry*, **1**: 149–153.

5. Crocq L. (1999) *Les Traumatismes Psychiques de Guerre*. Jacob, Paris.

6. Crocq L. (2001) Individual and collective behaviors in earthquakes, fire and manmade disasters. In G. Spinetti, L. Janiri (Eds.), *Psichiatria ed Ecologia*, pp. 37–45. CIC, Rome.

7. Marmar C. (1997) Trauma and dissociation. *PTSD Research Quarterly*, **8**: 1–3.

8. Green B., Lindy J., Grace M.C. (1989) Posttraumatic stress disorder. *J Nerv Ment Dis*, **173**: 406–411.

9. Bromet E., Dew M.A. (1995) Review of psychiatric epidemiologic research on disasters. *Epidemiol Rev*, **17**: 113–119.

10. Bouthillon-Heitzmann P., Crocq L., Julien H. (1992) Stress immédiat et séquelles psychiques chez les victimes d'attentats terroristes. *Psychologie Médicale*, **24**: 465–470.

11. Raphael B., Wilson J., Meldrum L., McFarlane A.C. (1996) Acute preventive interventions. In B. Van der Kolk, A.C. McFarlane, L. Weisaeth (Eds.), *Traumatic Stress. The Effects of Overwelming Experience on Mind, Body and Society*, pp. 463–479. Guilford, New York.

12. Griffin C. (1987) Community disaster and post-traumatic stress disorder: a debriefing model for response. In T. Williams (Ed.), *Post-traumatic Stress Disorders: A Handbook for Clinicians*, pp. 293–298. Disabled American Veterans, Cincinnati.

13. Horowitz M.J., Kaltreider N. (1980) Brief treatment of post-traumatic stress disorders. *New Direction for Mental Health Services*, **6**: 67–79.

14. Lindy J.D., Green B.L., Grace M., Titchener J. (1983) Psychotherapy with survivors of the Beverly Hills Supper Club Fire. *Am J Psychother*, **37**: 563–610.

15. Tuckman A.J. (1973) Disaster and mental health intervention. *Commun Ment Health J*, **9**: 151–157.

16. Klingman A., Eli Z.B. (1981) A school community in disaster. Primary and secondary prevention in situational crisis. *Professional Psychology*, **12**: 523–533.

17. Dunning C., Silva M. (1980) Disaster induced trauma in rescue workers. *Victimology*, **5**: 287–297.

18. Jones D.R. (1985) Secondary disaster victims: the emotional effects of recovering and identifying human remains. *Am J Psychiatry*, **142**: 303–307.

19. Lindy J. (1985) The trauma membrane and clinical concepts derived from psychotherapeutic work with survivors of natural disasters. *Psychiatr Ann*, **15**: 153–160.

20. Mitchell J.T. (1983) When disaster strikes: the critical incident stress debriefing process. *J Emergency Med Serv*, **8**: 36–39.

21. Armstrong K., O'Callahan W., Marmar C. (1991) Debriefing Red Cross disaster personnel: the multiple stressor debriefing model. *J Trauma Stress*, **4**: 581–593.

22. Dyregrov A. (1992) Traumatized kids, traumatized rescuers? *Emerg Med Serv*, **21**: 20–24.

23. Van der Kolk B., McFarlane A.C., Van der Hart O. (1996) A general approach to treatment of posttraumatic stress disorder. In B. Van der Kolk, A.C. McFarlane,

L. Weisaeth (Eds.), *Traumatic Stress. The Effects of Overwelming Experience on Mind, Body and Society*, pp. 417–440. Guilford, New York.

24. Turner S.W., Thompson J., Rosser R. (1995) The Kings Cross Fire: psychological reactions. *J Trauma Stress*, 8: 419–428.

25. Hagström R. (1995) The acute psychological impact of survivors following a train accident. *J Trauma Stress*, 8: 391–402.

26. Crocq L. (1998) La cellule d'urgence médico-psychologique, sa création, son organisation, ses interventions. *Ann Médico-Psychol*, 156: 58–64.

27. Shalev A., Schreiber S., Galai T. (1993) Early psychological responses to traumatic injury. *J Trauma Stress*, 6: 441–450.

28. Gökalp P.G. (2002) Disaster mental health care: the experience of Turkey. *World Psychiatry*, 1: 159–160.

29. Basoglu M., Salcioglu E., Livanou M. (2002) Traumatic stress responses in earthquake survivors in Turkey. *J Trauma Stress*, 15: 269–276.

30. Caldas de Almeida J.M. (2002) Mental health services for victims of disasters in developing countries: a challenge and an opportunity. *World Psychiatry*, 1: 155–157.

31. Shinfuku N. (2002) Disaster mental health: lessons learned from the Hanshin Awaji earthquake. *World Psychiatry*, 1: 158–159.

32. McFarlane A.C. (2002) Managing the psychiatric morbidity of disasters. *World Psychiatry*, 1: 153–154.

33. Boscarino J.A., Galea S., Ahern J., Resnick H., Vlahov D. (2003) Psychiatric medication use among Manhattan residents following the World Trade Center disaster. *J Trauma Stress*, 16: 301–306.

34. Crocq L. (2002) World Trade Center. Image sans parole, le trauma d'une communauté. *Revue Francophone du Stress et du Trauma*, 2: 3–6.

35. Cremniter D. (2000) La catastrophe du Concorde: intervention médico-psychologique. *Revue du Stress et du Trauma*, 1: 55–59.

36. Crocq L., Doutheau C. (1995) Psychiatrie de catastrophe. In J.L. Senon, D. Sechter, D. Richard (Eds.), *Thérapeutique Psychiatrique*, pp. 989–1001. Hermann, Paris.

37. Crocq L., Doutheau C., Louville P., Cremniter D. (1998) Psychiatrie de catastrophe. In *Encyclopédie Médico-Chirurgicale, Psychiatrie*, 37-113-D-10. Elsevier, Paris.

38. Koopman C., Classen C., Spiegel D. (1994) Predictors of posttraumatic stress symptoms among survivors of the Oakland/Berkeley, California firestorms. *Am J Psychiatry*, 151: 888–894.

39. Lundin T. (1987) The stress of unexpected bereavement. *Stress Medicine*, 4: 109–114.

40. Ursano R.J., Fullerton C.S., Kao T.C., Bhartiya V.R. (1995) Longitudinal assessment of posttraumatic stress disorder and depression after exposure to traumatic death. *J Nerv Ment Dis*, 183: 36–42.

41. Ursano R.J., Grieger T.A., MacCarroll J.E. (1996) Prevention of posttraumatic stress. Consultation, training and early treatment. In B. Van der Kolk, A.C. McFarlane, L. Weisaeth (Eds.), *Traumatic Stress. The Effects of Overwhelming Experience on Mind, Body and Society*, pp. 441–462. Guilford, New York.

42. Robertson C., Klein S., Bullen H., Alexander D.A. (2002) An evaluation of patient satisfaction with an information leaflet for trauma survivors. *J Trauma Stress*, 15: 329–332.

43. Crocq L. (2002) Special teams for medical/psychological intervention in disaster victims. *World Psychiatry*, 1: 154–155.

44. Dyregrov A. (1997) The process in psychological debriefing. *J Trauma Stress*, **10**: 589–606.
45. Crocq L. (2002) Historique critique du debriefing. In E. de Soir, E. Vermeiren (Eds.), *Les Debriefings Psychologiques en Question*, pp. 73–130. Garant, Antwerp.
46. Lebigot F., Gauthier E., Morgand D., Lassagne M. (1997) Le debriefing psychologique collectif. *Ann Médico-Psychol*, **155**: 370–378.
47. Lebigot F. (1998) Le debriefing individuel du traumatisé psychique. *Ann Médico-Psychol*, **156**: 417–420.
48. Damiani C. (2001) L'aide psychologique aux victimes. In R. Cario, D. Salas (Eds.), *Oeuvre de Justice et Victimes*, Vol. 1, pp. 175–188. L'Harmattan, Paris.

Mental Health Consequences of Disasters: Experiences in Various Regions of the World

7

The Experience
of the Kobe Earthquake

Naotaka Shinfuku

University School of Medicine,
Kobe, Japan

INTRODUCTION

People who visit Kobe now can hardly recognize the damages caused by the Hanshin-Awaji earthquake. Kobe appears as a busy, affluent and modern Japanese city. The Museum and the Memorial Park, however, as well as some newly built Research and Training Centers for the Mitigation of Earthquakes, remind the visitor of the event.

The earthquake killed more than 5,500 people in one day on January 17, 1995. One year after the event, Kobe City had lost almost 100,000 population due to migration to non-damaged areas. In recent years, the population of the city has gradually increased and has now reached the pre-earthquake level. However, the local business firms are still suffering from the damage caused by the earthquake. In particular, the port-related industry, once the vital line of Kobe's economy, lost its business to competitors such as Kaoshung of Taiwan and Pusan of Korea. Ships once lost to other ports are hard to attract back.

Kobe residents still live with the memory and the trauma of the disaster. I experienced the Hanshin-Awaji earthquake and have witnessed the changes of the city and the population since then.

THE EARTHQUAKE

The earthquake occurred at 5.46 a.m. The Richter-scale magnitude was 7.2 [1]. The epicentre was just below the major city areas of Hanshin, including Kobe City. The number of people affected by the earthquake was estimated

Disasters and Mental Health. Edited by Juan José López-Ibor, George Christodoulou, Mario Maj, Norman Sartorius and Ahmed Okasha.
©2005 John Wiley & Sons Ltd. ISBN 0-470-02123-3.

as 2.4 million. Immediately after the earthquake, the dead were counted as 5,502. The official number of the dead due to the earthquake was revised to more than 6,500 in August 1995, as some of the delayed death cases, for instance from pneumonia or suicide, were certified as resulting from the earthquake. Three-quarters of the immediate deaths were due to asphyxia. Other major causes were burns, multiple fractures including the cervical area, and traumatic shock.

SOON AFTER THE EARTHQUAKE

Many people were unable to realize what happened soon after the earthquake. This period is sometimes known as the "6-hour vacuum". When the earthquake struck, I was unable to realize that it was an earthquake. I thought that it was some kind of an explosion under my house. Also, it took a long time for many people in Kobe to realize that the epicentre of the earthquake was close to the city. Nobody expected an earthquake in the Kobe area. Many victims in the Kobe area could realize the magnitude of the event only after watching on television the scene of the nearby Nagata district on fire. It is important to know that the population affected by a disaster is sometimes the least informed on the magnitude and nature of the event [1].

HEALTH PROBLEMS IN THE ACUTE PHASE

Immediately after the Earthquake

At Kobe University Medical School, a considerable number of victims brought to emergency services were found to be DOA (dead on arrival). Many other cases were referred to orthopedic surgery. Several cases of crush syndrome were also reported. The forensic department was extremely busy for administrative autopsies and certifications of death [2].

Soon after the earthquake, most of the victims experienced emotional numbness. A friend of mine who lost his parents said that he felt out of touch with reality. He said that he could not feel sadness. I experienced a sort of depersonalization (possibly, a psychological protection from the disaster).

Two or three days after the earthquake, the majority of the victims became talkative and joyful. Some people even became hypomanic and showed signs of psychomotor excitement. These symptoms might be caused by the biological joy of survival. Major psychiatric problems in this early stage were recurrences of mental disorders and epileptic seizures due to the interruption of habitual medication. Loss of memory and disorientation were reported, particularly among the elderly. In general, manic-depressive patients turned manic [3].

In the First 2 Weeks after the Event

During the first week, everybody was anxious to secure food, water, and information. A kind of a battlefield friendship existed for a certain period. This resulted in mental excitement and friendship among victims. However, fear of after-shock and general anxiety were experienced at the same time. Survivor's guilt was strong for those who lost family members.

I experienced an abnormal sense of time: I felt one day was eternal, but I could not remember the events of the previous day.

After 1 week, the focus of health care was shifted from emergency medical care to care for chronic patients, including those with hypertension, diabetes mellitus, and mental disorders [4,5]. Care for demented elderly and mentally handicapped people in shelters posed difficult problems. Insomnia was common at crowded shelters. Acute stress responses and nightmares were reported. Psychiatric emergency care was established at some shelters. The Hyogo Prefectural Mental Health Center played a key role in coordinating mental health care to victims.

Volunteers, including physicians, psychologists and psychiatrists, flocked to Kobe and damaged areas. It is reported that almost 1.5 million volunteers from all over Japan, and some from abroad, came to the Hanshin area to assist after the earthquake.

After 10 days, the life in shelters became very stressful for many victims. An increase of acute stress responses, including serious stress peptic ulcer, was reported. The Department of Internal Medicine of Kobe University Medical School was busy with the treatment of many cases of extremely serious bleeding ulcers. Anxiety reactions and sleep disorders were common [6]. An increased occurrence of pneumonia and bronchitis was reported among the elderly (the earthquake took place in January, which was wintertime in Japan).

After 2 weeks, victims started facing reality and the loss of family members, housing and jobs. Depression became manifest among victims. A few suicide cases were reported. Acute symptoms of post-traumatic stress (ASD), such as flashbacks, continued among victims.

In the Following Months

After 1 month, a considerable number of the aged people became unable to cope with the continuing stress. Among elderly victims, dementia, disorientation and incontinence were often reported. The consumption of alcohol increased among victims, which led to an epidemic of alcohol-related problems in some shelters. Alcohol-related violence was sometimes reported. Some children showed regression. Burnout syndrome among volunteers became commonplace.

At one time, more than 320,000 people lived in shelters such as schools and public buildings. The government started the building of temporary houses which were similar to military barracks. In total, 47,000 temporary houses were built by public funding and almost 80,000 people lived in temporary housing.

Many victims lost their jobs and faced economic difficulties. In the process of rehabilitation and relocation, many victims faced degradation in social status which, in turn, caused depression.

Among the victims, the most disadvantaged population groups included the elderly who lost kin, families comprising a mother and children, the physically and mentally disadvantaged, and foreigners from developing countries.

After 2 years, victims moved gradually from temporary housing to condominiums built by the local government. Victims left their temporary houses one by one and by 1999 almost all temporary housing units became vacant [7].

LONG-TERM HEALTH CONSEQUENCES

A wide range of physical and psychological problems have been observed among victims even several years after the earthquake. These problems were mainly related to stressful experiences and conditions of the victims. However, other environmental factors and direct physical damage also played an important role. For example, hypertension among victims could be caused by several causes such as salty instant food, stressful living conditions, and nightmares. It will take a long time to obtain data on such possible effects of the earthquake as those on the psychosocial development of children, and those on the immune function (and on the incidence of allergy, cancer, etc.).

Long-Term Physical Effects

The isolated lifestyle increased alcohol use and cigarette-smoking, thus increasing the risk of hypertension and coronary heart disease. The lack of intake of fresh vegetables and the increased intake of "fast food" increased the risk of coronary heart disease among victims. Cold temperature and insufficient air-conditioning caused colds, bronchitis, and emphysema.

A small number of victims have been chronically disabled by the earthquake. They are suffering from head injuries and spinal cord injuries, and some have developed paraplegia. Pseudodementia has been suspected among a sizable number of elderly victims. Heavy drinking caused alcoholic hepatitis in some victims. A high-risk group for chronic stress disorders is elderly males who lost their family members. However, large-scale epidemiologic studies have yet to be completed for the victims of the earthquake.

Long-Term Psychological Effects

Among the major problems affecting the victims are psychological difficulties resulting from isolated life in temporary housing. This isolation and the loss of community sometimes have led to tragedies such as suicides and so-called solitary death (unattended death in temporary housing). More than 250 cases of solitary death have been reported among victims of the earthquake. This has become a major social concern among the population in Kobe and a reason to blame the local government. Lack of local health personnel was cited as one of the contributing factors for this tragedy. According to our study on schoolchildren, psychological effects have been marked among girls of a younger age who lost families and friends. Neurotic symptoms decreased after 6 months but depressive symptoms and physical complaints continued even after 12 months [7,8]. A few articles from the Kobe area report a relatively low prevalence of post-traumatic stress disorder (PTSD) among victims compared with data in other countries [9–11].

WHAT WE HAVE LEARNED

Stress-related physical symptoms have been the first to appear soon after the earthquake. Hemorrhagic ulcer and hypertension increased soon after the disaster, peaked at 2–3 weeks, and gradually decreased by 6 months. They were rather short-lived. Among psychological symptoms, anxiety symptoms were prevalent from the beginning and decreased with time. Guilt feelings appeared together with anxiety and decreased by 6 months. However, depressive symptoms did not decrease with time: they increased up to 6 months. Also, depressive symptoms were frequent among those who lost their home and family. Social problems became dominant after one year. Alcohol problems and interpersonal difficulties increased gradually with time, and they continue to exist as major problems among victims [12].

Post-Traumatic Stress Disorder

The concepts of ASD and PTSD are not adequate to cover the full range of trauma-related psychological problems [13]. Studies at the Psychological Care Center of Hyogo Prefecture have demonstrated that, among 1,956 cases seen at the Center after the earthquake, those with the full PTSD syndrome according to DSM-IV were 2.5%. However, the prevalence was 4.5% among those who lost their homes, and 13.1% among those who lost their family members [14]. The prevalence of PTSD was clearly related to the severity of damage such as loss of home and loss of family. However, the complete picture of PTSD so far has been fairly rare among the victims in Kobe.

There may be many reasons and possible interpretations for the low rate of PTSD among the victims in Kobe. One explanation is the low reporting of PTSD symptoms: victims might have had some reservations in reporting such symptoms as dissociation to medical professionals due to the stigma attached to mental symptoms. A second explanation could be the low recognition of PTSD by medical professionals: there was no particular motivation among medical professionals to ask about the existence of PTSD among victims. On the other hand, the PTSD concept became so popular soon after the earthquake that its widespread use contributed to reduce even the stigma attached to psychological problems in general. The media reported almost every day about PTSD. Almost all Japanese psychiatrists became familiar with the DSM-IV and its criteria for PTSD. A third explanation could be that Asians, including Japanese, tend to somatize rather than to develop psychological symptoms such as dissociation under a stressful situation [15]. However, there are no data supporting this explanation, which would invite discussion on the relationship between PTSD and somatoform disorder, and on the clinical validity of the current concept of PTSD among Asian victims. A fourth explanation could be that many victims in Kobe did not feel abandoned or neglected after the earthquake. The community-oriented Japanese society might have contributed to lower the incidence of PTSD in Kobe. Also, no political and financial incentives have been involved, for patients or doctors, in the diagnosis of PTSD in the Kobe area.

These explanations seem plausible. However, no rigorous epidemiological study on PTSD among the victims of the Hanshin-Awaji earthquake has been completed up to now. PTSD might increase with time. We have to continue careful observation regarding the psychological status of the victims in the Kobe area.

Volunteers

Soon after the earthquake, psychiatrists and mental health workers from all over Japan came to the Kobe area to provide mental health care. Some groups set up psychiatric clinics for the shelter population. However, very few victims visited. The care most valued by victims living at shelters was the help of housewives who could advise them about how to get food and information. Young volunteers who carried water and food and listened to the experiences of the victims were much valued. A group of psychiatrists prepared a simple manual for volunteers on basic rules on how to listen to victims. These rules included such topics as the importance of sharing experience, the need for informed consent, and how to keep confidentiality. These contacts might have been like briefing and debriefing sessions for many victims. They could feel that they were not abandoned. Also, victims could receive psychological support for 24 hours from their neighbors and volunteers, which was much more important than professional support. In summary, there were positive and negative aspects to professional mental health care in the Hanshin-Awaji earthquake: traditional psychiatric care, such as setting up psychiatric mobile clinics, was not at all useful; however, basic information on mental health care, distributed to volunteers through the mass media, was useful to the victims.

The usefulness of foreign volunteers was difficult to evaluate. A number of international experts on disaster mental health came to Kobe. They put a heavy burden on the small number of local experts, as they needed translators and someone to arrange their visits to the shelters. Some experts in Kobe developed burnout symptoms after meeting with so many foreign disaster experts. However, foreign experts were the ones who enlightened the Japanese media and professionals on the needs for psychological support to the victims. No one in Japan was prepared to cope with the mental health needs of the victims of the disaster. International experts surely contributed to increase the awareness of the importance of mental health care for the victims in Kobe.

WHAT WE SEE NOW 10 YEARS LATER

Social Issues Never End

For health professionals living in Kobe, the most important concern has been how to promote health among victims of the disaster and especially how to prevent so-called solitary death (unattended death) among victims. Immediately after the earthquake, there was a flood of volunteers to the Kobe area to take care of victims. Three years later, all volunteers had gone. Local governments mobilized public health nurses to visit temporary housing. However, the number of public health nurses was extremely limited. In each temporary housing community, autonomous committees have been set up to foster self-help among residents. These mechanisms have been working to prevent solitary death and long-term health problems.

It is very difficult for those who lost their homes, money, friends, and partners in old age to hold on to the meaning of life and hope. A minimum amount of compensation to rebuild homes and to start small-scale businesses will be indispensable for victims to find meaning in life.

We have to continue to promote public awareness of the long-term health consequences of the disaster and to find effective measures to reduce these problems.

From Victims to Supporters to Victims

In 1999, the Kobe University School of Medicine decided to organize an International Training Course on Comprehensive Health and Medical Care for Victims of Disasters, supported financially by the Japan International Cooperation Agency (JICA). Experts in disaster medicine from disaster-prone developing countries have the opportunity to study in Kobe for 8 weeks. The Kobe University School of Medicine felt that it was its duty and responsibility to share its experiences and to transfer the related technology to experts from developing countries. So far, we have had 30 doctors and nurses. They were from Turkey, Egypt, Bangladesh, Nepal, China, Thailand, Pakistan, India, Kenya, Peru and Nicaragua. The University dispatched emergency relief teams immediately after the earthquakes in Turkey and Taiwan.

Likewise, Hyogo Prefecture and Kobe City invited several United Nations agencies to set up research and training centers for disaster prevention in the Kobe area. It will be important for the victims of the Kobe earthquake to become supporters to victims of disasters. Through this process, Kobe City and its residents are trying to recover from their traumas.

From Kobe to Asia

Asian countries are constantly menaced by violent natural disasters. Up to now, little attention has been given to the impact of disasters on mental health. However, in the past decade, disaster mental health has gained an increased attention. In Japan, the Hanshin-Awaji earthquake marked the turning point in popularizing PTSD and the need for mental health care for survivors. This recognition has spread to mental health professionals in China and Taiwan after major disasters in their respective countries [16,17]. The Hanshin-Awaji earthquake was very tragic. However, the lessons learned in Kobe are being shared by mental health experts in Asia and in other developing countries.

REFERENCES

1. Baba S., Taniguchi H., Nambu S., Tsuboi S., Ishihara K., Osato S. (1996) Essay, the great Hanshin earthquake. *Lancet*, 347: 307–309.
2. Ueno Y., Nishimura A., Tatsuno Y., Yata K., Adachi J., Fujimoto S., *et al.* (1998) Analysis of the result of inquests in the Great Hanshin earthquake. In I. Kamae (Ed.), *Comprehensive Medical Studies on the Earthquake Victims*, pp. 27–34. Kobe University School of Medicine, Kobe.
3. Shinfuku N. (1999) To be a victim and a survivor of the Great Hanshin-Awaji Earthquake. *J Psychosom Res*, 46: 541–548.
4. Saito K., Kim J.L., Maekawa K., Ikeda Y., Yokoyama A. (1997) The Great Hanshin Awaji earthquake – aggravated blood pressure control in treated hypertensive patients. *Am J Hypertens*, 10: 217–221.
5. Inui A., Kitaoka H., Majima M.,Takamiya S., Uemoto M., Yonenaga C., *et al.* (1998) Effect of the earthquake on stress and glycemic control in patients with diabetes mellitus. *Arch Intern Med*, 158: 274–278.
6. Aoyama N., Kinoshita Y., Fujimoto S., Himeno S., Todo A., Kasuga M., *et al.* (1998) Peptic ulcer after the Hanshin-Awaji earthquake – increased incidence of bleeding gastric ulcers. In I. Kamae (Ed.), *Comprehensive Medical Studies on the Earthquake Victims*, pp. 45–52. Kobe University School of Medicine, Kobe.
7. Shinfuku N. (1998) Psychological consequences of the Great Hanshin-Awaji earthquake. In I. Kamae (Ed.), *Comprehensive Medical Studies on the Earthquake Victims*, pp. 189–193. Kobe University School of Medicine, Kobe.
8. Shinfuku N., Honda M., Uemoto M., Shioyama A. (1998) Epidemiological study of the Great Hanshin-Awaji earthquake's psychological consequences on affected school children. In I. Kamae (Ed.), *Comprehensive Medical Studies on the Earthquake Victims*, pp. 194–197. Kobe University School of Medicine, Kobe.
9. Kokai M., Takeuchi S., Ohara K., Morita Y. (1998) PTSD among victims of the Great Hanshin Awaji earthquake (in Japanese). *Sheishin-lgaku*, 478: 1061–1068.
10. Sharan P., Chaudhary G., Kavathkar S.A., Saxena S. (1996) Preliminary report of psychiatric disorder in survivors of a severe earthquake. *Am J Psychiatry*, 153: 556–558.
11. Coenjian A.K., Najarian L.M., Pynoos R.S. (1994) Posttraumatic stress disorder in elderly and younger adults after the 1988 earthquake in Armenia. *Am J Psychiatry*, 151: 895–901.
12. Araki K., Nakane Y., Ohta Y., Kawasaki N. (1998) The nature of psychiatric problems among disaster victims. *Psychiatry Clin Neurosci*, 52(Suppl.): 317–319.
13. Kokai M., Shinfuku N. (2000) PTSD in Asian Society. *Encyclopedia of Clinical Psychiatry*, S6: 309–318 (in Japanese).

14. Kato H., Asukai N., Miyake Y., Minakawa K., Nishiyama A. (1996) Post-traumatic symptoms among younger and elderly evacuees in the early stages following the 1995 Hanshin-Awaji earthquake in Japan. *Acta Psychiatr Scand*, **93**: 477–471.
15. Kokai M., Shinfuku N. (1998) Post-traumatic stress disorder and somatoform disorder (in Japanese). *Psychosom Med*, **2**: 193–197.
16. Chen C.C., Yeh T.L., Yang Y.K., Chen S.J., Lee I.H., Fu L.S., *et al.* (2001) Psychiatric morbidity and post-traumatic symptoms among survivors in the early stage following the 1999 earthquake in Taiwan. *Psychiatry Res*, **15**: 13–22.
17. Wang X., Gao L., Shinfuku N., Zhang H., Zhao C., Shen Y. (2000) Longitudinal study of earthquake-related PTSD in a randomly selected community sample in north China. *Am J Psychiatry*, **157**: 1260–1266.

8

The Experience of the Marmara Earthquake

Peykan G. Gökalp

Bakirkoy Teaching and Research Hospital for Psychiatry and Neurology, Istanbul, Turkey

INTRODUCTION

An earthquake (7.4 on the Richter scale) struck the Marmara region (north-western part of Turkey), unexpectedly, on 17 August 1999. The region – with the towns of Izmit, Gölcük, Adapazari and Avcilar/Istanbul – is the most heavily populated area of the country. 18,000 people were killed, approximately 50,000 were injured and thousands were left homeless, according to official records [1]. Almost 20 million people in the area needed support and a number of them professional help, because they experienced the first shock and the aftershocks, had losses from the epicenter, took part in rescue teams, or viewed the disaster and rescue scenes on TV.

Now, after 5 years, the inhabitants of Istanbul, almost 12 million people, are not comfortable at all. A probable earthquake, with a magnitude larger than 7.0 on the Richter scale, is expected in Istanbul within 30 years, as reported by geologists. This is one of the reasons why the majority of the population of the Marmara region is easily irritated by media releases about measures to be taken for a probable earthquake. Not all of the houses are built according to official requirements, owing to the high rate of migration to metropolises from rural areas. Earthquakes under these conditions can simply be classified as both a natural and a man-made disaster.

THE EARTHQUAKE

The earthquake took place at 3.02 a.m., when almost everyone was asleep, and lasted 45 seconds. The electricity was cut off within a few seconds and a

Disasters and Mental Health. Edited by Juan José López-Ibor, George Christodoulou, Mario Maj, Norman Sartorius and Ahmed Okasha.
©2005 John Wiley & Sons Ltd. ISBN 0-470-02123-3.

loud noise was heard from the ground which increased the degree of fear and horror. Then, the shaking, the collapse of the buildings and the screams all followed and added to the severity of the trauma. No one, even the governing bodies, completely realized how extensive the surface area affected was, nor what the extent of the losses was, until the next day. The main roads, telephone lines and other means of communication were interrupted, which caused the blockade of crucial information about the severity of the disaster. A large fire started in a huge oil plant near Izmit, which posed a threat to the nearby towns and caused great material loss. Major ecological problems arose because of the damage to several factories in the area. On the day after the disaster, there were millions of people shocked, injured and homeless, who had lost their loved ones from the family or the neighborhood, confused among the rubble.

THE IMMEDIATE POST-DISASTER PERIOD

On the first day, people were numbed. They showed hardly any reaction to the situation. Then, after the rescue teams arrived, there was an atmosphere of hope of saving those who were still alive. The media showed scenes from the disaster area in detail. The lack of distribution of sufficient supplies caused anger against official authorities.

Later, many donations from national and foreign organizations and individuals flowed to the area. There was an excess of many items in one tent camp, a shortage of the same item in the neighboring one. People tried to collect everything that was given out, without thinking whether they really needed it or not.

It was difficult to activate people for the fulfillment of their basic needs in tent camps. Men, who had a job to do before, were wandering aimlessly around; women, who were mostly housewives, had no house to clean any more. If their children were still alive, they were looked after by volunteer female students and/or psychologists in "game tents" in major tent camps. This inactivity might stem from intense feelings of helplessness due to the trauma, and regression caused by the circumstances, where "powerful others" did everything for them.

Rumors spread around about coming earthquakes with a larger magnitude, or other natural disasters, as well as mystic or supernatural explanations of why the earthquake had struck the region. These rumors increased the level of worry and dread among the survivors.

In the tent camps of the poorest people, support services for children and women were used enthusiastically. In most cases, this was the first time that children saw interesting and "expensive" toys, and women who had no formal education were able to learn new skills for coping with life.

Many volunteers, among them doctors, psychologists and nurses from large cities, rushed to the area in the first days without any organization. Members of private companies provided food, water, clothes and machines to remove the rubble. A volunteer rescue organization from Turkey, named Akut, started search and rescue efforts for the victims and became the symbol of the heroes of the disaster. International rescue teams reached the Marmara region from Japan, Israel, Greece, Hungary, the USA and many other countries, and saved the lives of many.

Psychiatrists went to the disaster area under the umbrella of the Turkish Medical Association, which established temporary health care units after the second day, and they mostly worked as general practitioners in the primary care units. Members of Chambers of Medicine from other cities were also organized by the Turkish Medical Association. The physicians also took part in the establishment of basic facilities for the survivors and volunteers.

The physicians and nurses worked without changing shifts to attend the severely injured. Those health care professionals who lived and worked in the area were themselves traumatized. Therefore, they were not able to attend to the needs of the survivors as efficient professionals, and they themselves needed help. Medical staff was mobilized from other regions of Turkey, to serve in the disaster area. Physicians and nurses had to be trained on "normal reactions to an abnormal event". Mental health teams conducted debriefing sessions for medical and rescue staff and survivors.

International medical staff joined the Turkish groups within a few days and established tent hospitals that served emergency patients as well as people who had chronic medical and psychiatric illnesses.

SOCIAL AND HEALTH CARE STATUS TWO YEARS LATER

According to the records of National Social Security System, 150,000 people lost their jobs after the disaster. The rate of jobless population was 16% for the population above the age of 14 years, which is significantly higher than the average rate of joblessness in Turkey (7.3%) from official records.

The average rate of using the health care services (primary care units, general hospitals and private services) in the disaster area was higher than the average rate for Turkey in general. 20% of the help-seeking population consisted of children younger than four years of age. 22% of those who sought medical help from health care facilities reported that their problem was not resolved. The reason for that was reported as not being able to obtain the medications due to financial reasons.

MENTAL HEALTH CARE

Injury care and support for people who had losses were the first duties of mental health workers. Outreach services were organized which served for several months in the area. The majority of mental health workers and organizations were not properly trained for trauma work. Therefore training programs, organized by the Psychiatric Association of Turkey and other Turkish and foreign professional organizations and non-governmental organizations (NGOs) went hand in hand with outreach services, especially in tent camps, in medical facilities and among the rescue staff.

The outreach services were organized by the Association of Turkish Psychologists, psychiatry departments of medical schools of major universities and teaching hospitals in Turkey, and foreign mental health professionals. The setting of the services was totally different from the settings under "normal conditions". Tents, open air, hospital wards, where many other injured and medical staff were also present, were used for interviews.

In my personal professional experience, I was used to people who came to the psychiatry department, because they needed help. The doctor–patient relationship was defined and had certain boundaries. On the disaster site, I served first in a temporary health station of the Turkish Medical Association in Golcuk, located in a park, among the rubble. The mental health team from my hospital consisted of a senior psychiatrist, a resident and a nurse, who took daily shifts in three different towns.

Messages were coming from newly established tent camps either about emergency psychiatric conditions or about those who needed psychiatric or psychological help, according to the physician. I or my colleagues used to visit the tent camps for these cases. We were directed to people who had losses from their families, but did not want any help. It was a difficult experience for us and for the survivors to establish a trusting and permanent relationship among the confusing conditions, where large changes took place every day both in the population of the tent camps and in their location.

There were numerous organizations and individuals who tried to help the survivors, including experienced professionals, and organized groups with appropriate supervision systems, but also students or individuals who did not know what to do but wanted to help. Foreign groups conducted sessions with the help of translators. A coordination meeting with the representatives of major mental health organizations was held in order to coordinate and establish a collaboration.

Motivating people who did not seek help to receive a psychiatric interview required new skills for mental health professionals. It was also difficult for the survivors to trust someone, where many other "helpers" approached them only for filling out questionnaires. Women expressed their feelings and applied for help more easily than men. The problem of trust was partly resolved after the mental health stations were located in the main tent camps in the area.

Looking back at this critical period, I would emphasize the need for keeping good records. Otherwise, it is not possible to learn the correct lessons from such a huge experience.

STUDIES ON THE MENTAL HEALTH CONSEQUENCES OF THE EARTHQUAKE

In one of the first studies on the earthquake survivors, the sample consisted of 42 injured survivors who were hospitalized at the surgery and orthopedics wards of a general hospital in Istanbul. The psychiatric assessment was made on the nineteenth day after the disaster. 40.4% of the subjects had lost a close relative in the earthquake, 26.1% had a diagnosis of acute stress disorder, 16.6% had adjustment disorder with anxious and depressed mood, and 11.9% had major depression [2].

A study of survivors evaluated at 4 to 6 months after the earthquake revealed a prevalence of post-traumatic stress disorder (PTSD) of 76% [3]. In another study conducted in the epicenter (Gölcük), 1,000 survivors were screened: PTSD was diagnosed in 43% of the group, and 31% were diagnosed as having major depression. Risk factors included high trauma exposure, great loss of resources, difficult post-disaster living conditions and the continuing experience of aftershocks [4]. In another study by the same group, 586 survivors were evaluated 20 months after the earthquake: the rates of PTSD and major depression were 39% and 18% respectively [5].

A study conducted at 6 to 9 months after the disaster in Kocaeli emphasized the importance of psychiatric conditions comorbid with PTSD: 38.3% of the subjects with a diagnosis of PTSD had another psychiatric disorder: major depression, generalized anxiety disorder and panic disorder were the three most frequent diagnoses [6]. Having this information about comorbidity in disaster survivors helps the professionals in implementing treatment strategies [7].

A study conducted in Avcilar/Istanbul explored the natural course of PTSD. In the first 3 months after the earthquake, 9,422 survivors were screened, of whom 62% met diagnostic criteria for PTSD. 15,453 people were screened at 6 and 10 months after the disaster, showing a prevalence of PTSD of 23.4%. The population screened at 18 months after the earthquake had a prevalence of PTSD of 8.1% [8].

Some other studies investigated the symptoms and the prevalence of PTSD in children who were either hospitalized after they were saved from the rubble, or who were living in tent camps after the earthquake [9]. The study by Berkem and Bildik reported that the reaction of children to the disaster and the presenting symptoms differed according to their age [10]. The study by Laor *et al.* [11] emphasized that the screening of children in the post-disaster period requires the detection of symptoms of PTSD, dissociation and grief.

A CLOSER LOOK AT A PREFABRICATED VILLAGE IN ADAPAZARI

Adapazarı is one of the cities most deeply affected by the earthquake. According to the Turkish Medical Association's *First Year Report on Marmara 1999 Earthquake*, 70% of the drinking water system in the city center was destroyed. There was a 33% reduction in the number of hospital beds and a significant reduction in the number of physicians and nurses [12].

The Psychological Support and Psychiatric Treatment Project for Psychological Problems Caused by the Earthquake in Adapazarı (ADEPSTEP) was started because of this inadequacy, 5 months after the earthquake, by a group of mental health professionals from two major psychiatric departments in Istanbul. The main objective of the project was to assess the traumatized population for their potential risks for psychiatric morbidity, and to provide treatment and follow-up for 12 months. The population that was assessed ($n = 350$) was severely traumatized. It was a low-income group, with a mean age of 38.4 years, and a high level of personal and material loss (39.4% had lost a close relative). In the clinician-assessed group ($n = 187$), 75.3% were diagnosed as having PTSD. In the PTSD group, 70.8% were female. The major problem in conducting the project was the difficulty in following up regularly the individuals who received a diagnosis of PTSD, since the population of the prefabricated village was mobile because of the instability of job, education and housing facilities.

The ADEPSTEP experience has provided valuable information on the long-term post-disaster phase. People with low socioeconomic status are reluctant to utilize mental health services. The improvement of community mental health services and education is a major issue in the pre-disaster period [13,14]. Training programs for primary care physicians are now being developed and implemented in different regions in Turkey [15,16].

LONG-TERM CONSEQUENCES OF THE EARTHQUAKE

In the comprehensive reports by the Turkish Medical Association on health care utilization, socioeconomic status and family structure 2 years after the earthquake, one can see the harmful effects of the disaster on the community [17]. Alcohol consumption has increased, as well as the rate of divorce and domestic violence.

Preparing for disasters in the future lies in the improvement of the housing and construction network of the urban areas, as well as the education of the public on general and mental health issues. Ethical concerns should be kept in mind in research and treatment efforts for disaster survivors, since this population is a group particularly vulnerable to instability of therapeutic relationships and abuse.

International relief efforts, which bring hope and fresh energy in the midst of a catastrophe, should be organized by a local crisis committee, since the needs of the people can be best evaluated by locals.

The experience of Turkey after the disaster was also an experience of solidarity with fellow citizens in the country and abroad, an experience for questioning authority and practicing NGO power during the reconstruction efforts.

ACKNOWLEDGEMENTS

The author would like to thank Professor Sahika Yüksel (Istanbul University, Istanbul Medical Faculty) for reviewing the manuscript and Dr Munevver Hacioglu for assistance in the search for the literature in Turkish.

REFERENCES

1. Istanbul Technical University (1999) www.itu.edu.tr/deprem.
2. Yücel B., Tükel R., Sezgin U., Ozdemir O., Polat A., Yüksel S. (2000) Efforts for psychiatric help for the survivors who had physical injuries: a clinical experience. *J Clin Psychiatry*, 3(Suppl. 3): 12–15 (in Turkish).
3. Yüksel Ş., Sezgin U. (2001) Lessons learned from disasters. Presented at the 7th European Conference on Traumatic Stress, Edinburgh, May 26–29.
4. Basoglu M., Salcığlu E., Livanou M. (2002) Traumatic stress responses in earthquake survivors in Turkey. *J Trauma Stress*, **15**: 269–276.
5. Şalcıoğlu E., Başoğlu M., Livanou M. (2003) Long-term psychological outcome for non-treatment seeking earthquake survivors in Turkey. *J Nerv Ment Dis*, **191**: 154–160.
6. Tural U., Aybar Tolun H.G., Karakaya I., Erol A., Yildız M., Erdoğan S. (2001) Predictors of current comorbid psychiatric disorders with PTSD in earthquake survivors. *Turkish J Psychiatry*, **12**: 175–183 (in Turkish).
7. Geyran P.Ç. (1996) Psychiatric disorders comorbid with PTSD. *Turkish J Psychiatry*, **7**: 58–62 (in Turkish).

8. Karamustafalıoğlu K.O., Bakım B., Guveli M. (2002) Preliminary findings of the RUDAM project: PTSD in survivors of 1999 earthquake in Turkey. Unpublished manuscript.

9. Yörbik O., Türkbay T., Ekmen M., Demirkan S., Söhmen T. (1999) Investigation of post-traumatic stress disorder symptoms related to earthquake in children and adolescents. *J Child Adolesc Ment Health*, **6**: 158–164 (in Turkish).

10. Berkem M., Bildik T. (2001) The clinical features of children who are hospitalized after the earthquake. *J Anatolian Psychiatry*, **2**: 133–130 (in Turkish).

11. Laor N., Wolmer L., Kora M., Yücel D., Spirman S., Yazgan Y. (2002) Posttraumatic, dissociative and grief symptoms in Turkish children exposed to the 1999 earthquakes. *J Nerv Ment Dis*, **190**: 824–832.

12. Turkish Medical Association (2000) *First Year Report on Marmara 1999 Earthquake*. www.ttb.org.tr.

13. ADEPSTEP Project Team (2000) Psychological support and psychiatric treatment project for psychological problems caused by the earthquake in Adapazarı. Presented at the 37th Turkish Congress of Psychiatry, İstanbul, October 2–6 (in Turkish).

14. Sezgin U.,Yüksel Ş. (2001) Survivors of Marmara Earthquake. Presented at the 7th European Conference on Traumatic Stress Studies, Edinburgh, May 26–29.

15. Gökalp P. (2000) *Post-Disaster Training Package for Physicians* (Part I): *Disaster Psychiatry Task Force*. Psychiatric Association of Turkey, Istanbul Branch (in Turkish).

16. Aker T. (2000) *Approach to Psychosocial Trauma in Primary Care (TREP)*. Mutludogan Ofset, Istanbul (in Turkish).

17. Turkish Medical Association (2001) *Second Year Report on Marmara Earthquake*. www.ttb.org.tr.

9

The Experience of
the Athens Earthquake

George N. Christodoulou, Thomas J. Paparrigopoulos
and Constantin R. Soldatos

*Athens University Medical School,
Eginition Hospital, Athens, Greece*

INTRODUCTION

Earthquakes constitute a rather frequent type of natural disaster in Greece, a country that occupies the sixth position in the worldwide rank of seismic activity. The earthquake which struck the Athens Metropolitan Area (AMA) on September 7, 1999 had a magnitude of 5.9 on the Richter scale and it was the second strongest over the last 20 years. Actually, because its epicenter was close to the surface, in certain residential areas, it caused large material and considerable human casualties. The main earthquake was followed by many aftershocks of a smaller magnitude that lasted for about a couple of weeks. The death toll rose to 152; in addition, more than 25,000 individuals were evacuated, mainly to tents close to their place of residence, and a few more thousands moved permanently elsewhere. Although much stronger earthquakes had hit Greece in the past [1,2], the fact that almost a third of the total population of the whole country resides in the capital city of Athens increases many fold the probability for any bio-psycho-social and material consequences caused by a seismic event of such a magnitude [3].

A strong earthquake was not expected in Athens at that time, because this area is considered to be less seismogenic than other regions of the country. Consequently, the central government was not prepared for such a catastrophic event. Needless to say, the population of the capital was far less prepared than the authorities. Fortunately, because the earthquake struck at the periphery of the AMA, heavy damage was limited to relatively sparsely populated residential areas, which border one of the industrial

Disasters and Mental Health. Edited by Juan José López-Ibor, George Christodoulou, Mario Maj, Norman Sartorius and Ahmed Okasha.
©2005 John Wiley & Sons Ltd. ISBN 0-470-02123-3.

zones of the capital. Thus, governmental rescue actions were fairly quickly and sufficiently implemented. Specialized rescue squads, firemen, military forces, emergency medical aid, and volunteers tried to provide support to the victims on the spot. Rescue work on the debris lasted for a couple of weeks.

IMPACT PHASE AND EARLY ACTIONS

During the first days following the 1999 earthquake in AMA, the prevailing feeling, mostly recorded through the mass media, was that the affected population had an increased need for psychological support. This need for psychological first aid, as well as for information dissemination, seemed to be multiplied many fold and to pertain also to people who were not directly affected by the catastrophic earthquake. This should be attributed to the overwhelming television coverage of the disaster, that has brought this devastating experience to the attention of practically everyone, leading to an increase in numbers of potentially traumatized individuals through close identification with the victims.

To meet these needs, most of the psychological support agencies of the public or other sectors rushed to the more heavily affected areas within the first 3 days. The special service for psychological support of earthquake victims of the Department of Psychiatry of the University of Athens was mobilized. Members of this service formed three psychosocial support units, two of them posted at the periphery of the AMA (within the most severely affected regions) and one centrally located in Eginition Hospital (main facility of the Department of Psychiatry in the downtown Athens area). Also, a telephone helpline unit started operating. These three units were staffed with psychiatrists, psychologists, and social workers who volunteered to provide their services to the victims [3].

Primary aims of these units were to provide pertinent information, relief from the traumatic experience and/or crisis intervention to the victims upon their request. The goal of intervention was not simply the prevention of post-traumatic stress disorder (PTSD), but also the management of acute stress reactions, grief, depression, and a host of other maladaptive psychological and behavioral responses according to the individual needs of the victims. Psychological care included mainly listening to the victims while they were referring to their personal experiences and ventilating their emotional overcharge, in addition to prescription of anxiolytic and/or antidepressant medication whenever needed. Also, particular emphasis was given to fostering resilience by providing coping skills training at an elementary level and education about the expected stress response, traumatic reminders and normal versus abnormal functioning. Anxiety reduction techniques to decrease physiological arousal were applied when feasible.

EARLY POST-IMPACT STRESS REACTIONS

During the 6 weeks of operation of the three psychological support units, 166 individuals sought help from those units, and 66 more had a telephone contact with our staff. The mean interval between the catastrophic event and the time of each subject's assessment was 8.2 ± 4.4 days (range: 3–22 days). The mean age of the subjects was 41.4 ± 14.9 years (range: 12–87). For the majority they were married women with children (males/females: 22% vs. 78%; married: 68%). 90% of the interviewees' houses had suffered repairable damages and 10% had been seriously damaged to the extent that they should be eventually rebuilt. In any event, at the time of the interview, all subjects were identified as evacuees temporarily settled in tents. The main reasons for seeking help were an intense apprehension of another impending earthquake (48.4%), diffuse anxiety (16.4%), and somatization of anxiety (15.6%).

In addition to properly addressing the aforementioned presenting complaints, 102 subjects were fully investigated through a checklist of sociodemographic variables and a semi-structured psychiatric interview focusing on the detection of acute stress reaction (ASR) and PTSD. This interview was devised according to the ICD-10 Research Diagnostic Criteria and consisted of 35 items pertaining to the ASR diagnosis and 10 items pertaining to the PTSD diagnosis. Items were ascertained dichotomously as either present or absent. More specifically, the 35 items assessing ASR were grouped into the eight symptom clusters described in the ICD-10 (i.e., autonomic arousal symptoms, symptoms involving chest and abdomen, symptoms involving mental state, general physical symptoms, symptoms of tension, dissociative symptoms, other "psychic" symptoms, and other non-specific symptoms of stress response), while the 10 items referring to PTSD assessed the presence of symptoms of persistent "reliving" of the stressor, symptoms of avoidance, selective inability to recall some aspects of the stressful event, and persistent symptoms of increased psychological sensitivity and arousal.

Acute Stress Reaction

In our sample of help-seekers, the majority of subjects (85%) fulfilled ICD-10 criteria for ASR within the first 48 hours following the earthquake. Even the remaining 15% had some symptoms of acute stress, particularly symptoms of autonomic hyperarousal, but they did not meet the criteria for a formal diagnosis of ASR. Among those who received a diagnosis of ASR, the most frequently encountered symptoms were "non-specific symptoms of stress response", i.e. exaggerated startle response, difficulty getting to sleep because of worrying and difficulty in concentrating, and symptoms of autonomic hyperarousal. These symptoms essentially constitute an immediate, potentially transient reaction to any traumatic experience and considerably overlap with the normally expected emotional and behavioral response to stress. It is noteworthy that symptoms of dissociation, which according to DSM-IV, but not the ICD-10, are purportedly cardinal symptoms of acute stress disorder, were rather scarcely reported by the interviewees. This observation raises an essential diagnostic issue regarding the prerequisites for the DSM-IV diagnosis of acute stress disorder.

In contrast to the findings of some previous studies, no significant differences were detected between those who developed ASR and those who did not, regarding most variables that have been reported to predict poor post-disaster adjustment [3–6]. Thus, no statistically significant age and gender difference was found in terms of the presence either of the diagnosis of ASR, or of the individual ASR symptoms. The same holds true for a series of sociodemographic variables, several factors related to the recent earthquake, and the pre-existence of a mental disorder. This lack of significant effects of various sociodemographic factors for the occurrence of ASR should be presumably attributed to the nature of the sample of this study, i.e. the fact that our subjects were help-seekers while those studied by other investigators were not.

The only statistically significant difference between the ASR group and the non-ASR group pertained to previous exposure to a similar stressful catastrophic event (81% in the ASR group vs. 50% in the non-ASR group, $p < 0.05$). This is in agreement with the findings of some other studies (7,8) and a recent large-scale epidemiological survey (9), which show that cumulative stress and previous exposure to stressful life events, rather than any single recent traumatic experience alone, are the significant risk factors for the development of post-traumatic syndromes.

Early Post-Traumatic Stress Disorder

Applying the ICD-10 criteria for PTSD, which set a 48-hour period as the lower time limit for the diagnosis of PTSD instead of the 1-month period required by the DSM-IV, we also assessed help-seekers for the presence of early PTSD symptoms, i.e. within the first month following the earthquake. Among addressees to our psychosocial support units, 43% were found to meet the ICD-10 criteria for PTSD; a highly significant association was observed between the occurrence of ASR and the development of early PTSD. Thus, within the group of help-seekers that developed early PTSD, almost everyone had been initially recorded as having suffered ASR, while this was not the case for individuals who did not eventually develop PTSD. A similar finding has been previously reported in several studies, demonstrating that the short-term reaction to stressful events is highly predictive of the occurrence of PTSD in the long run [10–13]. In our sample, one out of four individuals who did not develop early PTSD had not initially presented an acute stress reaction. Consequently, it is of paramount importance to identify, among victims who show signs of intense distress in the early aftermath of a disaster, those who are more likely to remain symptomatic.

Furthermore, we observed that self-reports of accelerated heart rate and feelings of derealization during the acute post-disaster phase, i.e. the first 48 hours following the earthquake, had a specific predictive value for the development of PTSD. This observation corroborates the findings that occurrence of dissociative symptoms [14–17] and increased autonomic responses [18,19] shortly after exposure to psychic trauma are associated with the subsequent development of PTSD. As a matter of fact, these particular symptoms of stress had been the main focus of attention and treatment by our mental health professionals who handled the psychological problems of the victims.

Longitudinal follow-up assessments are deemed necessary for monitoring the course of stress-related disorders. Unfortunately, in our study, this was hard to achieve, given the time-limited operation of our psychological support services and the difficulty in contacting the victims for follow-up visits.

CONCLUSIONS

Large-scale disasters have affected and even devastated communities of the Aegean region in the past and certainly will do so in the future. These are unpredictable events, which leave us powerless in preventing or controlling them. However, organizing and implementing pertinent pre- and post-disaster interventions can mitigate their impact on the individual and society at large. They present a challenge to mental health professionals, who should adequately prepare to assist the traumatized population in multiple ways. Although a considerable body of experience has been accumulated, many more issues should be also addressed, such as the identification of post-disaster psychological needs and priorities. Along these lines, defining the psychological profile of the victims is expected to be helpful in the early detection of ASR and the assessment of its severity by care providers, which may facilitate adequate case management, a prerequisite for the prevention of the more disabling chronic stress-related disorders, such as PTSD. Therefore, the recognition of highly symptomatic individuals – presenting in particular with "non-specific symptoms of stress response" and "symptoms of autonomic hyperarousal" – with a history of previous traumatic experiences might serve as a sensitive predictor in order to take appropriate actions both for prevention and intervention.

ACKNOWLEDGEMENTS

The following physicians are gratefully acknowledged for their invaluable contribution in the data collection: Drs G. Trikkas, V. Tomaras, D. Ploumbides, M. Economou, A. Pechlivanides, I. Zervas, A. Hatzakis, D. Pappa, and M. Theodoropoulou. Dr. D. Pappa also contributed to the handling of data.

REFERENCES

1. Soldatos C.R. (1987) Psychosocial consequences of the 1986 earthquake in Kalamata: study report. Organization for Earthquake Protection (OASP), Athens.
2. Bergiannaki J.D., Psarros C., Varsou E., Paparrigopoulos T., Soldatos C.R. (2003) Protracted acute stress reaction following an earthquake. *Acta Psychiatr Scand*, **107**: 18–24.
3. Christodoulou G.N., Paparrigopoulos T.J., Soldatos C.R. (2003) Acute stress reaction among victims of the 1999 Athens earthquake: help seekers' profile. *World Psychiatry*, **2**: 50–53.
4. McFarlane A.C. (1989) The aetiology of post-traumatic morbidity: predisposing, precipitating and perpetuating factors. *Br J Psychiatry*, **154**: 221–228.
5. Green B.L. (1994) Psychosocial research in traumatic stress: an update. *J Trauma Stress*, **7**: 341–362.
6. Paris J. (2000) Predispositions, personality traits, and posttraumatic stress disorder. *Harvard Rev Psychiatry*, **8**: 175–183.
7. McFarlane A.C. (1997) The prevalence and longitudinal course of PTSD: implications for the neurobiological models of PTSD. *Am NY Acad Sci*, **821**: 10–23.
8. Breslau N., Chilcoat H.D., Kessler R.C., Davis G.C. (1999) Previous exposure to trauma and PTSD effects of subsequent trauma: results from the Detroit Area Survey of Trauma. *Am J Psychiatry*, **156**: 902–907.
9. Kessler R.C., Sonnega A., Bromet E., Hughes M., Nelson C.B., Breslau N. (1999) Epidemiological risk factors for trauma and PTSD. In R. Yehuda (Ed.), *Risk Factors for Posttraumatic Stress Disorder*, pp. 23–59. American Psychiatric Press, Washington, DC.

10. Harvey A.G., Bryant R.A. (1988) The relationship between acute stress disorder and post-traumatic stress disorder: a prospective evaluation of motor vehicle accident survivors. *J Consult Clin Psychol*, **66**: 507–512.
11. Classen C., Koopman C., Hales R., Spiegel D. (1998) Acute stress disorder as a predictor of posttraumatic stress symptoms. *Am J Psychiatry*, **155**: 620–624.
12. Brewin C.R., Andrews B., Rose S., Kirk M. (1999) Acute stress disorder and post-traumatic stress disorder in victims of violent crime. *Am J Psychiatry*, **156**: 360–366.
13. Harvey A.G., Bryant R.A. (2000) Two-year prospective evaluation of the relationship between acute stress disorder and posttraumatic stress disorder following mild traumatic brain injury. *Am J Psychiatry*, **157**: 626–628.
14. Wilkinson C.B. (1983) Aftermath of a disaster: the collapse of the Hyatt Regency Hotel Skywalks. *Am J Psychiatry*, **140**: 1134–1139.
15. Spiegel D., Cardeña E. (1991) Disintegrated experience: the dissociative disorders redefined. *J Abnorm Psychol*, **100**: 366–378.
16. Marmar C.R., Weiss D.S., Schlenger W.E., Fairbank J.A., Jordan B.K., Kulka R.A., et al. (1994) Peritraumatic dissociation and posttraumatic stress in male Vietnam theater veterans. *Am J Psychiatry*, **151**: 902–907.
17. Harvey A.G., Bryant R.A. (1999) Dissociative symptoms in acute stress disorder. *J Trauma Stress*, **12**: 673–680.
18. Shalev A.Y., Sahar T., Freedman S., Peri T., Glick N., Brandes D., et al. (1998) Prospective study of heart rate responses following trauma and the subsequent development of posttraumatic stress disorder. *Arch Gen Psychiatry*, **55**: 553–559.
19. Bryant R.A., Harvey A.G., Guthrie R.M., Moulds M.L. (2000) A prospective study of psychobiological arousal, acute stress disorder, and posttraumatic stress disorder. *J Abnorm Psychol*, **109**: 341–344.

10

The Experience of the Nairobi US Embassy Bombing

Frank Njenga and Caroline Nyamai

Upperhill Medical Center, Nairobi, Kenya

INTRODUCTION

On August 7, 1998, at 10.30 a.m., a terrorist bomb exploded in downtown Nairobi. Prior to that a hand grenade had exploded, and many people had gone to their windows to investigate what was going on. Then the main explosion, consisting of 1 ton of TNT, and measuring 2.7 on the Richter scale, went off.

213 people died, 5,000 sustained injuries that took them to hospitals around the city, and many others had minor injuries that did not require medical attention. All these people, their friends and relatives, and many others who witnessed the event directly or indirectly through the extensive TV, radio and newspaper coverage were affected by the event.

According to estimates, Kenya lost 5–10% of its gross domestic product (GDP) as a result of the bombing [1]. 100 buildings and 250 businesses were wholly or partially damaged. Of the 5,000 wounded, 400 people will remain severely disabled.

IMMEDIATE RESCUE RESPONSES

Immediate issues arising included the challenges of the ensuing rescue process, first aid to the injured, transportation to hospital, the very large numbers with open and bleeding wounds, and the chaos that is usual following any major disaster. This was the first real test of the Kenya spirit *Harambee* (Let's Pull Together) following a terrorist attack. Like their counterparts would do in New York on September 11, 2001, Kenyans discharged themselves with honour and decorum. The traditional

Disasters and Mental Health. Edited by Juan José López-Ibor, George Christodoulou, Mario Maj, Norman Sartorius and Ahmed Okasha.
©2005 John Wiley & Sons Ltd. ISBN 0-470-02123-3.

boundaries of race, tribe, religion, class and creed were discarded in the face of disaster that did not itself make these distinctions as it killed and maimed. All Kenyans were equal before the terrorists. Their response was equal to the task.

THE MENTAL HEALTH RESPONSE

Amidst all this, however, it was quickly realized that there would be a lot of psychological, emotional and social issues that would need to be dealt with.

Operation Recovery was the project that was initiated by the Kenya Medical Association to respond to this need. The project brought together medical personnel, corporate firms, professional bodies, government agencies and individuals, with the prime goal of developing and implementing a coordinated psychosocial recovery assistance program for those affected by the bomb blast.

The Red Cross and other organizations put together other initiatives in different parts of the city. The churches were also actively involved. Each collaborating organization brought with it its own unique expertise and resources, and together helped make Operation Recovery the unique organization that it was.

The overall response was planned to alleviate human suffering resulting directly or indirectly from the bomb blast, and to assist the people of Kenya recover from the effects. It was also planned to offer psychological and emotional support through counselling to those injured in the blast, to relatives of those who died, to relatives of those injured, to rescue workers and to medical personnel, as well as to the general public.

THE MEDIA RESPONSE

The media was to prove to be an invaluable asset in the early stages of the tragedy [2]. The first of the media activities was a Cable News Network (CNN) appearance by the author in the afternoon of August 7. This was the first internationally televised statement from a medical doctor regarding the bomb attack. Most Kenyans were still not aware that terrorists had visited the country, resulting in catastrophic damage.

Later the same evening, a 3-hour phone-in program was broadcast on a local FM station. Details of the tragedy and its anticipated traumatic consequences were discussed with the listeners. The message was one of reassurance, that what Kenyans were experiencing at this time was a normal reaction to an abnormal event. The program was followed by several others in the days following and marked the beginning of what was to become an invaluable tool in the dissemination of information and awareness creation on the psychological effects of the bomb blast.

National and regional radio and TV stations generously gave airtime to mental health experts to disseminate information on the likely psychological sequelae. Question and answer sessions on the electronic media were an early and regular feature.

The purpose of this extensive media program thus became to educate the Kenyan people on what reactions to expect following this trauma, and to reassure them that theirs were indeed normal reactions to an abnormal event. The broadcasts also sought to help sensitize people to the possible mental health needs that could arise subsequently, and to let them know that help was available, and where it could be obtained.

PLANNING LONGER-TERM SERVICES

The planning of service provision proved most challenging. The knowledge base of the Kenyan mental health team was somewhat limited. This was, however, more than compensated for by the enthusiasm, empathy and desire to learn. On the Monday following the Friday event, the army of counselors equipped with varying degrees of knowledge converged at the medical association head office demanding training opportunities to be able to help fellow Kenyans. Some were lay counselors who had attended an afternoon of training in counseling while others (in the minority) were highly seasoned mental health experts. The first 10 days were very busy as the various players sought and found their niche in the novel organization.

By the time the US Secretary of State visited Kenya, the initial scenes of confusion were settling down, American disaster management experts were on the ground and played a crucial role in the planning of services.

CRISIS INTERVENTION

The greatest challenge in the first week was to provide a crisis intervention service to those in greatest need, while sorting out the ragtag army that was to prove so vital in the coming months. One of the collaborating agencies which was church-based organized the 1-day training that enabled the team to adopt a standard format on debriefing and reporting back to headquarters. Three church compounds became walk-in counseling centers in less than a week. We were set to go!

Debriefing, psycho-education and long-term counseling were some of the strategies put in place. A typical debriefing session would involve a group of 8 to 12 people and last between 1 hour and $1\frac{1}{2}$ hours. However, due to the large numbers of people being dealt with, groups as large as 25 people were held. Sessions as long as 3 hours were also held to give everyone an opportunity to speak. Two facilitators would run each group along the Mitchell model [3].

For many, particularly the men, hearing that other men also cried was very reassuring in view of the African view of men crying! (They simply don't!) It reassured them that such a reaction could indeed be found even in other "real men". This point was emphasized at the first formal session held for the senior officers of the Cooperative Bank, which was housed in the building next to the American Embassy.

For the women in the groups, the main issue was the fear for their families, particularly their children. "What would have happened to my children if I had died?...Who would have looked after them?" was a common question to be heard in such sessions.

Psycho-education was an integral part of debriefing sessions. After each group member had had the opportunity to share their experiences, the counselor facilitating the group session would then educate the group on the effects of trauma and what they could expect. This proved to be very useful, as most people experiencing the acute stress reaction signs and symptoms frequently feared that they could be "going mad". Learning this to be what it was – symptoms of the effects of the trauma they had gone through rather than an additional "illness" – was for many very reassuring.

CHILDREN'S PROGRAM

The government of Kenya requested Operation Recovery to provide counseling services to traumatized children in and around the city. 10% of the 360 schools in Nairobi were considered to be "high risk" due to their proximity to the blast. The project targeted 90 schools with a total population of 72,000. In the intermediate phase alone (November 1998 to April 1999), 2,730 children were seen. A special clinical assessment tool was developed with the help of Betty Pfefferbaum [4], modeled on her experience following the Oklahoma experience.

The children were severely traumatized by the bomb blast. More than 6 months after the blast, the children still remembered with horror the big bang, blood, burning cars, helicopters and many military men. Many feared going into the city in case it happened again, some had nightmares and others worried for their parents' safety whenever the parents came back late.

Different strategies had to be employed to suit different circumstances. Story-writing, discussion and drawing were important tools of communication. The counselors became increasingly creative and confident.

Different school authorities had to be approached with tact. Some were hostile; others were ignorant that children were in need; while some seemed to want a bribe to allow us to help the children! Always, however, whenever we got to children their needs were clear.

There was great variability in the character of schools visited. Kawangware Primary School had an average of 52 children per class. Some had a maximum of 25. Linguistic difficulties were encountered in the larger schools located in the slum areas of Nairobi. The differences in the level of education provided in the different areas of the city schools were very marked. For the different needs, different styles of approach and language were required.

Using young counselors for schoolchildren proved exceptionally effective in the program. The children identified with them easily as they spoke their slang language (Sheng).

OUTREACH SERVICES

Outreach services were provided for the affected communities. These were aimed at not only providing counseling services to the people where they lived and worked, but also increasing awareness of the possible psychological effects of a trauma of this magnitude and reinforcing the message that help was available.

Innovative ways of reaching people were used. Roadshows were an example, and were made possible by the contribution of one of the partners in the project. The large trucks normally used to advertise consumer products attract crowds of 5,000 to 10,000 people in urban and peri-urban centers through the medium of loud secular music. The message of the effect of trauma on normal humans was similarly conveyed through music and dramatization. Counselors were on hand for individual interactions. Many sessions of debriefing took place by the roadside, on Saturday afternoons in the middle of entertainment!

To our knowledge roadshows have not previously been used for medical purposes. They proved a very effective tool of reaching large numbers of people, and causing discussion in an informal atmosphere of mental health issues, something that does not happen very often. This outreach activity was truly creative and emphasized the need to utilize the available resources following disaster.

RESPONDING TO SPECIAL GROUPS

Children, rescue workers and medical workers, as well as the newly handicapped, comprised the special needs groups. Firefighters did not receive as much attention from the teams as we would have wished. We recognized them as a special high-risk group for the development of psychological sequelae of the trauma they experienced in the course of rescue work. We were, however, spread out thin on the ground and this inadvertently became one group that received less attention than would have been adequate for them. Debriefing was the only intervention given to a small number of the firefighters. Long-term effects of this omission can be expected.

The need for help for the helper was recognized from the beginning. Medical workers who had to deal with all the injured people as well as listen to the very horrific stories that many had to tell were exposed to this type of traumatization. Many experienced symptoms of the acute stress reaction.

The medical workers were, however, so busy attending to everyone else that it was not until much later that attention could finally get drawn to themselves. And even then only a very small number took advantage of the services offered. It was largely in the training sessions that contact was finally made with services, and it was common in the debriefing sessions that were held for some to break down and cry, in what was usually their first expression of how they truly felt.

The people who were blinded by the blast, or those who lost the use of their limbs so that they have had to be confined to wheelchairs following the blast, were people who had special needs specific to them. Their needs were scarcely met due to the shortage of resources.

EXTERNAL HELP

One consequence of a disaster of this magnitude is a sense of hopeless isolation and a need to engage informed professional colleagues in the response effort.

Specific requests were made to the American Psychiatric Association and the Royal College of Psychiatrists in the UK. As a result of this a US Federal Government Disaster Management Expert, Brian Flynn, who had experience in the Project Heartland that responded to the Oklahoma City bombing in 1995, came to Nairobi. From the Royal College of Psychiatrists we got David Alexander, who had led the mental health team following the *Piper Alpha* disaster. The US National Medical Association provided the rest of the overseas body of experts, highly valued by the Kenyans in their hour of need.

The team consciously defined the type of expert, his qualifications and experience before making the requests to the sponsoring bodies. Inexperienced volunteers and "experts" are to be avoided in disasters as they could get in the way of the disaster response before it becomes evident that they are in reality disaster tourists. We had a few such tourists to the disaster. Invited experts, however, were without exception qualified, experienced, and helpful and some have turned out to be "long-term" friends.

Following Brian Flynn's visit to Nairobi, he commended the team on its emergency response strategy, especially that of setting up the documentation unit as an integral part of the services. In his opinion, this response was way ahead of other response programs in the world. "I have never seen such a proactive response to trauma by an organization that can barely pay its telephone bills. Not even the response to the Oklahoma bombing was this fast and elaborate" [5].

Alexander [6] does justice to the hard facts of his visit, captures the spirit at the time, but does not do complete justice to the value of an external audit of our activities 3 months into the project. Following Brian Flynn's initial evaluation, we knew we were on track. We needed to hear it and see it in writing from another expert in the field. That the external auditor described Operation Recovery in the complimentary terms he did was a critical booster to morale at a time when all seemed so depressing, with no money and no promises of any. The value of a 3-month evaluation of a project of this nature is in its own right a morale booster and confirmation that all is well.

OTHER ACTIVITIES

As the end of the year approached, Operation Recovery realized that despair and hopelessness were beginning to take their toll on survivors, and the bereaved. Families that were used to sharing Christmas holidays with their loved ones found themselves empty and lonely as the season approached. Children came for school holidays to find their families dispirited. Christmas was never going to be the same again. The significance of the Christmas season in disaster survivors was driven home.

At the same time, the project was experiencing serious problems and doubt was being expressed regarding viability of the project. Serious cash problems are a constant feature of disaster work as, by their very nature, they are unplanned.

Simultaneous prayers were to signify the peace and unity between the USA and Kenya. A brilliant scheme was hatched and, in spite of significant planning problems, it took place to the satisfaction and excitement of many. Students in California were going to light 250 candles to signify the number of people killed in the blast. They had also organized the reading out of the 250 names of those killed in the blast.

Because of the time difference between the two cities, Nairobi held its program earlier. This involved a procession by over 40 children injured or orphaned as a result of the blast. Six children held two flags, those of Kenya and Tanzania. The third flag, that of the USA, was carried by a family who had lost one of their sons in the blast. The flag was unique in that it was the one that had been used to drape the casket bearing the remains of the son for burial in the USA. The central role played by symbolism in the recovery process is well documented in literature. There is abundant literature on the value of the spiritual in the recovery process of physical and psychological processes.

Nairobi is a small city and many of the mental health workers knew some of the survivors and readily identified with them. Special attention had to be paid to the team during the emergency and medium phases of the response.

As the team went through the recognized disaster phases (heroic, honeymoon, disillusionment and reconstruction) much energy was expended in holding the team together, as it often came close to disintegration because of various (often financial) constraints. And the process involved program planning and implementation.

Special and specific spiritual and secular activities were put in place for the counselors. A comedy night for the team was donated by the city comedy team and proved a very successful way of getting the team to laugh off their stress in the company of fellow counselors and their families, who, as it turned out, were themselves suffering much pain at the hands of the stressed counselors! The role of humour in alleviating stress in disaster workers is well documented [7].

PREGNANT WOMEN

During counseling sessions, some women reported spontaneous abortions, usually in the first trimester, while some reported spontaneously going into labour early, on the day of the bomb blast, or soon thereafter. Others reported the unanticipated occurrence of their menses while one complained that her breast milk had suddenly dried up.

A group of women who were pregnant at the time were brought together soon after the first anniversary of the bomb blast; 15 of them reported exaggerated startle response in their children, which was materially different from their other children at the same stage of development. They made the observation that their children seemed more nervous, startled more easily and slept worse. Whereas this could be a reflection of maternal hyperarousal, and part of maternal PTSD, it was an interesting observation as it was a spontaneous observation by experienced mothers. It raises interesting questions regarding maternal exposure to stress and PTSD in the offspring.

REACTIONS BY DIFFERENT GROUPS

Having initially acted with courage and solidarity, the bomb's victims moved to another phase. Anger permeated the culture, inside the embassy and out. Many Kenyans felt, understandably, that had it not been for the American presence, such death and destruction would not have been visited on their capital. Public and private criticism of the American reaction in the hours after the blast rained on them.

Kenyans and Americans were at each other, exactly as the terrorists had intended. The chaos and confusion in the early stages of the response were evident in many spheres, including the media.

The local press reported that the Americans were concerned only with their own people, ignoring the plight and suffering of the many Kenyans who were killed or injured. The horrific scenes of men, women and children lying in large pools of their own blood, freely mingling with pools of blood from others, began to haunt those who crashed into fitful sleep in the early hours.

Immediately after the disaster there was an enormous and sympathetic response, both locally and nationally, and offers of help came from many parts of the country and abroad. The organizers also needed to be able to make the best use of outside "experts" in a way, which did not create antagonism among the local helpers. The first groups of foreigners appeared in military gear, which proved most intimidating to the Kenyan medical teams.

LESSONS LEARNED

There are several lessons that can be learnt from the Nairobi bombing and the responses to it.

In Managing Disasters, Things Can and Do Go Wrong

As the Kenyans responded to the disaster in their own way, the American people who were the principal target of the attack were having problems of their own. The distance and time differences were to prove problematic. The response was occasionally chaotic and marred by a host of planning and logistical failures, especially in the area of military transportation. The Foreign Emergency Support Teams (FESTs) arrived in Nairobi and Dar es Salaam about 40 hours after the bombings, having experienced delays of 13 hours. There was disjointed liaison between the State Department, as the lead agency, and the Defence Department, FBI and other agencies. The personnel selection of the FESTs was ad hoc and not ideal. Medical and other emergency equipment was not always ready and available for shipment [8].

The chaos was not limited to the air and directly affected the medical care given to the survivors. Kenyan medical professionals at the Nairobi Hospital where the wounded Americans were receiving care claimed that US Air Force medical personnel were insensitive. This misunderstanding was to multiply against the background of allegations of looting at the embassy by Kenyans, who in turn accused the marines of protecting the Embassy grounds at the expense of the lives of Kenyans. Even as the digging in the rubble for survivors continued, sharp words were exchanged between frustrated well-meaning people united in their grief in the face of this tragedy.

As was to emerge later, there was confusion within the ranks of the seemingly organized American team. With the large influx of people from Washington and elsewhere into Nairobi, there were the inevitable coordinating problems with some personnel having to be reminded at times that the Ambassador was ultimately in charge [8].

The Role of Media

The role of media in disasters is well documented. In the Kenyan case, the media proved to be an invaluable asset [9]. In the early stages of the tragedy they provided factual information on what had happened, provided an outlet through which people could vent their feelings and discuss issues arising, and provided an avenue for messages of reassurance and education on the psychological effects to be expected following a tragedy of this magnitude.

Medical personnel in many cases shy away from the media. This can create a vacuum that gets filled with speculative messages. A key lesson from the Nairobi experience was that the media could play a positive role in disaster response. Another was that attention does need to be paid to the media personnel, who, like other people, also suffer the psychological effects of exposure to traumatic scenes [9].

The Importance of Effective Leadership

Kenya, like the rest of the African continent, was at the time a deeply traumatized country, by both natural and man-made disasters. Floods and politically motivated violence, had led to many deaths and much destruction to property [2].

This was the first time that Kenyans responded to any disaster with a mental health component. It was critical to have clear and decisive leadership, which was provided by the Kenya Medical Association.

Dealing with Different Reactions

Tragedy has a way of uniting people. In the Nairobi case there was initially great solidarity and courage demonstrated, with many pledges of help. Anger and harsh loud words blaming others were also notable. Chaos and confusion, especially in the early stages, were there in plenty. Terrorism destroys the sense of cohesion and safety and creates terror in the individual, in communities and in nations.

Anger gripped the people of Kenya, at first directed at Muslims, Arabs and any other groups thought to be even remotely connected with the terrorists. The Americans were the next "obvious" targets, firstly for being there, and secondly for their insensitivity to the Kenyans' needs and feeling in the face of the attacks. These are "normal" reactions to terrorism as the community searches for a scapegoat to heap its anger and frustration on.

The Honeymoon Effect of Disaster Response

This honeymoon phase has been described in disaster responses and was experienced first-hand after the Nairobi bombing. Immediately after the disaster there was an enormous and sympathetic response, both locally and internationally, and offers of help came from many parts of the country and abroad. Many offers of money and materials were made, most in the glare of cameras. Few kept their promises, not because they did not intend to, but because, before they could, other priorities engaged their attention.

The public did not forget the offers and kept calculating its value expecting that the project teams were suffocating under the weight of donations. Sadly, that was not the case.

Health care workers dealing with disaster need to be aware of this honeymoon phase, and to include it in their planning.

Research

Without research results, hypotheses cannot be tested, and well-intentioned approaches become confused with knowledge. Part of the heroic recovery effort was to collect data on those affected by the blast in order to inform treatment strategies in the short and the long term.

In the ideal world, researchers would have had to wait until survivors had finished with vital traditional activities like funeral rites. The sudden and unanticipated nature of the disaster followed by chaos severely challenged research planning. The team was driven by the realization that methodologically sound data are required to understand the mental health effects of terrorism in the region and to inform planning in the event of future disasters. The large convenience sample studied was predominantly educated professionals who witnessed the attack first-hand.

The analyzed sample consisted of 2,627 subjects. Of this group, 47% were female, 62% were married, and the mean age was 33.6 years (SD 9.7). 64 of the women were pregnant. 46% had completed secondary school and 40% had had some college education. The mean number of children per respondent was three (SD 2.1). 96% of the sample was Christian; the next largest religious group was Muslims, making up 2.5%. In all, this was a predominantly well-educated group of adults responsible for the care of many thousands of people.

Factors associated with post-traumatic stress syndrome (PTSS) (our approximation of post-traumatic stress disorder, PTSD), were: female gender, unmarried status, less education; being outside during the blast, seeing the blast, injury, not fully recovering from injury; feeling afraid, helpless, or threatened at the time of the blast; not talking with a friend or workmate about the blast; bereavement; experiencing or anticipating financial difficulty after the blast, inability to work because of injury, and receiving material or financial assistance. Notably, there was no significant association with PTSS symptomatology for age, number of children, religion; assessment of hospital care or immediate medical response; receiving counseling, or the relationship of the person mourned. The data show a strong link between injury and PTSS ($p < 0.0001$).

DISCUSSION

Many questions have been asked about the mental health response effort. Some have wondered what it achieved and what benefits came to the people of Kenya. There are no simple or accurate answers to these questions. However, as psychiatrists and mental health professionals, we live in a world where the challenges to our profession extend beyond our clinics and hospitals [10].

For this reason, post-disaster mental health response is an integral part of the duty of the mental health team. Controversy continues to surround the usefulness or otherwise of early intervention and in particular debriefing, since studies have shown diametrically opposed results. This valid academic discussion is, however, quickly thrown out in the face of real-life disaster. The community expects and demands help from the mental health experts.

Some of the interventions were as creative as they were untested and may have had little intrinsic long-term value. The roadshows are a good example of this. The people, however, seemed to respond positively to the initiatives, much as the team itself appreciated the comedy nights.

A strong and efficient mental health team came into being. Following other disasters in the region, the team was quickly assembled and was transported across the continent (Ivory Coast) to offer services to survivors of Flight KQ 101 on January 31, 2000.

The question of research following a major disaster is complex as it involves both moral and scientific considerations. Delay in initiating data collection limits opportunities to obtain early information needed to understand mental health effects of disaster. Secondly, if researchers do not act quickly, important data may be lost forever. It is for these reasons that we decided to put in place a research and documentation team, which among other things developed a 57-item self-administered questionnaire, capable of generating the DSM-IV diagnosis of PTSD. In so doing we were fully cognizant of the fact that conducting methodologically solid investigations of mental health is extraordinarily difficult in the chaotic and complex settings of disasters, particularly those associated with terrorism. Some might disagree.

CONCLUSION

Years after the attack, Kenyans continue to ask themselves the question: why us? Why did they pick on a peace-loving island of stability in a most traumatized continent? Has our suffering for our American friends been recognized? What caused this act of terrorism? What has the role of inequitable distribution of world resources to do with terrorism? Will they come again? These and many other questions may never find answers.

REFERENCES

1. Bushnell P. (2003) Leadership in the wake of disaster. In R.J. Ursano, C.S. Fullerton, A.E. Norwood (Eds.), *Terrorism and Disaster, Individual and Community Mental Health Interventions*, pp. 31–40. Cambridge University Press, New York.
2. Njenga F.G., Kigamwa P., Okonji M. (2003) Africa: the traumatised continent, a continent with hope. *Int Psychiatry*, 1, 4–7.
3. Mitchell J.T. (1983) When disaster strikes. The critical incident stress debriefing process. *J Emergency Med Serv*, 8: 36–39.
4. Pfefferbaum B. (1999) Posttraumatic stress responses in bereaved children after the Oklahoma City bombing. *J Am Acad Child Adolesc Psychiatry*, 38: 1372–1379.
5. Flynn B. (1998) Report on Operation Recovery. Submitted to the Kenya Medical Association.
6. Alexander D.A. (2001) Nairobi terrorist bombing: the personal experience of a mental health advisor. *Int J Ment Health*, 3: 249–257.
7. Palmer C.E. (1983) A note about paramedics' strategies for dealing with death and dying. *J Occupational Psychol*, 56: 83–86.
8. Accountability Board Report. Nairobi-Tanzania Bombings. January 1999.
9. Njenga F.G., Nyamai C., Kigamwa P. (2003) Terrorist bombing at the USA embassy in Nairobi: the media response. *East Afr Med J*, 80: 159–164.
10. Okasha A. (2002) Mental health in Africa: the role of WPA. *World Psychiatry*, 1: 32–35.

The New York Experience: Terrorist Attacks of September 11, 2001

Lynn E. DeLisi

New York University, New York, USA

INTRODUCTION

On September 11, 2001, at 8.52 a.m., the first of two large airliners deliberately crashed into the World Trade Center Twin Towers in New York City. Shortly afterwards, a third deliberately aimed for the Pentagon in Washington, and a fourth crashed in an open field in Pennsylvania. Approximately 3,000 people perished on this disastrous morning, and terrorists with Middle Eastern and Muslim backgrounds were found to be responsible.

September 11, 2001 was a day that will long be remembered by people from all cultures and countries. Anyone who had a TV saw the events of that day unfold with such rare and unimaginable horror. While this was an event with international repercussions, it was particularly a turning point for all Americans, many of whom were not yet born when the Japanese bombed Pearl Harbor, the last attack on American soil. It was a realization that geographic isolation could no longer render Americans immune to external attacks, which gave the issue of combating terrorism the highest priority in a newly formed "post 9/11" American foreign policy. The most affected individuals were those whose lives were seriously affected by the events and their aftermath: "New Yorkers". Many kinds of things are generally said about "New Yorkers", but the people who commute to this dense city of skyscrapers and those that live within the island of Manhattan were particularly distraught in the days and months to follow. Those who lived close to the World Trade Center site were forced to evacuate their homes, and many others, due to direct and indirect effects of this event, lost their jobs. Many knew someone who lost a friend or relative. US flags hung

Disasters and Mental Health. Edited by Juan José López-Ibor, George Christodoulou, Mario Maj, Norman Sartorius and Ahmed Okasha.
©2005 John Wiley & Sons Ltd. ISBN 0-470-02123-3.

from windows everywhere and were the most popular item one could purchase to decorate cars and even clothes. This first step in the collective grieving process seemed to be banding together with solidarity and obtaining solace from knowing one belonged to a nation that was stronger than each individual on his own, a nation that would help those who personally had lost so much.

In the first hours after the event, phone lines, cell phones, the internet and all methods of communication were lost in Manhattan. Television and radio re-gained transmission power the quickest; so those who did not happen to watch the events live (TV, in person or by internet) as they were unfolding, did see them when the scenes were repeated throughout the first day and for many days afterward. Many people felt glued to the television and could not take their eyes off the screen for fear of missing something. Afterwards, researchers concerned with post-traumatic stress disorder (PTSD) wondered what the effect of the news media repeating such an event over and over had on both children and adults.

In the first weeks following the disaster, smoke rose from the massive crater and tangle of hot steel ruins that was once the Twin Towers, and the smell of soot from the burning debris filled the air of most of the lower half of Manhattan. The country and New York City itself was on high alert for a repeat of these events. Pictures of "the missing" coated the walls of buildings, particularly the surrounding hospitals, with candles burning below. Many people who lost close relatives wandered the streets in grief and stood on lines at the quickly formed city Family Assistance Center to report their loved ones missing, in the hope of finding them alive somewhere or of eventually obtaining their remains. Police and the National Guard heavily guarded the streets. All entry points into Manhattan were closely inspected and guarded, with the bridges and tunnels in restricted use for many weeks. Several skyscraper and residential complexes were plagued daily in those early days with bomb scares.

Adding to the hysteria, some individual sent deadly anthrax spores in envelopes by the US Postal Service to highly visible personalities at news offices and other facilities, which secondarily infected anyone else who came in contact with the envelopes, from the postmen, to secretarial assistants, to even a child playing nearby. In October 2001, an American Airlines jet heading to the Dominican Republic crashed on take-off in a nearby residential neighborhood. Many thought that both of these subsequent events were connected to the September 11 terrorist attacks, leading to more fear and psychological trauma. A lone foreigner (now known as the "shoe-bomber") managed to travel on an international flight to the USA with a home-made bomb embedded in one of his shoes, only to be subdued by a gang of vigilant passengers who prevented him from setting himself on fire. Since that incident, most US airport checkpoints now require shoe removal and careful examination before each passenger is cleared to board an airline.

Most people in New York City and its surrounding suburbs in nearby states gathered in the city to volunteer in whatever way they could. More people donated their blood than was needed for storage and potential donors were eventually turned away. Many others persisted in arriving at the site of the disaster, soon dubbed "ground zero", despite rumors that the air was unsafe, to continue to search beneath the rubble for survivors, and then human remains, for months to come. Lawyers, restaurant owners, and others of all professions volunteered their services; physicians were no exception. However, despite the readiness of hospitals and all personnel, very few patients arrived. Either people survived with minimal physical injuries or were incinerated within the pile of hot steel. Early on, it became very evident that the physicians in most demand as a result of this event were psychiatrists. Particularly the emotional effects on families and children of those who died were of concern. However, anyone whose life was affected by the disaster in some way – job or home loss – was at high risk for psychological sequelae, as were individuals with pre-existing psychiatric conditions.

A very small non-profit organization, called Disaster Psychiatry Outreach, Inc. (DPO), was based in New York City. This group had been previously established by four young psychiatrists just completing their residency training, who had formed a common bond after their experience volunteering to help the relatives of victims of a couple of airline crashes two years prior to the September 11 event. This group met monthly in the living room of one of the doctors and planned how they would raise money and network to respond to more airline crashes, hurricanes, fires and other natural disasters. They spent many hours contemplating what was and was not by definition a disaster and even wrote a review paper on the topic during the pre-September 11 period that was not thought to be important enough to be published until afterwards [1].

On the morning of September 11, 2001, the first-hired administrative assistant to DPO, Olivia White, came to work having only been employed for two weeks. However, within a few days she had mobilized a large group of psychiatrists throughout New York who were willing to volunteer their services at the newly established Family Assistance Center (FAC) for September 11 victims. At first the FAC was housed in an armory in lower-mid Manhattan; then it moved to a large warehouse facility on a pier in the Hudson River. DPO managed to better cover the psychiatric support for the FAC than the psychiatry departments of the five major city medical schools, all of which were competing for the position to be the city's chief psychiatrists, yet never focused on organizing an efficient psychiatric care system. Everyone, including the mayor, who took on the role of the city's fatherly protector during the whole crisis, needed a psychiatrist [2]. The first estimates, however, of the prevalence of "September 11-caused psychiatric impairment" among New Yorkers was considerably inflated. So, funds poured in from many nationwide charities to the Federal Emergency Management Agency (FEMA), the Red Cross and to the City of New York. *Project Liberty* was formed by the Federal Government to give grants-in-aid; every organization that was eligible, including DPO, applied for these funds. Within a few days, DPO had expanded from someone's living room to a large grassroots organization that was supplying the city of New York with free psychiatric services as long as they were needed. It was Ms. White's role to schedule the 24-hour coverage and then, later, reduced-hour psychiatric care that was needed until the closure of the FAC.

RESEARCH STUDIES

As a full-time academic researcher, I immediately planned for and obtained human subjects institutional review board approval from New York University to conduct several surveys throughout New York City. The first of these protocols [3] was a systematic survey of randomly selected adults throughout New York City. These individuals were approached by psychiatrically trained interviewers who requested their participation in answering a questionnaire about their physical and mental health prior to and 3–6 months subsequent to the event. Various stresses were recorded, such as their proximity to and involvement in the events of September 11, whether they lost close relatives or friends, and specifically questions about anxiety, depression and the symptoms of PTSD. Each of the 17 items on the Davidson Trauma Scale [4,5] was scored from 0 to 4 for both frequency (0 = none to 4 = every day) and severity within the past week (0 = not at all distressing to 4 = extremely distressing). A total score was obtained by adding the frequency and severity scores for each item (range = 0–136). Three subscales were defined by using this scale: intrusion, avoidance/numbing, and hyperarousal. The intrusion score was calculated as the cumulative score of frequency and severity scores for five questions relating to this category, the avoidance/numbing score as the cumulative score for six corresponding questions, and the hyperarousal score as the cumulative score for four corresponding questions. A score of 8.0 on any one item was considered the highest level of pathology; while a score of 0.0 meant that the item was not present. On the basis of previous studies, Davidson considered a score of 24 or higher as suggestive of PTSD. A total of 1,009 adults (516 men and 493 women) were interviewed in person throughout

Manhattan. The results from this survey showed that a total of 56.3% had at least one severe (score greater than 8.0) or two or more mild to moderate symptoms and that the presence of these was correlated with the amount of time that had passed since September 11, 2001. Thus, over half of the individuals had some emotional sequelae 3–6 months after September 11, but the percentage was decreasing over time. Women reported significantly more symptoms than men. Loss of employment, residence, or family/friends correlated with greater and more severe symptoms. The most distressing experiences appeared to be painful memories and reminders; dissociation was rare. What appeared most concerning, however, was that only a small portion (26.7%) of those with severe responses (a score of 24 or greater) was seeking treatment.

The following are examples of experiences recounted to interviewers:

- One subject's relative broke all his fingers when evacuated from the World Trade Center. While the subject herself was not at the scene, her job was affected because the supermarket in which she served as a clerk received repetitive violent threats and business declined considerably because the owners were Arab.
- After seeing the second plane hit, one subject described seeing smoke coming from the World Trade Center towers and how he ran from the building just as it collapsed. He lost a close friend as well as a family member. After September 11, he also lost his apartment and his job as a building janitor.
- After the attack, a police officer allowed another interviewed subject and her husband to enter their apartment for 10 minutes to obtain essential items. They were not able to return for 8 weeks. She lost a friend (a fireman) and a professional client.
- A 49-year-old man agreeing to be interviewed had worked in the World Trade Center for 20 years. During the attack, he was on the Brooklyn Bridge on his way to work, and he later discovered that many of his close friends and colleagues were missing.
- A 47-year-old male worked in a bank next to the World Trade Center and lived near by. He survived only because on his way to work he saw the Towers from a distance collapsing in smoke and therefore ran back. He had not been allowed back to his apartment and at the time of the interview was still living with a friend's family.
- A 32-year-old female lawyer also worked in an office complex close by. She emerged from the subway just before the first building fell and then saw it fall. It "felt like an earthquake". She ran up the main street in front of a dust cloud and walked home to her apartment. Her first thoughts while fleeing on September 11 were of previous traumas. While living in Israel, she barely escaped injury in one bombing and had lost several

friends in another. At the time of this interview she was having flashbacks of these previous events.

- A 45-year-old Asian-Indian male stated that he was self-employed as a plumber, but his work was currently scarce because of new prejudice against Muslims on the part of his previous clients.
- One subject was a 24-year-old male restaurant manager. At the time of the interview, he stated that he set his alarm for 9.11 a.m. each day because, he stated, "It's very important to me that I don't forget how angry and upset I was that day." He described September 11 as "a wake with a closed casket". He felt the loss of the buildings that were part of the view from his apartment across the river in New Jersey as if he had "lost a family member".
- A 53-year-old interviewed male who was a technology manager was walking into Tower 1 when he found out what was occurring. He saw the building on fire and later stood watching until the second plane hit. He lost seven friends and 75 colleagues in the disaster.
- One subject was a 32-year-old female director of a daycare center six blocks away from the World Trade Center. Subject spoke about the daycare center, which was located next to a police precinct. The children were evacuated by police to nearby Chinatown where the parents were able to pick them up. One of the children's parents died; he was a police officer. Subject states that the staff had meetings for 3–4 weeks afterwards about how to approach the issue with the children and it was agreed that they would not talk about it unless the children specifically asked questions. There were some workshops where the children drew pictures and made paper airplanes to tell what happened. About 10 of them had seen the burning buildings. The daycare center was not fully operational for 6 weeks (no phones or fax). There were no psychiatrists on site to be able to tell these workers how to handle the children's questions.
- One subject, a 26-year-old female administrative assistant, worked in Tower 1 on the 27th floor. She managed to escape down the staircase before the building collapsed. However, she lost 10 colleagues and friends. Subject remained quiet during the interview and said that there were parts of the evacuation that she does not remember and parts that she does not want to remember. She did not want to talk about the experience.
- A 27-year-old male interviewee had previously been in the Marine Corps and had seen similar disaster and acts of violence throughout the world. He claimed to be largely unaffected by the events of September 11.

Despite statements of how well they were coping, all of the above had various degrees of anxiety, depression and other symptoms that prevented them from working and socializing up to the time of the interviews. Many others described failed relationships, had difficulty concentrating and acknowledged occasional thoughts of death and suicide.

The second survey focused on patients at the New York City Bellevue Hospital who had serious psychiatric disorders and were hospitalized at the time of the terrorist attacks. Medical records for 156 psychiatric inpatients were examined to evaluate their psychiatric condition during the time prior to and subsequent to September 11, 2001. For 5 of these patients, no diagnosis could be ascertained. Of the subjects, 100 were males (66.7%) and 51 females (33.3%). 44 were Caucasian (28.2%), 62 African-American (39.7%), 25 Hispanic (16%), 17 Asian (10.9%) and 8 of other ethnic origins (5.1%). All diagnostic categories were represented: bipolar disorder ($n = 15$, 9.6%), schizophrenia ($n = 54$, 34.6%), schizoaffective disorder ($n = 52$, 33.3%), depression ($n = 8$, 5.1%), primary substance abuse ($n = 5$, 3.2%), miscellaneous ($n = 17$, 9.9%). 39 patients (29.8%) had increases in their medication the week following September 11, while only 3 had decreases in medication. 37 patients (24.5%) improved. 55 patients (36.4%) worsened after September 11 in the following diagnostic categories: bipolar disorder ($n = 3$, 20.0%), schizophrenia ($n = 28$, 51.8%), schizoaffective disorder ($n = 17$, 32.7%), depression ($n = 1$, 12.5%), substance abuse ($n = 1$, 20.0%), miscellaneous ($n = 5$, 35.7%). It has generally been thought that in the face of a disastrous environmental event, whether natural or man-made, patients with a psychotic illness may actually improve, while patients with pre-existing depression might actually worsen. In the present study of the effects of the New York City World Trade Center terrorist attacks on seriously ill hospitalized patients, we did not find evidence that patients' condition improved in response to the events. Surprisingly, few patients with depression on admission worsened. While some patients across diagnoses were in need of medication for anxiety or sleep in the week following the event, the majority was not. In addition, there were no differences across diagnostic categories, symptoms or medication changes for those patients on wards facing the World Trade Center ($n = 40$) compared with those who were not ($n = 110$). It is thus assumed that the secure environment and reassurance of mental health professionals covering the inpatient units at this time provided a therapeutic effect that prevented patients from deteriorating, but we found no evidence that psychotic conditions resolved based on the reality of the disastrous events.

Some descriptions from the records are as follows:

- In a group therapy session, therapists explored the patients' feelings and ideas regarding the terrorist attack in New York City. Patients were encouraged to talk and express their emotions. One patient who was quiet during most of the session, expressed confusion and her speech remained disorganized.

- One patient verbalized that he thought his teacher from Pluto was responsible for the World Trade Center disaster, not Osama Bin Laden.
- One patient was withdrawn and spent most of the morning watching TV news and drawing pictures about the event. In a support group meeting, this patient focused on paranoid and grandiose delusions of FBI/CIA intelligence he "knew", drawing loose references to himself and his responsibility for the events that happened.
- Another patient incorporated the terrorist attack into a delusional system in which he believed that the US government had done this as a part of a conspiracy to gain world domination.

Our third set of surveys involved questionnaires to medical students and physicians of all types who aided the victims for the first 6-month period subsequent to September 11, 2001, particularly at the FAC [6]. One study was performed to investigate the emotional impact of this involvement on medical students from a major medical school in New York City, the Mount Sinai School of Medicine. 157 students responded to a mail survey with a set of questions about their personal and professional involvement in the disaster as well as their psychiatric symptoms in the week after the event and at a time 3–4 months later. This study found, similarly to the survey of randomly selected New Yorkers, that there was a greater emotional impact on female students than male and that those students involved in less-supervised and more-stressful activities were more prone to emotional sequelae. However, the intense experience of aiding victims going through profound emotional trauma did not contribute to psychiatric symptomatology per se in the volunteers and, if anything, was associated with enhanced professional self-esteem.

The fourth survey focused on physicians who volunteered to help victims. Very few of them were in fact interested in responding to a survey. In general, they wanted to put the experiences behind them and not to reactivate their emotions by recalling the events. We suspect that they too had lasting effects, but could not find the time or the willingness to express it. However, of the ten physicians that did respond to advertisements throughout New York City about 1.5 years after September 11, 2001, five were male and five female (mean age 46). Nine of the ten wished they could have had some type of psychiatric support system during and after their work with the victims. One felt doctors should be able to "handle these things themselves". The following are examples of some of the experiences encountered:

- One physician went to a building close to ground zero to volunteer his services for one day, but stated that other than "washing out a few firemen's eyes, there was nothing to do. Those people who were physically unharmed had fled, while the others were deceased. It was that extreme".
- One particular physician, a female psychiatrist, was extremely vocal and felt that she needed to speak about the event. She had volunteered for 1 month after September 11 at the FAC, made referrals, wrote prescriptions, offered general counseling, and staffed a hotline for medical/ psychiatric referrals. She also experienced survivor guilt, and that she needed to be doing more. At the time of the interview, she still felt somewhat removed from other people and irritable, and had upsetting reminders that lingered.
- At the time of the disaster, one physician felt like she could not talk about the events. She did not know anyone in the city who could relate to how she was feeling and what she was going through. She felt isolated, especially when the phones were not working for a few days after September 11. When she finally felt like she could discuss her experiences, all of her friends wanted the events "behind them" and were at a different stage than she was. She only felt comfortable talking about September 11 at conferences, but that was a professional setting so she felt that her expression of emotion had to be limited. She relayed that she spent such intense time helping others that she could not deal with the tragedy herself and experienced feelings of guilt that she could not do more.
- Another physician said he drank twice as much alcohol after September 11 than before. He worked at a triage unit close to the World Trade Center site volunteering about 10 hours per day. His apartment was very close to the World Trade Center, and he and some neighbors formed a group where they would get together over drinks and discuss the events. He stated that his worst memory was seeing people jump out of the towers.
- One psychiatrist volunteered at a professional school located near ground zero. She offered general counseling to both students and firemen. The tragedy helped her obtain a research grant on emotional memory and thus she actually gained professional status because of the events. Yet she reported survivor guilt for the month subsequent to September 11 and developed asthma. She lost weight, had problems sleeping and lost her appetite.
- One physician was a staff psychiatrist on an inpatient unit who worked longer hours after the attacks. His alcohol intake increased after the attacks and at the time of the interview he still admitted to being preoccupied with painful images intruding on his thoughts. He still avoided participating in activities that would remind him of the events.

DISCUSSION

Currently, over 2 years since the terrorist attacks on New York City, a literature search on MEDLINE has resulted in approximately 100 relevant publications on the psychiatric/emotional responses to the disaster of the general public, of previously treated psychiatric patients, and of health care workers. Reactions in children, adolescents, young adults, previous drug and alcohol abusers and others of special needs have been described [7–12] and not only in people of New York City [3,13], but in others throughout the world (e.g., 14,15).

September 11, 2001 brought change in the attitudes and lifestyles of people throughout the USA. A new era of suspicion and anxiety began that was reminiscent of the "Cold War" in the 1950s, when many citizens built bomb shelters and stocked them with food. Following September 11, 2001, Americans were told to be prepared for a mass terrorist attack by knowing an escape route, arranging with family members a site to meet, and stocking one's car with water and at least a week's supply of canned food. Duct tape was sold in large quantities in stores because it was deemed necessary to seal door and window cracks from outside air, should nuclear or other chemicals be released in the air. Keeping large supplies of batteries was also recommended, so that radios and portable TVs would be available should electric power be disrupted by terrorists.

The emotional consequences to all involved were many. Although it is not surprising, the most vulnerable people were those with pre-existing depression and anxiety disorders, and women. Those with a psychotic illness, such as schizophrenia, were already too disabled to fully notice the reality around them and some brought the world events into their limited delusionary systems, although there were individual cases where this was not so. However, these patients were already in treatment situations that gave them added support, whereas the random citizen was not, and many times did not have support when it was needed. Rather, he or she required continual encouragement to seek treatment for preoccupation with a persistent emotional response that prevented him/her from resuming pre-existing life and relationships.

There have been many natural and man-made disasters periodically worldwide and the documentation that exists of psychiatric sequelae as a consequence has been reviewed in Katz et al. [1]. What has emerged from September 11, 2001 and these many research studies is the notion that psychiatrists can play an important role in the aftermath of a disaster and that prevention of chronic emotional debilitation as a result of having been a victim of a disastrous event is a challenge in psychiatry worth taking up. Ultimately, early detection of those at high risk of PTSD and treatment that has been known to be successful will enable individuals who have acutely suffered to quickly go back to and maintain a normal life.

The effect this event had on the people of New York City and the American government has been lasting. Although, 2 years later, super-ficially life seems to have returned to its pre-September 11 state, this is clearly not the case. Many programs have been funded to treat both physical and mental problems of not only the adult survivors who lost spouses or siblings, but also the children who lost a parent, and the firemen and policeman who survived. Even the former mayor, Mr. Giuliani, despite his public demeanor of a man in control who at all hours comforted those who had losses, wrote in a subsequent book about his private moments to express emotional responses and at the Carter Center in Atlanta, Georgia – a few months later, in a meeting addressing disaster response – he emphasized the importance of the psychiatric counseling he obtained [2]. In the several months afterwards, several disaster-training drills were called, new organizations for disaster response and networks for physicians and psychiatrists were instituted by national organizations and the federal government, including the President's creation of a new cabinet post for the Office of National Security. Many personal freedoms guaranteed in a democratic society have been currently forfeited as the government now focuses on combating terrorism. The bridges and tunnels entering New York City are still heavily guarded and it is more difficult for foreigners, particularly of Middle Eastern origin, to enter the USA or become immigrants. For Americans, air travel particularly has become traumatic in itself, with detailed searches including shoe and belt removal.

Unfortunately, there are also secondary negative aspects to any such devastating event, such as the focus on obtaining the huge amounts of funds that were donated for the rebuilding and care of victims and the fact that much of these funds were not used for what they were intended. Research dollars were diverted to academic institutions to perform large studies such as those described here, but with more sophisticated tools available, and some funds remain still frozen and unusable because of the restrictions placed on them or the bureaucracy necessary to obtain a portion of them.

This was and still is the New York experience of a man-made disaster and its consequences in the 2 years that followed.

ACKNOWLEDGEMENT

The author wishes to thank Tiffany Cohen, Andrea Maurizio, Olivia White and Marla Yost for their help in gathering and discussing aspects of the surveys. Andrea Maurizio performed all statistical analyses.

REFERENCES

1. Katz C.L., Pellegrino L., Pandya A., Ng A., DeLisi L.E. (2002) Research on psychiatric outcomes and interventions subsequent to disasters: a review of the literature. *Psychiatry Res*, **110**: 201–217.
2. Giuliani R.W. (2002) *Leadership*. Hyperion Press, New York.
3. DeLisi L.E., Maurizio A., Yost M., Paparozzi C.F., Fulchino C., Katz C.L., *et al.* (2003) A psychiatric survey of the people of New York City 4–5 months subsequent to the September 11, 2001 terrorist attacks. *Am J Psychiatry*, **160**: 780–783.
4. Davidson J. (2003) *Davidson Trauma Scale (DTS)*. Multi-Health Systems, North Tonawanda.
5. Davidson J.R., Book S.W., Colket J.T., Tupler L.A., Roth S., David D., *et al.* (1997) Assessment of a new self-rating scale for post-traumatic stress disorder. *Psychol Med*, **27**: 153–160.
6. Katz C.L., Gluck N., Maurizio A., DeLisi L.E. (2002) The medical student experience with disasters and disaster response. *CNS Spectrum*, **7**: 604–610.
7. Adinaro D.J., Allegra J., Cochrane D.G., Cable G. (2003) Increased rate of anxiety related visits to selected New Jersey emergency departments following the September 11, 2001 terrorist attacks. *Acad Emerg Medicine*, **10**: 550.
8. Ford C.A., Udry J.R., Gleiter K., Chantala K. (2003) Reactions of young adults to September 11, 2001. *Arch Pediatr Adolesc Med*, **157**: 572–578.
9. Factor S.H., Wu Y., Monserrate J., Edwards V., Cuevas Y., Del Vecchio S., *et al.* (2002) Drug use frequency among street-recruited heroin and cocaine users in Harlem and the Bronx before and after September 11, 2001. *J Urban Health*, **79**: 404–408.
10. Zywiak W.H., Stout R.L., Trefy W.B., LaGrutta J.E., Lawson C.C., Khan N., *et al.* (2003) Alcohol relapses associated with September 11, 2001: a case report. *Substance Abuse*, **24**: 123–128.
11. Baker D.R. (2002) A public health approach to the needs of children affected by terrorism. *J Am Med Womens Assoc*, **57**: 117–118, 121.
12. Halpern-Felsher B.L., Millstein S.G. (2002) The effects of terrorism on teens' perceptions of dying: the new world is riskier than ever. *J Adolesc Health*, **30**: 308–311.
13. Galea S., Ahern J., Resnick H., Kilpatrick D., Bucuvalas M., Gold J., *et al.* (2002) Psychological sequelae of the September 11 terrorist attacks in New York City. *N Engl J Med*, **346**: 982–987.
14. Austin P.C., Mamdani M.M., Chan B.T., Lin E. (2003) Anxiety-related visits to Ontario physicians following September 11, 2001. *Can J Psychiatry*, **48**: 416–419.
15. Schuster M.A., Stein B.D., Jaycox L., Collins R.L., Marshall G.N., Elliot M.N., *et al.* (2001) A national survey of stress reactions after the September 11, 2001 terrorist attacks. *N Engl J Med*, **345**: 1507–1512.

12

The Experience of the Chornobyl Nuclear Disaster

Johan M. Havenaar[1] and Evelyn J. Bromet[2]

[1]Altrecht Institute for Mental Health Care, Utrecht, The Netherlands
[2]State University of New York at Stony Brook, NY, USA

INTRODUCTION

With the possible exception of the largely unknown 1957 Kysjtym accident in the Urals, the Chornobyl nuclear power plant disaster has by far been the largest peacetime nuclear disaster ever. On the night of April 26, 1986, one of the four blocks of the Ukrainian nuclear power plant at Chornobyl exploded as a result of a breach of safety procedures by the plant's staff during a routine shut-down operation. That night, at 01.24 hours, eyewitnesses outside Chornobyl Unit 4 observed two explosions, one after the other. Burning debris and sparks shot into the air above the reactor, some of which fell on the roof of the machine room and started a fire. The explosions left a gaping hole in the roof, exposing the reactor core to the outside air. Hundreds of tons of radioactive dust were dispersed all over Europe. Initially the Soviet authorities tried to keep the accident hidden from the public, while at the same time mounting an extensive operation to control the damage. A 30-km exclusion zone was declared and everyone living within it, including the entire population of the city of Pripyat (population approximately 50,000), was evacuated in a matter of days. During the evacuation, pregnant women were strongly advised to have an abortion although they were not given the true reason, and most reportedly complied. The cities and towns in which evacuees were resettled were at first unreceptive and even hostile.

To maintain the impression that everything was normal, the government did not cancel the First of May parade in Kyiv, the capital of the former Soviet republic Ukraine, situated 160 kilometers from Chornobyl. However, as rumors spread, shortly thereafter an exodus of women and children

Disasters and Mental Health. Edited by Juan José López-Ibor, George Christodoulou, Mario Maj, Norman Sartorius and Ahmed Okasha.

fleeing from Kyiv took place. Only when alarming background readings of radioactivity in the Scandinavian countries made further denial impossible did the first public announcements appear in the Soviet press. Even then no protective actions were undertaken. For example, no iodine tablets were distributed, which could have prevented the uptake of radioactive iodine and thus reduced future thyroid cancer risks. According to some informants, the authorities were afraid that distribution would cause too much unrest among the population.

At the same time, a radioactive cloud containing predominantly short-lived radio-iodine was dispersed over Ukraine, the adjacent republics of Belarus and Russia, and the rest of Europe, raising concerns in many countries. Governments imposed protective measures for the safety of the population in areas as remote from the reactor site as the Netherlands and Italy. The resources allocated by the governments of the three affected republics of the former Soviet Union to assess and monitor the consequences of the accident make it probably one of the greatest operations ever put in place in response to a human-made disaster [1].

In assessing the damage after more than 15 years, it is clear that "Chornobyl" has affected and continues to affect the lives of millions of people, especially the roughly 4 million people who are living in areas officially designated as contaminated (see Table 12.1). In total about 50 million curies of radioactive material were released, about two hundred times greater in magnitude than the atomic bomb dropped on Hiroshima. Some 135,000 people have been evacuated and an additional 270,000 have been offered assistance to be evacuated if they request it. An unknown number of people have by now taken up this offer. Territories in the region have been divided into four zones according to the levels of contamination and the response measures taken: a strict control zone (115,000 people); a constant control zone (270,000 people); a periodic control zone, requiring special monitoring (580,000); and a periodic control zone, requiring regular monitoring (4,000,000 people). In addition, between 600,000 and 1 million people were involved in the clean-up of the nuclear plant site and the surroundings. The 30-kilometer zone around the nuclear plant is now still a forbidden area, although elderly people who want to live and die in their home villages are allowed to do so. Nearly 300,000 persons live in "strict control zones", where continuous monitoring of the level of radioactive contamination takes place.

In retrospect, the wisdom of some aspects of the evacuation and of the implementation of permanent versus periodical control zones has been questioned. The highest exposure took place in the early hours and days after the accident. Evacuation after more than a few weeks could do little to reduce lifetime exposure. In the case of the periodic control zones, the

TABLE 12.1 Estimates of average exposure rate and number of people exposed by level of contamination from the Chornobyl nuclear power plant catastrophe

Geographic area	Levels of surface contamin-ation with ^{137}Cs (kBq/m²)	Estimated average exposure	Population exposed	Response measures taken
Strict control zone (>40 Ci ^{137}Cs/km²)[a]	>1,480	>5 mSv/year	115,000	Approximately total evacuation
Constant control zone (15–40 Ci ^{37}Cs/km²)[a]	555–1,480	<5 mSv/year	270,000	Assisted to relocate if requested
Periodic control zone (5–15 Ci ^{137}Cs/km²)[a]	185–555	<2 mSv/year	580,000	Special health monitoring
Periodic control (<5 Ci ^{137}Cs/km²)[a]	37–185	<1 mSv/year	4,000,000	Regular health monitoring
Clean-up workers ("liquidators")[b]	—	10%: >250 mGy 40%: 100–250 mGy 50%: <100 mGy	600,000	Regular health monitoring

[a]1 Ci ^{137}Cs/km² = 37 kBq/m². In this study the >40 Ci and 15–40 Ci zones are combined and referred to as "severely contaminated"; 5–15 Ci zones as "moderately contaminated" and <5 Ci as "mildly contaminated". Source: World Health Organization (1995) [28].
[b]Source: Bard et al. (1997) [3].

exposure levels did not exceed the level of natural background radiation and remained well below the accepted exposure limits of 1 mSv/year for the general population and 5 mSv/year for people living near nuclear plants. Another point of criticism has been the fact that different exposure limits were adopted in different republics over time, and that evacuation advisories were only partly implemented because of lack of financial resources.

In this chapter we review the literature about the mental health consequences of the Chornobyl disaster. Special attention will be given to one of the most typical features of this accident: the complete breakdown in communication of information and the credibility gap which started with the initial denial and which continues up to this very day. We will argue that this feature is quite typical for nuclear accidents in general and carries important lessons for future similar events, not only for other radiological accidents, but also for the eventuality of a terrorist attack with a radiation dispersal device or "dirty bomb".

SOCIAL, CULTURAL AND ECONOMIC CONTEXT OF THE DISASTER

In order to understand the reactions of the inhabitants to the Chornobyl disaster, it is essential to realize the social and historical context in which the accident occurred. President Gorbachev had recently officially declared Glasnost ("openness") and perestroika ("restructuring" or "renovation"), but the government had been unable to put these concepts into practice to gain credibility. The secrecy with which the government of the Soviet Union and the official press initially handled the Chornobyl disaster confirmed the inhabitants' distrust in official information. In the years that followed, information remained scarce. It was acknowledged that many of the 200 firefighters involved in the clean-up of the nuclear reactor suffered from radiation disease, but other health problems were denied. Until 1989 the official position was that the problems were under control. This policy, however, did not ease the worries of the exposed populations. Around 1989, the inhabitants became more and more upset and tensions started to build. Rumor had it that women had more miscarriages and that babies with monstrous deformities were being born. In many cities demonstrations were held [2]. In the end the government had no other choice than to release more factual information on the consequences of the disaster. Maps showing the extent of contamination of the land were made publicly available. In the city of Gomel in Belarus, an illuminated sign showing day-to-day background radiation readings was installed on the main square. This new policy of providing massive information was met with as much distrust as the previous lack of it had been.

In addition to the health concerns and other societal strains raised by the accident and the response measures that were put in place, the disaster had serious socioeconomic consequences. In Belarus, the most seriously affected of the three adjacent republics, 38,000 square kilometers, or 18% of the land area of this republic, was more or less severely contaminated, especially by radioactive cesium-137, which has a half-life of 30 years. In this republic, 300,000 hectares of farmland were taken out of production for this reason. Some 1 million hectares of the forests were contaminated to varying degrees [1]. The population was advised not to eat mushrooms or berries from these forests, thereby depriving them of an otherwise welcome dietary supplement and favorite pastime. In addition to losses in agricultural production, the market for food products from the region was completely lost, as was tourism, another major source of income in some districts. The affected parts of Ukraine and Russia experienced similar consequences. More importantly, these troubles coincided with and were worsened by the simultaneous total political and economic collapse of the former Soviet

Union. In the local press, this political and economic breakdown was referred to as "the second Chornobyl".

PHYSICAL HEALTH EFFECTS

The extent to which the radioactive fall-out from Chornobyl has caused physical disease varies according to the source. This is most clearly illustrated by reports about the disaster's death toll. In 1986, only days after the accident, the *New York Post* reported 15,000 deaths. In April 1992, the Russian press agency ITAR-TASS claimed that over a hundred thousand people died as a result of the accident. 6 years later, in April 1998, Reuters reported that 12,519 of the 350,000 Ukrainian firefighters and relief workers involved in the clean-up had died as a result of the accident.

However, official reports by the World Health Organization (WHO) and the scientific literature in general paint an entirely different picture. According to these sources, 500 people were hospitalized for symptoms of acute radiation syndrome. The diagnosis was confirmed in 237 cases, of whom 28 died. In addition, 3 other deaths were caused by accidents or burns [3]. Unofficial sources such as the Chornobyl Union, a citizen's lobby, estimates that 256 clean-up workers died because of the accident [4]. Direct deaths occurred primarily among the firefighters who were there during the first hour.

In later years a sharp increase of thyroid cancer among children was observed. More than 600 new cases were found, where only a handful would have been expected under normal conditions [3]. In almost all cases, they were successfully treated by thyroidectomy [5]. The expected epidemic of leukemia or other cancers has not occurred [6], and the anticipated increase in the number of stillbirths and congenital malformations has not been substantiated [7,8].

MENTAL HEALTH FINDINGS

Population Studies

Psychiatrists from the Soviet Union were involved in the enormous civil operation that was mounted immediately after the nuclear catastrophe and an assessment of the psychological damage was made [9]. Unfortunately, most of these early Eastern European studies, as well as most of those that followed in later years, used non-standardized methodology and had other methodological shortcomings [10,11]. Rumyantseva *et al.* [12] assessed psychological adjustment and mental health in the first year after the event and found higher rates of psychological distress among people in the exposed areas. The clean-up workers (called "liquidators" in the Russian vernacular) were at greatest risk, with 84% showing signs of psychological disorder.

Later studies by Western investigators, using internationally accepted methodology and instruments, by and large confirmed these initial findings. Viinamäki et al. [13] reported higher rates of psychological distress as measured with the General Health Questionnaire (GHQ) in an exposed compared to an unexposed population 6–7 years after the accident. The highest rates were found among women. Havenaar et al. [14,15] confirmed these findings in a large-scale population-based study in the severely polluted Gomel region in Belarus and a non-affected but socioeconomically comparable area of Russia (the Tver region). Using the GHQ, these authors also found elevated rates of psychological distress among evacuees but not among liquidators. Importantly, this study also showed that the differences in mental health problems were limited to self-report measures of psychological distress. Differences in the prevalence of psychiatric diagnoses in terms of DSM-III-R, particularly anxiety disorders, were only found among evacuees (odds ratio, OR 3.78; 95% confidence interval, CI 1.09–13.14) and mothers of young children (OR 2.84; 95%CI 1.64–4.92).

More recently, other Eastern European studies have investigated the mental health impact of the disaster. Rahu et al. [16] reported that suicide was the leading cause of death among Estonian clean-up workers. However, methods of registration of causes of death among the heavily monitored clean-up workers group differed substantially from those used in the general population, thereby making comparison with the general population risky. Another report suggested that there was an increase in the rates of schizophrenia and dementia in clean-up workers [17], but this finding has not been verified. More likely, selection bias, non-blind evaluations, confounding variables (especially alcoholism), and other methodological factors explain these implausible findings.

Subjective Physical Health and Health-Related Behavior

Apart from psychological distress, it seems clear that the Chornobyl disaster caused considerable subjective physical health problems among the affected population. In the study by Havenaar et al. [15] described earlier, large differences were found between exposed and unexposed populations in subjective evaluations of overall health. In the exposed region, 74.5% of the population rated their physical health as "moderate" or "poor", in contrast to 56.5% in the unexposed region. These differences in subjective health could not be accounted for by differences in actual clinical health status as assessed with a standardized physical examination by a Dutch medical team with considerable diagnostic resources [18]. Subjects from the exposed region reported significantly more visits to doctors (OR 1.31; 95%CI 1.14–1.50) and a higher consumption of prescribed medications (OR 1.52; 95%CI 1.30–1.78). Cognitive variables, such as perception of risk and sense of control over the situation, appeared to be important explanatory factors for both the subjective health ratings and service utilization [19].

Several other authors have reported changes in health-related behavior following the Chornobyl accident. Allen and Rumyantseva [20] showed that adherence to safety advisories and ingested dose of radionuclides by villagers in the area was modified by psychological variables such as fatalism. Fatalistic attitudes and behaviors were observed most frequently among elderly people and among women. The authors believe the latter finding may reflect the fact that women are faced more directly with the need to compromise and accept local foods in the absence of alternatives.

A number of studies report on changes in reproductive behavior. Rachmatulin *et al.* [21] reported a 240% increase in induced abortions in factory workers in an area partly contaminated by fall-out from Chornobyl. Bertollini *et al.* [22] reported a reduction of births in Italy 9–12 months after the Chornobyl disaster, followed by a catch-up increase in the ensuing months. In some Italian regions, there was an increase of induced abortions in the first 3 months following the disaster. Lower pregnancy rates and a rise in the number of induced abortions in the year following the disaster were observed in the Scandinavian countries [23–25]. Although a direct link between these changes in reproduction behaviors and the accident remains speculative, Knudsen [23] concluded, on the basis of these data, that the fear of radiation from this disaster probably caused more fetal deaths than the released radioactivity itself.

Mothers and Children

There have been conflicting reports about the effects on young children, especially on children who were exposed during gestation. Ukrainian researchers have reported that children exposed *in utero* have higher rates of borderline intelligence and mental retardation than controls [26,27]. In contrast, an earlier study conducted under the auspices of WHO [28] failed to find significant signs of brain damage. Also Kolominsky *et al.* [29], while finding similar differences in average IQ between exposed and non-exposed children, did not find a significant dose–response relationship. It has been postulated that the observed intellectual differences may be related to other environmental influences, such as endemic thyroid deficiencies. In general these studies are fraught with methodological problems involving sample selection and assessment procedures.

A systematic study of the long-term psychological effects on children who were evacuated from exposed areas to Kyiv was conducted by a collaboration of Ukrainian and American researchers [30]. A random sample of 300 evacuated children and their mothers as well as their teachers were interviewed using an extensive battery consisting of cognitive and intelligence tests, and standardized psychological assessments. The children were also given a physical examination and basic blood test. The evacuated children were compared with gender-matched classmates from the same school who did not have the evacuation experience. The study found no significant differences in physical health, school performance, self-reported symptoms, or performance on neuropsychological tests of non-verbal intelligence, memory, and attention [31]. Also no differences were found in subjects (about one-third of the evacuee sample) who had been exposed *in utero*. Interestingly the mothers did report significantly more memory problems in their children as well as more physical health problems. Moreover, the evacuee mothers reported more somatic complaints, and more anxiety and depression, than the classmates' mothers [32,33]. The authors hypothesized that familial, medical and psychosocial supports may have acted as protective factors, thereby buffering the children from the influence of chronic maternal anxiety and maternal belief that Chornobyl had significantly compromised their family members' health [30].

Emigrants

After the Soviet Union opened up its borders, about 700,000 people emigrated from the Soviet Union to Israel. It is estimated that about a quarter of them came from areas surrounding the Chornobyl power plant. Several Israeli studies have looked into the mental health status of immigrants from the former Soviet Union. Cwikel *et al.* [34–36] followed up one such group of immigrants who had sought an evaluation at a university specialty clinic in southern Israel. Compared to immigrants from other parts of the former Soviet Union, those from areas contaminated by Chornobyl had higher rates of mental health problems and marital problems. Also, the immigrants exposed to radiation from Chornobyl had significantly higher systolic blood pressure. Remennick [37] also found poorer self-reported post-immigration adjustment among these immigrants.

By 1998, more than 500,000 people had emigrated from the former Soviet Union to the United States, according to the US Immigration and Naturalization Service. One study reported higher levels of anxiety and post-traumatic stress symptoms among Russian immigrants from near Chornobyl, than from other parts of the former Soviet Union [38].

SERVICE DEVELOPMENT

Large-scale population relocations, hundreds of thousands of more or less seriously exposed people and continuing concerns about possible long-term health effects made population-scale interventions necessary. In the early days, the Soviet health authorities focused on setting up a system to control the safety of food products and to organize periodical medical check-ups for the most seriously contaminated people. To achieve this, a series of specialized polyclinics were organized throughout the Soviet Union. Even though Soviet psychiatrists were involved in the early rescue operations, and despite the fact that the first International Red Cross fact-finding mission mentioned mental health needs as a priority area [39], it took many years before any form of mental health support was organized. Pioneering efforts to address the mental health situation were launched in the framework of a Dutch humanitarian support project. In Gomel, a provincial capital in one of the most severely contaminated regions in Belarus, a health information center was organized. The center provides health information to the general public and especially to opinion leaders, such as doctors and teachers. It also offers psychosocial counseling to the population and organizes periodical health promotion campaigns [40].

A second major effort to address such problems was launched by the United Nations Education, Scientific and Cultural Organization (UNESCO). Working closely with local and national governmental and non-governmental organizations, nine "Community Development Centers for Social and Psychological Rehabilitation" were established across Ukraine, Belarus and Russia. The centers were located in places where large concentrations of evacuees or clean-up workers lived [41]. The centers focus their attention on community development with various activities for different age groups. Among the services offered are individual and family counseling, support groups, day-care, play therapy and art therapy, a variety of workshops and classes, information services, and radiation and ecology education. Thousands of people have made use of the services provided by the centers since their opening in 1993–1994 [42].

DISCUSSION

This review of the literature about the psychological consequences of Chornobyl demonstrates a number of important points. First of all, not surprisingly, it shows that the accident had a serious impact on mental health and well-being. Importantly, however, it appears that this impact is demonstrable mainly at a sub-clinical level. Increased rates of psychiatric disorders in a stricter sense have only been observed among high-risk groups, notably mothers with young children and evacuees. The massive fear that arises in a population after exposure to radioactive radiation was referred to by some as "radiophobia" or "mass psychosis", concepts that have been strongly criticized by Drottz-Sjöberg and Persson [43]. The empirical studies reviewed here do not support a view that the public anxiety caused by the Chornobyl nuclear disaster bears a resemblance to clinical psychiatric disorders such as phobia or psychosis. However, the experience of Chornobyl does show that radiation exposure incidents, whether accidental or as a result of terrorist action, have a tremendous propensity to induce fear among the affected population. It shows that the psychological impact of disaster is not limited to mental health outcomes. It also has ramifications for other areas of subjective health and health-related behavior, especially reproductive health and medical service utilization. It furthermore may influence people's willingness to adopt safety guidelines issued by the authorities.

Even though the Chornobyl disaster is unique in many respects, especially because of its political and socioeconomic backdrop, there are many points of similarity with other radiation exposure events, e.g. the public reactions to the near-accident at the Three Mile Island (TMI) nuclear power plant in 1979 [44]. Indeed, using comparable stress and symptom data obtained from mothers of young children after the TMI and Chornobyl accidents, Bromet and Litcher-Kelly showed remarkable parallels in the effects of these events. Another example is the Goiania incident in which children found a piece of radioactive cesium from a demolished hospital in Brazil [45]. This incident, which in itself was limited in scale, disrupted the economy of the entire state for many years. Finally, the long-term psychological impact of the bombings in Japan during World War II have also been documented [46]. These examples seem to suggest that cultural factors have a limited impact on the consequences of such events. In all cases there is a massive concern for future health effects, which by far exceeds the actual reality of the health threats and which affects a far larger number of people than those who had actually been put in harm's way. Underlying this pattern is probably the fact that radioactivity is potentially very harmful to the human body, but it cannot be detected directly through the senses. Some of the possible health effects have long latency periods, even extending to future generations. These qualities all contribute to the sense of dread which surrounds radiation exposure incidents. The Chornobyl disaster and other experiences show that, after a radiation exposure incident, a massive increase in demand of medical services (check-ups) and health information may be expected, a situation for which health services in most countries will find themselves poorly prepared. Also it is important to be prepared for substantial indirect effects, especially socioeconomically, because buyers will avoid products from an affected area.

The observed consequences of the Chornobyl accident are in agreement with contemporary theories on the role of cognitive factors in the occurrence of health complaints under conditions of stress [47]. In this model, apprehension invoked by the exposure and the subsequent concerns about future health stimulate people's awareness of physical sensations, which may be harbingers of exposure-related illness. The neuro-vegetative manifestations of anxiety and depression may be one source of these sensations, while unrelated health conditions may be another. In the context of a serious health threat caused by fall-out from Chornobyl, people are more likely to be alarmed by physical complaints and more inclined to attribute them to the effects of ionizing radiation. This will also influence their readiness to report complaints and to seek medical care.

What the Chornobyl disaster has clearly demonstrated is the central role of information and how it is communicated in the aftermath of radiation or toxicological incidents [48,49]. The Chornobyl experience presented the world with a worst-case scenario for information management. Even though, at first glance, this may appear to be typical for the Soviet Union as it functioned at the time, nuclear activities and especially nuclear accidents in Western countries have also tended to be shrouded in secrecy. The Chornobyl experience has raised the awareness among disaster planners and health authorities that the dissemination of timely and accurate information by trusted leaders is of the greatest importance [50,51].

REFERENCES

1. Shigematsu I. (1991) *The International Chernobyl Project. An overview. Assessment of Radiological Consequences and Evaluation of Protective Measures. Report by an International Advisory Committee.* International Atomic Energy Agency, Vienna.
2. Young M.J., Launer M.K. (1991) Redefining Glasnost in the Soviet media: the recontexualization of Chernobyl. *J Communication*, **41**: 102–124.
3. Bard D., Verger P., Hubert P. (1997) Chernobyl, 10 years after: health consequences. *Am J Epidemiol*, **19**: 1–18.
4. Feshbach M., Friendly A. Jr (1992) *Ecocide in the USSR. Health and Nature under Siege.* Basic Books, New York.
5. Rybakov S.J., Komissarenko I.V., Tronko N.D., Kvachenyuk A.N., Bogdanova T.I., Kovalenko A.E., et al. (2000) Thyroid cancer in children of Ukraine after the Chernobyl accident. *World J Surg*, **24**: 1446–1449.
6. Alexander F.E, Greaves M.F. (1998) Ionising radiation and leukaemia potential risks: review based on the workshop held during the 10th Symposium on

Molecular Biology of Hematopoiesis and Treatment of Leukemia and Lymphomas at Hamburg, Germany on 5 July 1997. *Leukemia*, **12**: 1319–1323.

7. Dolk H., Nichols R. (1999) Evaluation of the impact of Chernobyl on the prevalence of congenital anomalies in 16 regions of Europe. EUROCAT Working Group. *Int J Epidemiol*, **28**: 941–948.

8. Castronovo F.P. Jr (1999) Teratogen update: radiation and Chernobyl. *Teratology*, **60**: 100–106.

9. Alexandrowski J.A., Rumyantseva G.M., Jurow W.W., Martjuschow A.N. (1992) Dynamik der psychischen Desadaptionszustände unter chronischem Stress bei Bewohnern der Gebiete, die beim Gau im KKW Tschernobyl in Mitleidenschaft gezogen wurden. *Psychiatrische Praxis*, **2**: 31–58.

10. Yevelson I.I., Abdelgani A., Cwikel J., Yevelson I.S. (1997) Bridging the gap in mental health approaches between East and West: the psychosocial consequences of radiation exposure. *Environ Health Perspect*, **105**: 1551–1556.

11. Bromet E., Dew M.A. (1995) Review of psychiatric epidemiologic research on disasters. *Epidemiol Rev*, **17**: 113–119.

12. Rumyantzeva G.M., Matveeva E.S., Sokolova T.N., Grushkov A.V. (1993) Psychological maladjustment and its relationships with the physical health of the population residing in territories contaminated due to the Chernobyl disaster (in Russian). *Socialnaya Psihiatriya*, **4**: 20–25.

13. Viinamäki H., Kumpusalo E., Myllykangas M., Salomaa S., Kumpusalo L., Kolmakov S., *et al.* (1995) The Chernobyl accident and mental wellbeing – a population study. *Acta Psychiatr Scand*, **91**: 396–401.

14. Havenaar J.M., van den Brink W., Kasyanenko A.P., van den Bout J., Meijler-Iljina L.I., Poelijoe N.W., *et al.* (1996) Mental health problems in the Gomel Region (Belarus). An analysis of risk factors in an area affected by the Chernobyl disaster. *Psychol Med*, **26**: 845–855.

15. Havenaar J.M., Rumyantseva G.M., van den Brink W., Poelijoe N.W., van den Bout J., van Engeland H., *et al.* (1997) Long-term mental health effects of the Chernobyl disaster: an epidemiological survey in two former Soviet Regions. *Am J Psychiatry*, **154**: 1605–1607.

16. Rahu M., Tekkel M., Veidebaum T., Pukkala T., Hakulinen A., Auvinen A., *et al.* (1997) The Estonian study of Chernobyl clean-up workers: II. Incidence of cancer and mortality. *Radiation Res*, **147**: 653–657.

17. Loganovsky K.N., Loganovskaja T.K. (2000) Schizophrenia spectrum disorders in persons exposed to ionizing radiation as a result of the Chernobyl accident. *Schizophr Bull*, **26**: 751–773.

18. Havenaar J.M., Rumyantzeva G.M., Kasyanenko A.P., Kaasjager K., Westermann A.M., van den Brink W., *et al.* (1997) Health effects of the Chernobyl disaster: illness or illness behaviour? A comparative general health survey in two former Soviet Regions. *Environ Health Perspect*, **105**(Suppl. 6): 1533–1537.

19. Havenaar J.M., de Wilde E.J., van den Bout J., Drottz-Sjöberg B.-M., van de Brink W. (2003) Perception of risk and subjective health among victims of the Chernobyl disaster. *Soc Sci Med*, **56**: 569–572.

20. Allen P.T., Rumyantseva G. (1995) The contribution of social and psychological factors to relative radiation ingestion dose in two Russian towns affected by the Chernobyl NPP accident. *Society for Risk Analysis (Europe)*, pp. 1–9.

21. Rachmatulin N.R., Karamova L.M., Dumkina G.Z., Girfanova L.V. (1992) The results of clinico-hygienic research in the region of the Mozyr (in Russian). *Gigiena Truda I Professional 'Nye Zabolevaniia*, **5**: 3–5.

22. Bertollini R., Di Lallo D., Mastroiacovo P., Perucci C.A. (1990) Reduction of births in Italy after the Chernobyl accident. *Scand J Work Environ Health*, **16**: 96–101.
23. Knudsen L.B. (1991) Legally-induced abortions in Denmark after Chernobyl. *Biomed Pharmacother*, **45**: 229–231.
24. Irgens L.M., Lie R.T., Ulstein M., Skeie Jensen T., Sjærven R., Sivertsen F., *et al.* (1991) Pregnancy outcome in Norway and Chernobyl. *Biomed Pharmacother*, **45**: 233–241.
25. Ericson A., Källén B. (1994) Pregnancy outcome in Sweden after the Chernobyl accident. *Environ Res*, **67**: 149–159.
26. Nyagu A.I., Loganovsky K.N., Loganovskaja T.K. (1998) Psychophysiologic aftereffects of prenatal irradiation. *Int J Psychophysiol*, **30**: 303–311.
27. Igumnov S., Drodovitch V. (2000) The intellectual development, mental and behavioral disorders in children from Belarus, exposed in utero following the Chernobyl accident. *Eur Psychiatry*, **15**: 244–253.
28. World Health Organization (1995) *Health Consequences of the Chernobyl Accident. Results of the IPHECA Pilot Projects and Related National Programmes*. World Health Organization, Geneva.
29. Kolominsky Y., Igummnov S., Drozdovitch V. (1999) The psychological development of children from Belarus, exposed in the prenatal period to radiation from the Chernobyl atomic power plant. *J Child Psychol Psychiatry*, **40**: 299–305.
30. Bromet E.J., Goldgaber D., Carlson G., Panina N., Golovakha E., Gluzman S.F., *et al.* (2000) Children's well-being 11 years after the Chernobyl catastrophe. *Arch Gen Psychiatry*, **57**: 563–571.
31. Litcher L., Bromet E.J., Carlson G., Squires N., Goldgaber D., Panina N., *et al.* (2000) School and neuropsychological performance of evacuated children in Kiev eleven years after the Chernobyl disaster. *J Child Psychiatry Psychol*, **41**: 219–299.
32. Adams R.E., Bromet E.J., Panina N., Golovakha E. (2002) Stress and well-being in mothers of young children 11 years after the Chernobyl nuclear power plant accident. *Psychol Med*, **32**: 143–156.
33. Bromet E.J., Gluzman S., Schwartz J.E., Goldgaber D. (2002) Somatic symptoms in women 11 years after the Chornobyl accident. *Environ Health Perspect*, **110**(Suppl. 4): 625–629.
34. Cwikel J., Abdelgani A., Goldsmith J.R., Quastel M., Yevelson I.I. (1997) Two-year follow-up study of stress related disorders among immigrants to Israel from the Chernobyl area. *Environ Health Perspect*, **105**: 1545–1550.
35. Cwikel J., Rozovski U. (1998) Coping with the stress of immigration among new immigrants to Israel from Commonwealth of Independent States (CIS) who were exposed to Chernobyl: the effect of age. *Int J Aging Hum Develop*, **46**: 305–318.
36. Cwikel J., Abdelgami A., Rozovski U., Kordysh E., Goldsmith J.R., Quastel M.R. (2000) Long-term stress reactions in new immigrants to Israel exposed to the Chernobyl accident. *Anxiety, Stress and Coping*, **3**: 413–439.
37. Remennick L.I. (2002) Immigrants from Chernobyl-affected areas in Israel: the link between health and social adjustment. *Soc Sci Med*, **54**, 309–317.
38. Perez Foster R. (2002) The long-term mental health effects of nuclear trauma in recent Russian immigrants to the United States. *Am J Orthopsychiatry*, **72**: 492–504.

39. Revel P. (2001) Meeting psychological needs after Chernobyl: the Red Cross experience. *Military Med*, **166**(Suppl. 2): 19–20.
40. Nijenhuis M.A.J., van Oostrom I.E.A., Sharshakova T.M., Pauka H.T., Havenaar J.M., Bootsma P.A. (1995) *Belarussian-Dutch Humanitarian Aid Project: "Gomel Project"*. National Institute for Public Health and Environmental Protection, Bilthoven.
41. UNESCO (1996) *Community Development Centres for Social and Psychological Rehabilitation in Belarus, Russia and Ukraine: Achievements and Prospects*. United Nations Educational, Scientific and Cultural Organization Chernobyl Programme, Paris.
42. Becker S.M. (2002) Responding to the psychosocial effects of toxic disaster: policy initiatives, constraints and challenges. In J.M. Havenaar, J.G. Cwikel, E.J. Bromet (Eds.), *Toxic Turmoil: Psychological and Societal Consequences of Ecological Disasters*, pp. 199–216. Kluwer Academic and Plenum Press, New York.
43. Drottz-Sjöberg B.M., Persson L. (1993) Public reaction to radiation: fear, anxiety, or phobia? *Health Physics*, **64**: 223–231.
44. Bromet E.J., Litcher-Kelly L. (2002) Psychological response of mothers of young children to the Three Mile Island and Chernobyl nuclear plant accidents one decade later. In J.M. Havenaar, J.G. Cwikel, E.J. Bromet (Eds.), *Toxic Turmoil: Psychological and Societal Consequences of Ecological Disasters*, pp. 69–84. Kluwer Academic and Plenum Press, New York.
45. Petterson J.S. (1988). Perception vs reality of radiological impact: the Goiânia model. *Nuclear News*, 84–90.
46. Yamada M., Kodama K., Wong F.L. (1991). The long-term psychological sequelae of atomic bomb survivors in Hiroshima and Nagasaki. In R. Ricks, M.E. Berger, R.M. O'Hara (Eds.), *The Medical Basis for Radiation Preparedness, III: The psychological perspective*, pp. 155–163. Elsevier, New York.
47. Salkovskis P.M. (1996) The cognitive approach to anxiety: threat beliefs, safety-seeking behavior, and the special case of health anxiety and obsessions. In P.M. Salkovskis (Ed.), *Frontiers of Cognitive Therapy*, pp. 48–74. Guilford, New York.
48. Prince-Embury S., Rooney J.F. (1997) Perception of control and faith in experts among residents in the vicinity of Three Mile Island. *J Appl Soc Psychol*, **17**: 953–968.
49. Havenaar J.M., Cwikel J.G., Bromet E.J. (2002) Epilogue: Lessons learned and unresolved issues. In J.M. Havenaar, J.G. Cwikel, E.J. Bromet (Eds.), *Toxic Turmoil: Psychological and Societal Consequences of Ecological Disasters*, pp. 259–272. Kluwer Academic and Plenum Press, New York.
50. Sjöberg, L. (1998) Worry and risk perception. *Risk Analysis*, **18**: 85–93.
51. Sjöberg L. (1992) *Risk Perception and Credibility of Risk Communication*. Center for Risk Research, Stockholm.

The Experience of the Bhopal Disaster

R. Srinivasa Murthy

National Institute of Mental Health and Neurosciences, Bangalore, India

INTRODUCTION

The Bhopal gas leak disaster is the greatest industrial disaster in human history. On the night between 2 and 3 December 1984, about 40 tons of methyl isocyanate (MIC) from tank 610 of the Union Carbide India Limited (UCIL) factory at Bhopal, in central India, leaked into the surrounding environment. This leak of an "extremely hazardous chemical", which occurred over a short span of a few hours, covered the city of Bhopal in a cloud of poisonous gas. The gas spread and covered an area with about a 7-kilometer radius round the plant, affecting about 200,000 people. More than two thousand persons died on the night of the disaster.

The disaster was the result of a combination of factors. The cause is thought to have been the entry of water into the tank with MIC or the spontaneous polymerization of the liquid of MIC, which had been in storage for over a month, a longer period than normal. In addition to this, the gauges measuring the temperature and pressures were not functioning properly; the refrigeration unit for keeping the tank of MIC cool had been shut off for some time; the gas scrubber had been shut off for maintenance; and the flare tower which could have burned off the escaping MIC was not functional. Thus, the disaster was the result of a combination of negligence and poor operational procedures.

Though the estimated number of persons who died immediately was around 2,000, it is estimated that more than 10,000 persons were killed in the following years. In addition, the population of 200,000 who were exposed to the gas leak and survived have a wide variety of health problems and disabilities.

During the last 20 years, the Bhopal disaster has continued to be an important public health and legal issue. The major milestones in the legal

Disasters and Mental Health. Edited by Juan José López-Ibor, George Christodoulou, Mario Maj, Norman Sartorius and Ahmed Okasha.
©2005 John Wiley & Sons Ltd. ISBN 0-470-02123-3.

responsibility were the passing of the Bhopal Gas Relief Act in 1985 and the settlement of the Government of India and the company for the one-time compensation of $470 million. However, the legal battles for the rights of and relief to the survivors continues and occupies much public space. The issues of the damage to the population, the legal liability of the company and the continuing needs of the affected population continue to be active in India.

By coincidence the Advisory Committee on Mental Health of the Indian Council of Medical Research (ICMR) was meeting on December 12–14, 1984. The experts in the meeting recognized the needs of the affected population as follows [1]:

> The recent developments at Bhopal involving the exposure of "normal" human beings to substances toxic to all the exposed and fatal to many, raise a number of mental health needs. The service needs and research can be viewed both in the short-term and long-term perspectives. The acute needs are the understanding and provision of care for confusional states, reactive psychoses, anxiety-depression reactions and grief reactions. Long-term needs arise from the following areas, namely, (i) psychological reactions to the acute and chronic disabilities, (ii) psychological problems of the exposed subjects, currently not affected, to the uncertainties of the future, (ii) effects of broken social units on children and adults, and (iv) psychological problems related to rehabilitation.

STUDIES OF MENTAL HEALTH CONSEQUENCES OF THE DISASTER

In spite of this early recognition of the need for mental health interventions, there was a delay of 6–8 weeks before mental health professionals were involved. An important reason for this was the lack of mental health professionals in the state of Madhya Pradesh and the city of Bhopal. At that point of time, none of the five medical colleges had a psychiatrist on their faculty.

The first assessments of mental health effects were made in the first week of February 1985 (2 months after the disaster) by psychiatrists visiting affected people at home and examining those attending the general medical facilities [2–4]. Following this, people seeking general medical care were studied. Subsequently, a 5-year prospective study of the general population, which included annual population surveys for mental health effects, was completed [5,6]. In addition, a number of general population studies to understand the health effects also covered mental health aspects [7].

From June 1985, the Lucknow team, funded by the ICMR, conducted a detailed community-level epidemiological study. This study included recording of the complaints of subjects, and the record of illnesses and deaths in 100,000 people in the different areas of Bhopal. A fresh census of the total population was undertaken prior to the study. The sampling frame was drawn in such a manner that populations variously exposed to the disaster were included, along with a control group located far away from the gas-exposed area, but from the city itself. The methodology used for the screening of the households was an interview with the householder for the presence of symptoms from a standardized checklist. Those found to have symptoms were further seen by a qualified psychiatrist who administered the Present State Examination, 9th edition (PSE-9) and arrived at an ICD-9 diagnosis. Each year a new set of families were sampled and studied in addition to follow-up of the patients diagnosed in the previous years.

The first-year survey involved 4,098 adults from 1,201 households. A total of 387 subjects were diagnosed to be suffering from mental disorders, giving a prevalence rate of 94/1,000 population. Most of the population consisted of females (71%); 83% were in the age group 16–45 years. 94% of the patients received a diagnosis of neurosis (neurotic depression, 51%; anxiety state, 41% and hysteria, 2%) having a temporal correlation with the disaster. Detailed case vignettes and descriptive accounts of the patients were prepared. The relationship between rates of psychiatric morbidity and severity of exposure to the poisonous gas was maintained throughout the 5 years of the survey. At the end of this period, the number of fully recovered subjects was small and large numbers continued to experience the symptoms along with significant disability in functioning.

MENTAL HEALTH INTERVENTIONS

The provision of psychiatric services to the affected population was a very significant challenge. For a total population of 700,000 and an affected population of about 200,000, there was no psychiatric help available in the city. A number of measures were taken to meet this challenge. Firstly, some experienced psychiatrists worked to prepare clinical vignettes of patients to sensitize the medical professionals and the administrators. Because of the issue of compensation, the majority of the administrators and medical professionals believed that the complaints, especially the psychiatric symptoms, were factitious. This misconception was corrected by demonstrating the real nature of the symptoms and the universality of the effects of disasters on the mental health of the affected populations. Secondly, starting from February 1985, teams of psychiatrists, clinical psychologists and psychiatric social workers from Lucknow were located in Bhopal for periods of 2–4 weeks to provide psychiatric care to the affected population. The third measure was to train the general medical officers working with the affected population with the essential skills for mental health care. This was indeed very challenging, but it was a rapid way of improving mental health care in the city. In view of its importance and the fact that it was carried out for the first time in India, and possibly in a developing country, this training will be described in detail.

Soon after the disaster, additional medical officers were moved to the city and located in the different gas-affected areas to provide general medical care to the population. In April 1985, about 50 medical officers were working in the various health facilities in the gas-affected areas. Most of the doctors had no training in mental health care as part of their initial medical training, as there were no teachers of psychiatry in the state medical colleges. This lack of training was reflected in their poor perception of the emotional needs of the disaster-affected population. The basic orientation of these doctors was highly medical/biological. In the pre-training interviews, most of them expressed the view that distribution of monetary compensation would solve the physical complaints of a large number of their patients. Some expressed the view that the free rations (food grains and other essentials) provided by the state was the reason for the complaints of weakness and inability to work reported by most patients. The medical officers believed that the "lethargy" of their patients would disappear not by treatment from doctors or by the use of drugs but by "stopping the free rations and distribution of compensation money".

The basic aim of the training was to enhance the sensitivity of the medical officers to the emotional needs of individuals and to provide the skills to recognize, diagnose, treat and refer (when required) the mental health problems [2]. The period of initial training was 6 working days. It was decided that the training should be as practical as possible and should be imparted to groups not exceeding 20 persons. The methodology of training took into account principles of "adult learning", i.e. an open learning environment in which participants were free to share their needs and experiences, with greater stress on interaction. The predominantly lecture approach was changed to case studies and group discussions facilitated by audio-visual materials with maximum learner involvement. A total of 38 medical officers took part in the training.

Training was carried out in two batches by two consultant psychiatrists. A manual was prepared for this training on the basis of experience of training primary care physicians at the National Institute of Mental Health and Neurosciences (NIMHANS), Bangalore. Additional sections on emotional reactions to sudden severe stress, emotional reactions of children to stress and emotional reactions to physical problems were written and incorporated in the manual. A revised manual incorporating the experience of the training and the needs of the medical officers was prepared subsequently and distributed to all the doctors working with the gas-affected population [1].

Some of the comments of the participants in the post-training evaluation supported the usefulness of the training. Some doctors mentioned that earlier they used to give the patients only symptomatic treatment, but after the training they were able to diagnose the condition in terms of a psychological approach. Some doctors mentioned that, earlier to the training, they were not aware of any psychiatric problems and were of the opinion that the patients were malingering and giving vague symptoms to evoke sympathetic response and get more medicines. All the doctors who took part in the training agreed that there was a need for privacy for interviews, support from psychiatrists for difficult cases, and a regular supply of psychotropic drugs.

UNRESOLVED ISSUES

There are a number of unresolved issues concerning the Bhopal disaster. Firstly, there is an international debate about the right to know. The Bhopal disaster jolted activist groups around the world into renewing their demands for right-to-know legislation granting broader access to information about hazardous technologies. Secondly, the need for continuing study of the effects of the disaster on the health of the population has been voiced by a number of researchers and human rights activists. However, except for limited efforts, large-scale systematic studies are not forthcoming. Long-term monitoring of the affected community has to be done for at least the next 50 years. Formal studies of ocular, respiratory, reproductive, immunological, genetic and psychological health must be continued to elucidate the extent and severity of long-term effects. Thirdly, the need to provide appropriate medical services to the affected population has been emphasized. 20 years after the disaster, thousands of men, women and children are still suffering from respiratory illnesses, precocious blindness, cancers and many other related ailments for which they receive no treatment. The efforts to date are to set up specialized centers without a clear link to community services. It has been repeatedly emphasized that a health-care-pyramid approach should be adopted to deal with health problems resulting from the gas leak. Community-level health units should be developed to serve only a maximum of 5,000 people. Local hospitals with specialized departments may be used to provide secondary care. A specialized medical center should be established, dedicated to research into the more serious problems arising from the gas leak. There is clearly an urgent need to develop standard protocols of treatment for the unique problems of the gas-affected population.

A striking aspect of the Bhopal disaster was that the community participation in post-disaster rebuilding remained a goal largely unattended. The state took the parent role, literally taking away the regenerative and reorganizing capacity of the community. The affected population, instead of helping each other, compared who got more support and developed feelings of jealousy amongst each other. The support from the primary group tended to decrease as the population received free rations, money or houses from the state. However, in the rebuilding process, human relations are more important than material benefits. There cannot be community participation without community empowerment.

Moreover, in India, we do not have a framework for rehabilitation with a long-term perspective. In all disasters there is a massive upsurge of goodwill and material support during the acute phase. However, much of this is in terms of charity. People are seen as problems rather than individuals with needs. The situation with regard to care on a long-term perspective is abysmal. Even in Bhopal, where availability of funds was not the issue, no credible system for rehabilitation, health care, jobs etc. has arisen even after two decades [8]. The mental health professionals need to develop such a framework and demand that this be part of the care program from the government and non-governmental organizations.

Finally, it is well recognized that disaster mental health care cannot occur only with outside professionals or resources. Most of the care has to arise from within the community. The need is for all professionals in general, and mental health professionals in particular, to develop methods of care and interventions that can be adapted to the community. There are some beginnings in terms of training, information-sharing, and development of audio-visual aids, but a comprehensive and effective system of care has not been developed to date. This is an urgent need.

REFERENCES

1. Srinivasa Murthy R., Issac M.K., Chandrasekar C.R., Bhide A.V. (1987) *Bhopal Disaster – Manual of Mental Health Care for Medical Officers*. NIMHANS, Bangalore.
2. Srinivasa Murthy R., Issac M.K. (1987) Mental health needs of Bhopal disaster victims and training of medical officers in mental health aspects. *Indian J Med Res*, 86(Suppl.): 51–58.
3. Bharucha E.P., Bharucha N.E. (1987) Neurological manifestations among those exposed to toxic gas at Bhopal. *Indian J Med Res*, 86(Suppl.): 59–62.

4. Sethi B.B., Sharma M., Trivedi J.K., Singh H. (1987) Psychiatric morbidity in patients attending clinics in gas affected areas in Bhopal. *Indian J Med Res*, 86(Suppl.): 45–50.
5. Srinivasa Murthy R. (2002) Bhopal gas leak disaster – impact on mental health. In J.M. Havenaar, J.G. Cwikel, E.J. Bromet (Eds.), *Toxic Turmoil: Psychological and Social Consequences of Ecological Disasters*, pp. 129–148. Kluwer Academic and Plenum Press, New York.
6. Indian Council of Medical Research (2003) *Mental Health Studies of Bhopal Disaster*. ICMR, New Delhi.
7. Cullinan P., Acquilla S.D., Dhara V.R. (1996) Long term morbidity of survivors of the the 1984 Bhopal gas leak. *Natl Med J India*, 9: 5–10.
8. Srinivasa Murthy R. (2000) Disaster and mental health: responses of mental health professionals. *Indian J Soc Work*, 61: 675–692.

The Latin American and Caribbean Experience

José Miguel Caldas de Almeida and Jorge Rodríguez

Pan American Health Organization, Washington, DC, USA

INTRODUCTION

Natural disasters in Latin America and the Caribbean are not only occurring with increasing frequency, but also with greater destructive potential, making this a significant problem in terms of its social, economic, and health impact. After the major disasters of 1985 in Mexico and Colombia, the governments of the Americas met in Costa Rica in 1986 and laid the foundations for a common policy to make health care more efficient and more compatible with the needs of the population. Since then, great progress has clearly been made. Instead of responses that were largely improvised, organized national policies are now in place.

In the first phase, responses to emergencies have focused above all on immediate medical care, problems related to communicable diseases, environmental sanitation, and damage to the health infrastructure. In recent years, however, responses have begun also to pay attention to the psychosocial component that is always present in these human tragedies. In addition, the approach to emergency management has evolved toward a new perspective that goes beyond the response to damages to focus on risk management, seeking to eliminate or reduce the probability that damages will occur.

In Latin America, in addition to natural disasters, political violence and civil wars have produced a significant number of deaths and injuries, accompanied by a great deal of grief and suffering. They have also contributed to the rising tide of refugees and displaced persons. As in other parts of the world, the experience in the region has shown that, in both natural disasters and emergencies produced by wars and conflicts, psychosocial needs are high, especially in the more vulnerable groups. It

Disasters and Mental Health. Edited by Juan José López-Ibor, George Christodoulou, Mario Maj, Norman Sartorius and Ahmed Okasha.
©2005 John Wiley & Sons Ltd. ISBN 0-470-02123-3.

has also shown that an increase in psychological disorders is to be expected in these situations.

The 1985 disasters in Armero, Colombia [1] and in Mexico [2] were especially important, because in those cases it was possible to perform an evaluation of psychiatric morbidity and to implement strategies to enable primary health care professionals to manage mental health problems. These disasters also underscored the importance of teamwork and of community-based interventions.

The town of Armero, in the Colombian Andes, was destroyed on 13 November 1985 by a volcanic eruption that produced an avalanche of ash, boiling mud, rocks, and tree trunks. The landslide killed 80% of the town's 30,000 inhabitants and left almost 100,000 inhabitants of the adjoining region homeless.

It was an unusual tragedy in that survivors lost not only their family members and property, but the entire town in which they had lived, with the destruction of social support networks and many cultural reference points.

The impossibility of recovering the bodies, the vast majority of which were swept away by the avalanche and buried under tons of sand and rubble, made it impossible to hold the traditional ceremonies dictated by local culture. It also meant that, for months afterward, family members were deceived by rumors that one of the dead had been spotted wandering around, like a crazy lost person, in nearby or distant areas. Each such false report awakened new hopes, always followed by disillusionment. For as long as 2 years after the tragedy, each discovery of a body that could be identified spurred families to seek the remains of their relatives to perform the customary religious and cultural rites.

In Armero, the disaster killed 37 mental health professionals and workers and destroyed the regional psychiatric hospital, where 87% of the psychiatric beds in the Department of Tolima had been located. Thus, the general health sector, especially at the primary care level, had to address most of the area's psychiatric needs, both normal, everyday needs, as well as those created by the disaster. Despite all the difficulties found after the disaster, it has been possible to confirm that in this kind of situation effective mental health care can be provided by primary health care workers.

The experience of the earthquake in Mexico showed the limitations of some of the conceptual models previously used to understand psychological processes, both individual and collective, related to disaster situations. It highlighted three main issues: (a) the importance of identifying symptoms associated with post-traumatic stress; (b) the recognition of the limitations of strict psychodynamic models for understanding and treating this type of psychosocial process; and (c) the affirmation of a new paradigm that considers symptoms as reactions to the disaster and that emphasizes the importance of facilitating the creation of settings where collective experiences can be reworked within self-help groups.

Simultaneously with these new experiences in the management of disasters, the 1990s saw an evolution in the understanding of and approaches to mental health in Latin America, with significant consequences for the organization of mental health care in the majority of the countries of the region. The Declaration of Caracas [3] and subsequent resolutions of the Directing Council of the Pan American Health Organization (PAHO) in 1997 [4] and 2001 [5] called for the development of community-based, decentralized mental health services. Under this model, the psychiatric hospital ceases to be the main locus of mental health care provision; rather, such care is provided mainly by primary health care services and specialized community services and programs.

The restructuring of psychiatric services and the inclusion of a psychosocial component in primary health care (PHC) have made it possible to change work patterns in many countries, improving the conditions for responding to natural disasters and other emergencies.

The main trends observed in the fields of mental health and emergencies in Latin America over the last 15 years can be summarized as follows [2]:

- Mental health: (a) development of national mental health programs; (b) insertion of a psychosocial component in PHC; (c) decentralization of psychiatric services; (d) displacement of the psychiatric hospital as the fundamental axis of mental health care; (e) evolution from a medicalized model of care focused on illness, to another more comprehensive and community-based model.
- Emergencies: (a) focus on risk management, representing a preventive approach aimed at eliminating or reducing the possibility of damage; (b) development of organizational plans and structures in the health sector for emergency management; (c) health care that is efficient and compatible with the needs of the population; (d) recognition of a mental health component as part of the response to emergencies.

PSYCHOSOCIAL CONSEQUENCES OF DISASTERS AND EMERGENCIES IN LATIN AMERICA

Two recent research projects sponsored by the PAHO have helped to improve our knowledge about the predominant psychosocial impacts of disasters and emergencies in the region. The first is a study of the prevalence of psychological disorders in Honduras during the period immediately following Hurricane Mitch. The second is a qualitative research study providing a description of the psychosocial dynamic among populations affected by the domestic armed conflict in Guatemala, which lasted more than three decades.

Research findings on psychological disorders in the adult population of Tegucigalpa, Honduras, in the aftermath of Hurricane Mitch [6] show that 19.5% of the population experienced episodes of major depression. The high-exposure areas had a rate of 24.2%, compared with 14.2% in the least-exposed neighborhoods.

Post-traumatic stress (PTS) was found in 10.6% of the general population, in 7.9% of the low-exposure group and 13.4% of the highly exposed sample. However, the rate of hurricane-related PTS symptoms was much higher (23.0%) when the criteria for duration and disability were excluded. The comorbidity rate (PTS and episodes of major depression) was 6.9% overall, 8.9% in the high-exposure group and 4.9% in the low-exposure group.

Alcohol-related problems were significantly higher in the high-exposure, low socioeconomic group living in shelters.

Significant risk factors for morbidity included the following: high exposure; female gender; low socioeconomic status; divorced, separated, or widowed status; low levels of education; and having had "previous problems with nerves".

Research on utilization of health services showed that 26.5% of the sample consulted the health services after Hurricane Mitch. In the same sample, 8.9% reported consulting someone or requesting assistance after the hurricane because of "nerves". Women consulted the health services at a higher rate than men and more often sought assistance for "nerves".

Approximately one-third of the respondents were exposed to violence after the hurricane, and 6.2% reported that they had been assaulted. 7% of the interviewees admitted to perpetrating acts of violence. The poorest people were the most affected by violence.

In the qualitative study conducted in Quiché and Alta Verapaz on psychosocial consequences for the population affected by the war in Guatemala [7], the most significant results were the following:

- Mental health problems – the majority agreed – developed or increased during and after the 36-year armed conflict.
- Today, the majority of the people, especially in rural and indigenous areas, experience a sense of frustration and despair.
- The most common mental health problems in children included anxiety, depression, irritability, aggressiveness, timidity and isolation, behavior problems, conflicts with authority, sleep disorders, and enuresis. Young people in rural areas show an increase in addictions, mainly to alcohol and tobacco, but also, on a smaller scale, others such as sniffing glue or

gasoline. Suicidal behavior in young people is a relatively new phenomenon that was observed in Nebaj.

- During the armed conflict, family life was disrupted, and there was a great deal of mistrust among the people; communication was poor and fear pervasive. People witnessed or experienced traumatic situations such as death, violence, torture, massacres, disappearances, and so forth. People lost their small landholdings and became further impoverished. Religious sects (mainly evangelical Protestant) proliferated at the expense of traditional Mayan practices and the Catholic faith. The natural environment was neglected and even destroyed as a result of the war.

- It was reported that, since the armed conflict, many traditions and cultural values of Guatemala's indigenous population have been lost, because "the elders could not transmit their culture". The influence of urban "customs from the capital" and the mass media are considered harmful. Today, individualism prevails instead of solidarity, and many people say that having so many religions has worked to divide the population. Others, however, insist on the need to rely on the "Word of God" in facing current social problems. It is said that many people are still wary and afraid to speak.

- With regard to coping mechanisms, respondents emphasized that, before and during the armed conflict, their most important supports were spiritual or religious help and assistance from family members or friends. There is currently less reliance on customs and traditions.

The studies in Honduras and Guatemala confirm that three major groups of psychosocial problems must be confronted in disasters and emergencies:

- Fear and grief, resulting from damage and losses and/or fear that the traumatic situation will recur.
- Psychopathological symptoms or obvious psychiatric illnesses.
- Social unrest, violence, and substance abuse. This includes crime and acts of vandalism, uprisings, exaggerated demands, sexual abuse, domestic violence, etc.

This reality has several consequences for the planning of interventions for populations affected by disasters and emergencies [2,8]. First, it is not enough to consider psychopathological conditions; it is also necessary to consider a wide range of problems with significant social content. Moreover, the need to expand the area of expertise of mental health professionals cannot be ignored. Finally, it must be taken into account that psychosocial problems can and should be handled, in large part, by non-specialized personnel.

Crisis theory has provided a conceptual framework that makes it possible to consider psychological reactions as normal responses to critical situations, thus facilitating a systemic, multidimensional approach within the sociocultural context.

It is clear that depressive and anxiety disorders, acute stress reactions, and alcohol abuse are the problems most commonly cited during the acute phase of disasters.

Recovery can be hindered by secondary stress factors, including poverty and exposure to violence. Individuals subjected to secondary stress are perhaps more vulnerable and have higher rates of PTS, depression, disability, and psychological distress. The individuals at risk and the factors that can influence this must be identified so that appropriate services and interventions can be implemented.

MENTAL HEALTH PROTECTION IN DISASTERS AND EMERGENCIES: LESSONS LEARNED IN LATIN AMERICA AND THE CARIBBEAN

Experiences from Latin America and the Caribbean show that, even in countries with very few resources, the development of mental health services for disaster victims and disaster preparedness can be significantly improved if the right strategies are used. In the first phase, most of the support was provided or at least coordinated by international mental health teams sent to the site of the disaster. While this strategy has proved useful in meeting the immediate needs of the country, especially when well integrated in the larger relief plan, it has not helped the countries to prepare fully for future disasters. To meet this latter objective, additional strategies have been used in the past few years [9].

The first is the formulation of a national plan to address mental health in the context of disasters, or the integration of a specific disaster response component in the national mental health plan. This plan usually defines: (a) the agency responsible in a disaster situation for developing a rapid assessment of the psychosocial needs of the affected population, setting priorities and coordinating actions; (b) the roles of non-specialized personnel (primary care professionals, schoolteachers, community workers, among others) in providing psychosocial care to disaster victims, and the mechanisms to ensure their participation; (c) the services – psychiatric hospitals, general hospitals, community-based services, emergency teams, non-governmental organizations (NGOs) – responsible for providing direct psychiatric treatment to affected persons and how these services are integrated into the general response plan; (d) the mechanisms to provide intensive mental health training to professionals and community workers in disaster situations; (e) the mechanisms to educate the community and promote its participation in the social recovery process.

International cooperation also began to address new needs of the countries. A manual on mental health for victims of disasters and guidelines for trainers and professionals were recently published, with PAHO sponsorship [10,11]. In addition, in 2001 PAHO held two workshops on mental health interventions in natural disasters and wartime situations to produce guidelines on this issue, which were published in 2002 [2]. These initiatives integrate the new strategies with the old: the training of experts who can participate in emergency interventions in the future, and the dissemination of knowledge and capacity building at the country level. Finally, in 2003, a mental health plan for disasters in Central America was prepared, through cooperation between the Central American countries and PAHO.

Notwithstanding all these efforts, certain problems are still common in Latin America:

• The absence, in many cases, of a national mental health program, as well as a mental health component in emergency health plans.
• The difficulties encountered by affected populations in gaining access to specialized care, since this one is frequently based in distant psychiatric hospitals.
• The inadequate preparation of PHC workers to deal with the psychosocial impact of disasters.
• The lack of coordination among government institutions, NGOs, and community organizations.

It is clear that, in disasters and other emergency situations in developing countries, psychiatric hospitals cannot meet the vast majority of the population's mental health needs. They can, in fact, make it even more difficult to meet these needs, by adding the stigma associated to them and by being culturally and geographically distant from the place where the people who need help are located.

The lessons learned point toward the development and/or strengthening of a community mental health care model that can offer timely services with broad coverage and coordination of the various social actors involved in emergency care. In addition, the personnel who participate in emergency programs should have at least a minimum level of training on psychosocial issues.

A major effort has been under way in recent years to reorient psychiatric services, a necessary and important step for achieving continuity and the sustainability of action taken in response to emergencies.

In some countries, mental health work undertaken as part of the health care provided to people affected by emergencies has helped make the authorities more aware of the need to include a mental health component in public policies, strengthen the network of services, and improve institutional coordination.

Another lesson is that after a large-scale disaster, especially an earthquake, there is a need to provide community education and guidance about the emotional insecurity caused by the fear of new disasters or aftershocks.

In designing intervention strategies, it is important to consider the values, traditions, and customs of the population, as well as other characteristics specific to groups defined by age, gender, place of residence, etc. Also significant is the specific psychosocial vulnerability of populations that live in extreme poverty. The active participation of the community in identifying its own problems and devising ways to resolve them should be promoted.

Providing direct assistance in shelters, schools, and other community venues appears to be an essential strategy, permitting the early identification of psychosocial problems and an active response to them, instead of limiting the role of the health sector to the passive reaction to demands.

Nevertheless, placing victims in shelters or refugee camps should be considered a last resort. Experience has shown that populations living in shelters for extended periods experience greater psychosocial problems.

No advance preparation can completely eliminate the possibility that a person who works with victims will experience symptoms of post-traumatic stress disorder (PTSD) (compassion syndrome). People who do such work for an extended period or even for just one incident are vulnerable because of the situations they experience [2,12,13]. For this reason, the members of response teams are themselves a risk group that should be a priority for mental health care [2].

It has been shown that mental health surveillance and care for children affected by disasters is very important for their future psychosocial development. One of the challenges in caring for children has been to promote a shift from the traditional psychological approach toward community-based actions, giving priority to work with groups rather than with individuals.

The intervention strategy should basically relate to the daily lives of the affected children. With this age group the goal is to facilitate the expression of feelings, redefinition of the traumatic facts, and working through affective or physical suffering to enable the child to adopt new approaches to reality. The school has proven to be an excellent place for mental health activities with children and their families.

There should also be no fear of involving adolescents who themselves have experienced violence in the effort to provide psychosocial assistance. Some young people in the communities can be selected as volunteers, even though they themselves have also been affected, since the child-to-child method will enable them to help themselves through this work.

In the psychosocial approach, it seems that there are no major differences between what is done in the case of natural disasters and actions in response to armed conflicts and population displacements, or what is called a "complex emergency".

The lessons learned offer some conclusions and guidelines for carrying out interventions in these situations [2,8]:

- The first priorities should be to provide immediate assistance to people affected and to establish safe places.
- It is very important to emphasize a return to "normalcy" as soon as possible, avoiding revictimization.
- Victims must not be separated from the rest of the community. Community-based services that meet the needs of all should be developed; this does not preclude people at greater risk from receiving prioritized care.
- Interdisciplinary intervention teams that include indigenous elements are especially important. These teams must be well-trained and familiar with the local culture. They should be provided with the necessary resources so they can be transferred to various areas and remain self-sufficient.
- The presence of groups at significant times, such as exhumations, is a community approach that complements clinical interventions. This is important for coping with death within the context of the community's own traditions and customs.
- Psychosocial care for children and adolescents, utilizing the school as part of the intervention strategy, should be prioritized.
- Development of educational activities with community groups is an obligatory component of an intervention strategy.
- In extended armed conflicts it has been shown that, to a greater or lesser extent, the entire population experiences stress and suffering. Children are especially vulnerable and, on many occasions, are involved as direct actors (as guerrilla fighters or soldiers).
- It has been shown that the psychosocial impact of armed conflicts affects several generations.
- Measures aimed at institutionalizing actions within the health sector, with a medium- and long-term vision, are of particular significance.

The January 2001 Earthquake in El Salvador

The main difficulties during the first week were: lack of skilled human resources, lack of a mental health program, lack of a specialized team at the central level, lack of adequate transportation for reaching the affected areas, and lack of coordination among institutions [14].

Prior to the earthquake, the only place in the country offering mental health services was a National Hospital in San Salvador, where 98% of the country's specialized human resources were concentrated.

The event served as a learning experience for professionals at the hospital, who recognized that better results could be achieved by working where the people live rather than expecting them to come to the facility. The creation of self-help groups was also promoted, but these professionals recognized their own lack of preparation for that task.

The very specific characteristics of this event (a series of earthquakes and repeated aftershocks within a short period) led to a population reaction similar to the response of someone subjected to a continuing pattern of suffering, more than that of a typical person affected by an earthquake. The population's reactions to the first and subsequent tremors were different, because confidence in scientific explanations had already been lost; religious beliefs, notions of divine plans, and myths came into play.

This disaster produced victims from different social strata in the population. The majority of the fatalities from the first earthquake in January were middle-class residents in the Las Colinas neighborhood of Santa Tecla; in the second earthquake in February, most of those affected lived in rural settlements with very limited resources in the central part of the country. A significant number of indigenous campesinos suffered considerable damage to their lands through loss of livestock and the destruction of irrigation systems, houses, and access routes. These communities have habits and customs that are very different than those of other affected communities, meaning that they needed special mental health approaches consistent with their psychosocial characteristics. However, these differences were not taken into account.

Effects of Hurricane Mitch on Nicaragua. The Landslide in Las Casitas

It was found that the country had no mental health plan for dealing with natural disasters. As a result, many institutions provided services to the same people in the area of the landslide. Not until 6 months after the catastrophe did organizations coordinate their efforts by organizing and dividing up responsibility for assistance [15].

Assistance in the mental health field consisted basically of the contributions of specialized human resources (psychiatrists, psychologists, and other professionals) from more than 30 governmental organizations and NGOs. Afterwards, mental health services continued for 2 years.

The mental health services focused on three aspects: (a) identifying survivors and providing crisis intervention, (b) identifying those who were disturbed and unresponsive to initial psychological assistance, in order to refer them to health centers, and (c) providing direct assistance in shelters, schools, and community centers.

The agencies that provided assistance focused on people who had lost their homes and were located in temporary shelters. However, it was shown that the entire population was traumatized in one way or another; accordingly, interventions should have been directed to the entire community.

The majority of the survivors were treated – by the government and the agencies – as victims, thus creating a second victimization and dependency on these institutions. Service providers were also overwhelmed and felt themselves impotent to respond to the situation. The model that functioned positively was one that involved the community in its own recovery process through seed-planting and construction projects.

Return of Joy (UNICEF, Colombia)

In this case it was possible to work comprehensively with an approach that included children, parents, schools, health workers, and the community [16].

The children were divided by age group, encouraging them to play openly, taking advantage of alternative environments in the area. The children were helped to express themselves through drawings, written expression, dramatizations, puppets, and stories to release their emotions. The "Therapy Briefcase or Dream Backpack" contained resources for promoting self-expression and play.

In order to facilitate the process, young people of both sexes between 14 and 20 years of age were linked up voluntarily, with preference given to members of organized youth groups. This group of young people was given training, a process that not only empowered them but also helped them to acquire skills in education for life and the practice of values.

Community support groups made up of adults were also trained to observe and take note of the concerns voiced by children. The organization of workshops, educational talks, and discussions with parents allowed room for questions about patterns of child-rearing and relationship systems, making it possible to raise awareness for preventing and/or diminishing abuse within the family.

A psychologist was assigned to follow the process. The "Return of Joy" methodology was used to treat 115,901 children in Colombia from 1996 through 2000.

Guatemala: Mental Health Care and Recovery after a 36-Year Armed Conflict

In Guatemala, mental health problems are multiple and complex. They are aggravated by the armed conflict that the country experienced for more than three decades, and by the existence of violence, poverty, uprooting, and discrimination. The toll of dead and disappeared from the fratricidal conflict came to more than 200,000; some 669 massacres have been documented. Estimates of the number of internally displaced persons and refugees in other countries range from 500,000 up to 1.5 million [17].

The indigenous population was forced to live far from its places of origin and in communities where several ethnic groups coexisted under military control. The conflict is known to have caused serious disturbances in the traditional structures of community and family life. Almost all children in the regions most affected by armed conflict have lived in a "culture of fear".

In Guatemala, mental health services were nonexistent in the country's interior until 1997. That year, after signing of the peace agreements, the Ministry of Public Health, with technical cooperation from PAHO, prepared and began implementation of a mental health program, targeted especially on care and psychosocial recovery for populations affected by the armed conflict.

Currently, mental health units have been set up in 17 departments and 16 health centers in the capital city. Moreover, the program has worked over these years to provide training for PHC workers, teachers, and community leaders. A methodology for psychosocial care was also developed for school-age children.

SPECIFIC PROBLEMS RELATED TO THE HANDLING OF LARGE NUMBERS OF BODIES IN DISASTERS AND EMERGENCIES

Even though the number of dead and missing caused by some disasters (earthquakes, hurricanes, floods, volcanic eruptions, and man-made accidents) has been declining, thanks to more efficient alert and control systems, as well as better community preparedness, there are still times when the number of fatalities can be very high.

The presence of a large number of dead bodies after a disaster creates uncertainty and fear in the population. This is sometimes exacerbated by inaccurate information about the danger of epidemics that these bodies represent. There is simultaneously stress and widespread grief; the prevailing chaos and the emotional climate can also lead to behaviors that are difficult to control. This type of situation requires appropriate psychosocial interventions at both the individual and community levels.

However, this phenomenon of mass deaths occurs not only in natural disasters or man-made accidents; it is also a frequent problem in wars. Many Latin American countries in recent decades have experienced domestic armed conflicts characterized by massive human rights violations and indiscriminate massacres of civilians. In addition, most of these massacres have resulted from processes that also involved earlier psychological manipulation.

The handling and disposal of bodies is a problem with serious psychological implications for the families of the dead as well as other survivors and has other political, sociocultural, and health consequences that cannot be ignored.

Any form of mass burial always has a very negative psychosocial impact at the individual and community levels; it denies the very understandable universal desire to give a proper farewell to family members and friends. Another problem in mass burial is the failure to identify the bodies, which heightens the pain and uncertainty and complicates the grieving process for survivors.

The fire that occurred in Lima, Peru, on the night of 29 December 2001 [18] is a good example of these problems. It broke out in the commercial area known as "Mesa Redonda" in the historical central city of Lima, causing approximately 270 deaths. Many of the bodies were charred, which made identification very difficult.

The first response was the responsibility of the fire department, which labored for more than 14 hours to control the fire and encountered significant problems due to the number of people requiring assistance. Many of the firefighters were affected emotionally by the large number of bodies they had to see and handle.

On 31 December there was still no clear idea in the Central Morgue of how to organize the identification of the bodies. A slow process was foreseen to allow for an autopsy on each. This led to confusion and frustration among the family members who were waiting to receive their dead. Rumors began to circulate, provoking verbal violence, demands, and protests among these people that began to spread. Another difficulty was that once a body was identified, family members still had to wait a long time before they could take it away.

Psychosocial interventions at the morgue were divided into two major groups. Outside the morgue, psychologists met with people in groups of 6 to 8 to give them factual and up-to-date information. Catholic priests were also present.

Inside the morgue, people were taken in groups of 20; they received orientation and were shown where to go, with a psychologist or a volunteer assigned as a companion. On the second day, given the popular pressure, access was also permitted to an area where bodies that were unrecognizable had been placed; in some cases, people succeeded in making positive identifications. A medical post was set up within the morgue for crisis response. A government agency responsible for offering free funeral services also set up in a tent.

Bodies that in the end were unrecognizable were sent to a pavilion in the cemetery. This decision calmed anxiety and fears among many family members who thought that the bodies might be cremated or placed in a single "mass grave".

CONCLUSIONS

The psychosocial impact of a disaster results from several factors that need to be properly considered, such as the nature of the event, how the individual is involved, and the kind of losses incurred. Moreover, continuous monitoring is required to determine the impact in the medium and long term.

Coping with a disaster or emergency is not only a problem for the health sector: other actors, such as government institutions, NGOs, local authorities, and the community itself are also involved. Some of the more general, immediate measures that help to create a climate of order and emotional calm are:

- A proper orderly response by the authorities.
- Factual and timely information.
- Encouraging interinstitutional cooperation and community participation.
- Guaranteeing basic health services and prioritizing mental health care for survivors.
- Prioritizing care for the most vulnerable groups, considering differences based on sex and age.
- Anticipating an increase in the number of people exhibiting exaggerated grief or psychiatric disorders and facilitating adequate care for them.
- Guaranteeing the careful and ethical handling of bodies by relief workers, as well as establishing an orderly individualized mechanism for providing reports of deaths and disappearances.

- Avoiding burials in mass graves. Promoting identification and appropriate record-keeping for bodies, as well as handing them over to family members.

Traumatic experiences and grief necessarily take on different forms of expression, depending on the culture. Carrying out the farewell rites for loved ones is important for the processes of acceptance and reworking of what has happened.

It is still true, however, that the most frequent institutional responses are based on individual psychiatric care and serve only a small fraction of the people affected.

In the case of massacres, the emphasis should be on the need for medium- and long-term measures to reconstruct the social fabric:

- Compensation (material and financial).
- Humanitarian care and respect for the human rights of survivors.
- Rebuilding of the collective memory and honoring the victims.
- Exhumations that can help to clarify the facts and facilitate the process of family and community mourning.
- Active role of different actors (state and civil society).
- Promoting peaceful coexistence.
- Social and political changes that contribute to the general well-being and to the consolidation of peace and democracy.

Many Latin American countries have been historically affected by multiple traumatic events such as armed conflicts and natural disasters, within a context of marked socioeconomic adversity. The human and material losses have been enormous. Urgent steps must be taken to make the psychosocial recovery of these populations a state policy within the framework of a comprehensive health service.

REFERENCES

1. Lima B.R., Gaviria M. (Eds.) (1989) *Consecuencias Psicosociales de los Desastres: La Experiencia Latinoamericana*. Programa de Cooperación Internacional en Salud Mental Simón Bolivar, The Hispanic American Family Center, Chicago.
2. Organización Pan Americana de la Salud Protección de la salud mental en situaciones de desastres y emergencias (2002) *Serie de Manuales y Guías sobre desastres No.1*. Organización Panamericana de la Salud, Washington, DC.
3. Gonzalez Uzcátegui R., Levav I. (Eds.) (1991) *Organización Panamericana de la Salud Reestructuración de la Atención Psiquiátrica: Bases Conceptuales y Guías para su Implementación*. Organización Panamericana de la Salud, Washington, DC.

4. Organización Panamericana de la Salud/Pan American Health Organization (1997) Resolution CD 40.R19. Pan American Health Organization, Washington, DC.
5. Organización Panamericana de la Salud/Pan American Health Organization (2001) Resolution CD 43/15. Pan American Health Organization, Washington, DC.
6. Kohn R., Levav I. El Huracán Mitch y la salud mental de la población adulta: un estudio en Tegucigalpa, Honduras. Submitted for publication.
7. Rodríguez J., Bergonzoli G., Levav I. (2002) Violencia política y salud mental en Guatemala. *Acta Psiquiátrica y Psicológica de América Latina*, **48**: 43–49.
8. Rodríguez J. (2001) *Principios Básicos y Organizativos de la Atención en Salud Mental en Situaciones de Desastres. Taller Latinoamericano sobre atención en Salud Mental en Casos de Desastres.* Organización Panamericana de la Salud, Guatemala.
9. Caldas de Almeida J.M. (2002) Mental health services for victims of disasters in developing countries: a challenge and an opportunity. *World Psychiatry*, **1**: 155–157.
10. Cohen R. (1999) *Salud Mental para Víctimas de Desastres. Guía para Instructores.* Organización Panamericana de la Salud, Washington, DC.
11. Cohen R. (2000) *Salud Mental para Víctimas de Desastres. Manual para Trabajadores.* Organización Panamericana de la Salud, Washington, DC.
12. Fullerton C.S., Ursano R.J. (2002) Mental health interventions and high risk groups in disasters. *World Psychiatry*, **1**: 157–158.
13. Jarero I. (1998) *Primeros Auxilios Emocionales.* Asociación Mexicana para la Ayuda Mental en Crisis, México.
14. Cohen R. (2002) Mental health services for victims of disasters. *World Psychiatry*, **1**: 149–152.
15. Prewitt J., Saballos M. (2001) *Salud Psicosocial en un Desastre Complejo: El Efecto del Huracán Mitch en Nicaragua.* American Red Cross, Regional Office for Central America, Guatemala.
16. Quiros N., Romero C. (2001) *Experiencias de UNICEF en la Recuperación Psicoafectiva de los Niños en Situaciones de Emergencia. Talleres sobre Atención en Salud Mental en Casos de Desastres y Emergencias.* Organización Panamericana de la Salud, Guatemala.
17. Rodríguez J., Ruiz P. (2001) *Recuperando la Esperanza.* Organización Panamericana de la Salud, Guatemala.
18. Valero S. (in press) *El Afronte de la Muerte.*

15

The Israeli Experience

Arieh Y. Shalev

Hadassah University Hospital, Jerusalem, Israel

INTRODUCTION

In thinking about civilian casualties of the continuing conflict in Israel, one often focuses on the years 2000–2004. However, the wave of terror that started in October 2000 was not the first to have been experienced by Israelis. Quite to the contrary, this problem has been with residents of Israel for decades, and very intensely so, though intermittently, since the early 1970s. The latter were marked by salient events such as the hostage-taking and assassination of the Israeli delegation at the Berlin Olympics Massacre (September 5, 1972); the hostage-taking and killing of 26 ninth-grade high school students in Maalot (May 15, 1974); the hijacking of the Air France Tel Aviv–Paris flight 139 to Entebbe, Uganda (July 4, 1976); a bus hijacking and killing of 34 passengers on the Haifa–Tel Aviv highway (1978); and terrorist bombing in Jerusalem and elsewhere. The latter truly started to accumulate in the early and late 1990s, often linked with specific political instances, such as the 1996 elections, which followed Prime Minister Itzhak Rabin's assassination, and the elections that followed the collapse of the Camp David negotiations in year 2000. At these two time points, terrorism significantly affected the vote, and ultimately the outcome of the elections. But even between such salient "waves" of terror, attacks against civilians were frequent.

Yet the wave of violence experienced since 2000 is very different. Firstly, the incidence of terrorist acts increased by an order of magnitude (Table 15.1). Civilian deaths from terrorism rose from an annual average of 17 before the Oslo agreement (1988–1993), and an annual average of 42 in 1993–2000, to 190 yearly (October 2000–February 2004), with the year 2002 representing a peak of 297 civilian fatalities, of which 77 occurred within a single month (March 2002). Within this wave, suicide bombs became the

Disasters and Mental Health. Edited by Juan José López-Ibor, George Christodoulou, Mario Maj, Norman Sartorius and Ahmed Okasha.
©2005 John Wiley & Sons Ltd. ISBN 0-470-02123-3.

TABLE 15.1 Causes of civilian deaths in Israel, September 2000–March 2004

Type of attack	N
Suicide bombing	402
Bombings	24
Car-bomb	15
Shooting	93
Shootings at vehicle from an ambush	62
Shootings at towns and villages	15
Drive-by shooting	28
Lynching	17
Rocks	2
Stabbing	6
Running over	1
Other	1
Total	666

most deadly of all weapons, causing about 60% of all civilian deaths in the years 2000–2004 (402 of 666), followed by shooting incidents (198, or 30% of all civilian deaths). Suicide bombs characteristically give rise to a larger number of psychological casualties. Civilian casualties (666 deaths and 4,447 injuries) outnumbered those of security forces (276 dead and 1,843 injured) by a factor of 2.4.

Secondly, terrorism has ceased to be seen as sporadic and specifically targeted, and has progressively shaped itself into a full-fledged, unselective campaign. Contrasting with previous years, in which violence preferentially targeted those living in the West Bank, most casualties from 2000 onwards were within towns and cities inside Israel. Additionally, there seemed to be no guiding logic in the choice of targets – other than the ease of access – and these could include, side by side, a disco on Tel Aviv beach, a neighborhood of foreign manual workers, a university campus, or buses serving an ultra-orthodox community in Jerusalem.

Thirdly, and most importantly, peace talks, which continued, despite terrorist acts, throughout the 1990s, virtually stopped, leaving the entire Israeli–Palestinian scene to violence and terrorism. Many opinions about the reasons for this change have been expressed by Israelis and by the media in Israel. These range from pointing to Israel and the Israeli occupation as source of all violence to total denial of the Palestinians' right for sovereignty. Whatever the reason, by its sheer volume, and by the breaking of all previous – if unspoken – assumptions, terrorism and defending against its consequences became a problem of survival.

With such a background, the mental health care community in Israel was burdened with two important tasks: catering for direct survivors of terrorist acts and addressing distress within entire communities. Additionally, the state of Israel implemented a series of steps and established structures, routines and ad hoc dispositions, which, as a whole, came to constitute a supportive network for survivors and communities. The psychological effect of the latter cannot be overestimated and will be addressed below. So, this chapter first considers the network of care, then addresses community and individual responses and finally discusses patterns of resilience and the occurrence of mental disorders.

A NETWORK OF CARE

Medical care in Israel is free of charge. Additionally, the National Insurance Institute of Israel (NII), a government agency responsible for most types of disabilities, supports the medical, financial and rehabilitation costs related to trauma emanating from terror. The NII provides extensive coverage, including medical care, disability compensation, dependants benefits, vocational rehabilitation and other forms of assistance (e.g., loans and grants for housing). These benefits extend to psychiatric casualties: indeed, the NII has been very active in reaching out for casualties following major acts of terror, and has provided psychological debriefing sessions to groups of survivors. The NII also follows widows and dependants, starting from the first days of grief and escorting some individuals for years. Despite individual complaints about red tape and the slow process of recognition, the NII provides a safety network for all physical and psychological casualties of terrorism, so that injury – including mental injury – is not followed by social drift.

Other technical steps were taken to reduce the effect of terrorist attacks on communities. First amongst these is the allocation of resources for immediately repair, amendment and rebuilding of the physical environment following terrorist act. Sites of terror bombing are immediately tended to; all gruesome reminders are carried away and repair of buildings and even replacement of trees start within hours of an event. Consequently, Israeli towns and cities do not bear traces of terrorism – except for symbolic icons. This effort was joined by officials, voluntary organizations (such as Zedaka – a group of orthodox volunteers who painstakingly collected body parts from sites of explosions), businesses (such as the public transportation companies or shop owners) and the public at large, which, following a few days of alarm, returns to streets, shopping malls and buses. From a mental health perspective, the absence of visual evidence of past events significantly facilitates the healing of traumatized survivors by reducing their exposure to reminders of trauma. Thus, when, during exposure therapy, a patient goes back to the street in which he had been affected, he or she finds no reminders – indeed he or she sees that life is back.

Several other steps may reduce the stressfulness of the early aftermath of terrorist attacks. For example, receiving hospitals routinely open large communication centers, staffed by trained social workers, and lists of casualties are shared and continuously updated across receiving institutions. Consequently, relatives can access reliable and comprehensive information with one telephone call, without having to wander between hospitals. Additionally, family centers are opened in receiving hospitals, and dedicated personnel take care of families' anxieties and needs, as they arise – from facilitating interaction with treating physicians to accompanying the family to unfortunately recognize a body. In line with this trend, the Institute of Forensic Medicine developed special expertise in rapid identification of human remains. Following the Jewish rule, which requires rapid burial of the dead, the Institute endeavors to provide unequivocal identification within 24 hours of terrorist acts. This greatly alleviates the agonizing pain of expectation.

Finally, public broadcasting agencies, as well as government and local officials, compete to provide the public with accurate and reliable information. Indeed, each act of terrorism constitutes an implicit test of these agencies' reliability and accuracy: within minutes of a terrorist act, and throughout the following hours and days, they must provide accurate descriptions of sites of trauma, casualty rates, road access, receiving hospital, etc. The public readily translates the information into concrete and necessary knowledge about routes to take or avoid, relatives to be worried about or reassured about, and sources of help and advice. This very concrete meaning of mass media broadcasting might differ from the purely informative tasks of the media, and of opinion leaders, in larger countries. So far, the record is good, even in the eyes of skeptical Israelis, who are quick at spotting mistakes and misinformation. This is extremely important psychologically, since for most of the population the information provided signals the absence of proximal threat, and therefore constitutes a safety signal.

TREATING DIRECT SURVIVORS

Acute Psychological Responses

In the immediate aftermath of a terrorist act, civilians who, on site, show symptoms of acute distress are likely to be evacuated to general hospital emergency rooms (ERs), along with other casualties. This practice is justified by the potential for blast injuries following bombing in closed spaces (e.g., buses, shopping malls) and by the risk of subtle injuries by small metal fragments, which can easily be overlooked at initial examination. The proximity of ERs to most urban centers in Israel is another argument for performing the initial triage in these rooms rather than on site.

This has brought numerous psychological casualties to ERs. Indeed, their number often exceeds that of physical injuries. Statistics from Hadassah University Hospital's ER, which has taken care of more terror victims than any other hospital in Israel, show that 60% of terror-related ER admissions in the first 24 hours of a terrorist attack are psychological. A similar trend was documented during the 1991 Gulf War [1], where 72% of all ER admissions following missile attacks were psychological casualties, including unnecessary self-injections of atropine.

Hospitals in Israel undergo systematic training for mass casualty disasters, pertaining to the simultaneous evacuation of hundreds of casualties. Few hospitals, however, have ever activated that contingency plan, given the smaller numbers of casualties evacuated following attacks by "traditional" explosives (tens to a hundred). Many have, however, developed routines for interventions in psychological casualties, which mainly consist of first making a differential diagnosis with physical injury, secondly reducing the stressfulness of the ongoing event (by responding to urgent and concrete needs, supporting survivors' contact with family members, helping them gain control and recover their sense of mastery and orientation and attending to their need to narrate, if they so wish, their recent experience) and thirdly identifying survivors with extreme reactions (e.g., recurring dissociation) and addressing their distress. The latter is mostly done by psychological means (e.g., suggestion, reality orientation, modeling and structuring verbal and bodily communication despite distress).

Systematic debriefing has been attempted in some settings but is far from being accepted by all. Help at this early phase is generally conceived as "stress management" and mainly consists of optimizing early recuperation, reducing secondary stressors and providing soothing human contact and support for natural helpers (e.g., families). There are no data showing any relationship between these interventions and subsequent rates of post-traumatic stress disorder (PTSD), and the general belief is that early stress management and the prevention of PTSD are two separate matters. Survivors are often provided with advice and contact phone numbers, often to the same therapist or group of therapists that saw them in the ER. Criteria for release from ERs consist of having attended to and reduced uncontrollable dissociative states, assuring continuity of care by informed family members and having provided contact information and resources for further psychological help [2].

Early Post-Traumatic Stress Disorder and Clinical Treatment

Whilst many distressed survivors are evacuated to ERs, smaller but yet unknown numbers require clinical interventions and even fewer might require or be willing to attend formal therapy. Few Israeli hospitals provide systematic reaching out for traumatized survivors. Patient-initiated help-seeking is, therefore the key for receiving professional help in the aftermath of terrorist attacks (though help centers are regularly advertised). The NII offers a network of free consultations for identified direct survivors.

A recent outreach program, conducted at Hadassah University Hospital in Jerusalem, indicates that 311 (36%) of 862 trauma survivors have clinically significant distress within 5 days of ER admission. Of those, 183 (59%) have accepted an offer to see a psychologist for clinical consultation; 91 of the latter (50%) were found, by clinicians, to require early treatment and 62 (68%) started early treatment. This brings the number of potential patients for early clinical interventions to about 10% of those exposed.

On the basis of these data, and of clinical experience across the country, one can safely assume that a significant proportion of psychological casualties go undetected and might never come for formal therapy. Two community surveys (see below) indicate that much help is sought from other community resources (e.g., general practitioners, religious authorities) and most help is received within families. An estimate based on 7 years of ER admissions in Jerusalem shows that the rate of PTSD following terrorist attacks is twice as high as that observed in other traumatic events. However, recovery from early PTSD symptoms during an era of terror (2000–2003) is similar to that observed before the current wave of hostilities [3]. Thus, as might be the case in other areas of the world, the interface between the acute response and prolonged disorders is not entirely covered, and there might be a gap in the management of victims during that transition.

COMMUNITIES UNDER STRESS

Beyond direct victims, terrorism affects communities at large. Published work by Bleich et al. [4] suggests that almost half of Israeli residents have been exposed to traumatic events emanating from terrorism, either directly or via friends and relatives (Table 15.2). About 60% felt that their lives were in danger and 58% disclosed being depressed. Nonetheless, and

TABLE 15.2 Traumatic events emanating from terrorism: telephone survey of a representative sample of 512 Israelis [4]

Exposure	
Personal exposure	16.3%
Friends and relatives	28.0%
No close exposure	55.6%
Appraisal	
Life in danger	60%
Depressed	58%
Optimistic about personal future	82%
PTSD symptoms	
Re-experiencing (at least 1)	37.1%
Avoidance (at least 1)	55.5%
Hyperarousal (at least 1)	49.4%
PTSD by symptom criteria alone	9.4%
PTSD by symptoms and distress/impairment	2.7%

PTSD: Post-traumatic stress disorder.

paradoxically so, 82% were optimistic about their personal future. The rate of clinically significant PTSD was surprisingly low (2.7%), and mostly consisted of females (87.5%). The study found no association between PTSD symptoms and objective threat.

The extent to which PTSD symptoms are the right identifiers of population in distress has been debated (e.g., 5). In the reality of continuous terrorism, many such symptoms represent normal and eventually protective responses (e.g., avoiding dangerous places and situations; being emotionally reactive to reminders, vigilant and tuned). Additionally, PTSD assumes past trauma, whereas reactions under continuous terror comprise an element of anticipation. Nonetheless, PTSD symptoms have been used by most current studies and therefore offer convenient comparisons across populations.

A survey of two suburbs of Jerusalem during the current hostilities [6] has addressed the relationship between PTSD symptoms in the community and PTSD as a disorder. As in Bleich *et al.* [4], the survey showed that proximity to the sites of hostilities did not affect the likelihood of expressing PTSD symptoms. It also showed that adding measures of impairment and distress to merely assessing PTSD symptoms significantly reduces the prevalence of the disorder (5.5% in this study). Contrasting with Bleich *et al.* [4], however, the survey did not find higher responses or higher prevalence of PTSD in women. Importantly, however, within affected communities, a significant minority (23%) expressed high levels of symptoms – both PTSD and other psychological symptoms – whereas most others' reactions were within the peacetime adult norm. This prompts the conclusion that, under continuous strain, a subset of those exposed becomes highly distressed, whereas the majority is mildly affected.

How did Israelis cope with terrorism? The two studies mentioned above suggest that much of the coping consists of actively seeking relevant information (e.g., about relatives exposed, about sources of threat), better structuring the situation and thereby reducing personal distress. Additionally, the study of two suburbs of Jerusalem found that residents with higher exposure to terror (e.g., to roadside shooting, stoning, road blocks and snipers) tended to use diverting coping strategies (e.g., reframing, humor and acceptance). Thus, it would seem that, in order to successfully endure continuous traumatization, one has to sometimes ignore it. Another pertinent finding is that apprehensions, amongst the highly exposed, remained circumscribed and focused on actual sources of threat, rather than expanding to any threat. Importantly, anxieties about family members' exposure were higher than those concerning self-exposure, which should shift our attention from addressing individual distress to distress within families and social groups.

UNCHARTED, YET VERY COMMON WAYS OF COPING

Empirical research into coping with terror falls short of providing sufficient explanations of the obvious discrepancy between the pervasiveness of the threat and the limited prevalence of mental disorders. Clearly, humans are more resilient than current risk-averse culture leads us to assume. Not that most humans are heroes, or otherwise extremely well trained for missions and fighting: resilience is probably an attribute of ordinary people. Resilience *of the normal type* (as opposed to the often-depicted heroic resilience under combat-stress or during captivity) might be the best lesson we have learned from the response to terrorism in Israel.

Yet this *is* an uncharted area. After 3 years of intense terrorism in Israel, several patterns of resilience emerge, which defy (or have escaped) systematic research. Following is a short comment on each.

Shifting Expectations

A frequent way of adjusting to terrorism has been to progressively shift expectations, in ways that have enabled most people to *successfully* live another day, and another week. When living without terror became an illusion, people would be encouraged if terrorist acts did not happen for a week, or a month. When terror occurred, a small number of casualties would be a good sign. When one could not go out without risk, returning home unharmed would be a small victory. Thus, Israelis, as much as, supposedly, most other populations under strain, created, and re-created adequate expectations: adequate in the sense that they were plausible and could be materialized – in which case they immediately became sources of satisfaction and pleasure.

Shifting Priorities

Similarly, people came to appreciate non-conflictual areas of living and to re-prioritize life accordingly. For many, the family became the focus of attention. Feeling safe was more important than being entirely free. Overcoming difficulties superseded risk-aversion etc. Importantly, for those who managed to cope well, the new priorities were chosen such that they were achievable and within reach, such that relative satisfaction could follow.

Creating Routines of Living

Consequently, most people developed a routine of living under terror. This was particularly obvious in residents of highly threatened areas who, for example, had to plan their entire day on the basis of roadblocks and other constraints. Within days, people found new "arrangements" for getting their children back from school, leaving work earlier or carefully planning previously spontaneous activities, such as driving to work or shopping.

Territorializing Threat, Identifying Patterns

Another prevalent way of coping was to re-structure space and time into threatening and non-threatening components. This was often done by assigning degrees of threat to situations and places and organizing one's behavior accordingly. Thus, each of us had his or her virtual *map of fear*, which, for some, forbade travel to East Jerusalem, for others (e.g., residents of Tel Aviv) excluded visits to Jerusalem at all, and for yet others allowed visiting local groceries but excluded shopping malls.

These virtual maps seem to have kept people in an illusionary but functional control pertaining to the risk they were ready to take. As long as they were proven stable and reliable, fear maps worked to reduce distress and apprehension. But, as soon as the reality defied one's virtual map, there was distress and concern. For example, it was believed, at some point, that

Fridays were relatively safe because of their meaning for Islam. When a terrorist bomb exploded on Friday this particular map was betrayed and distress followed. The same distressing shift happened when a bomb hit the Frank Sinatra cafeteria, at the Hebrew University, a should-be safe place that hosted Jews and Arabs in the presumed sanctuary of academia. Similarly, when a suicide bomber exploded in the midst of a large Pesach celebration in a hotel, readjustment had to be made and strong emotions emerged. The case of the "Moment café" in Jerusalem is similar: this hub of left-wing liberals and the international media crowd was supposedly safe, and many Jerusalemites were utterly shocked by its being targeted by terror.

But virtual safety maps took a few days to reconstruct, and within such time most people regained a sense of orientation and relative mastery over their acts and whereabouts. In that sense one might say that terror did not succeed in creating prolonged havoc and fear, mainly because of the simple, unintended, day-by-day capacity of ordinary people to adjust.

Proceeding with Life

The necessities of daily living were another obvious reason for people's perseverance and persistence. One had to work. One had to have one's children go to school. Exams were waiting for students, investments for businessmen, babies were born and weddings planned in families. None of these could be stopped or critically postponed. No one could seriously afford to stop living.

The Unyielding Attraction of Life

Ultimately, the major resilience factor, in Israel, and probably elsewhere, is the attraction of life. For as long as one is not depressed or pathologically anxious, life is fundamentally appealing, pleasure and satisfaction are found – or invented – and terrorism, at least at the dimension in which it was present in Israel, does not stop it.

Mental Disorders, Breakdown of Families, Broken Lives and Post-Traumatic Conditions

Yet a few have paid the price for most others: direct survivors who became afflicted with PTSD; survivors maimed by physical injury; grieved, decimated and bereaved families. For them, each act of terror reinforced and restated profound anxieties and fears. In their lives, fear ceased to have a territory. Terror invaded their days and nights, perverted the safety of their homes, disturbed the silence of falling evenings, spoiled their sleep. They could not develop adaptive routines of living, nor could they proceed with life. Their utmost priority became avoiding inner and external tension. They were thenceforth alienated from the pleasures of living. Their life was shattered.

Possibly the most consequential lesson from years of terror in Israel is that, despite leaving communities relatively untouched, more and more individuals come to pay the full price. When all this comes to solution, these affected survivors, and their counterparts on the other side, will bear the full consequences of current follies. They will eventually become more and more alienated, when societies will reach solutions, hence the need to remain vigilant and adamant about their rights and their destiny. This would be the ultimate sign of a healthy response to terrorism.

ACKNOWLEDGEMENT

This work was supported by the US Public Health Service/National Institute of Mental Health grant MH 50379.

REFERENCES

1. Bleich A., Dycian A., Koslowsky M., Solomon Z., Wiener M. (1992) Psychiatric implications of missile attacks on a civilian population. Israeli lessons from the Persian Gulf War. *JAMA*, **268**: 613–615.
2. Shalev A.Y., Addesky R., Boker R., Bargai N., Cooper R., Freedman S., *et al.* (2003) Clinical intervention for survivors of prolonged adversities. In R.J. Ursano, C.S. Fullerton, A.E. Norwood (Eds.), *Terrorism and Disaster, Individual and Community Mental Health Interventions*, pp. 162–186. Cambridge University Press, Cambridge, UK.
3. Shalev A.Y., Freedman S. PTSD following terrorist attacks: a prospective evaluation. Submitted for publication.
4. Bleich A., Gelkopf M., Solomon Z. (2003) Exposure to terrorism, stress related mental health symptoms and coping behavior among a nationally representative sample in Israel. *JAMA*, **290**: 612–620.
5. North C.S., Pfefferbaum B. (2002) Research on the mental effects of terrorism. *JAMA*, **288**: 633–636.
6. Shalev A.Y., Tuval Mashiach R., Hadar H. (2004) Posttraumatic stress disorder as a result of mass trauma. *J Clin Psychiatry*, **65**(Suppl. 1): 4–10.

16

The Palestinian Experience

Eyad El Sarraj and Samir Qouta

Gaza Community Mental Health Programme, Gaza Strip, Palestine

INTRODUCTION

The state of mental health in Palestine is bound up in a combination of factors so interlinked that it is difficult to consider their effects separately. Therefore, they remain indivisible when their impact on the human psyche, on individual lives and on the community as a whole is considered. Behind the specific traumatic upheavals of the past decades (1948 uprooting, 1967 War, Occupation, the first Intifada, Al-Aqsa Intifada, etc.) lies the amalgamation of the stressors, frustrations and humiliations present in everyday life in Gaza and the effect that this constant tension and frustration has had on the mental health of its population.

The disaster of uprooting left a strong influence on the Palestinian community and it is known from the literature that traumatic events are harmful for the development of the individual. For this reason it is important, when exploring the impact of specific types of human rights abuses on victims and on Palestinian society, always to take into consideration the global context in which they are occurring and to which they are adding a new element of suffering. It follows, naturally, that any intervention designed to improve mental health, and to prevent further human rights abuses, must acknowledge and incorporate the significance of the intertwined elements of past and present experience, as well as attitudes towards the future. Even the impact of the peace process on Palestinians cannot be comprehended without understanding the initial meaning of the Oslo Agreement itself and what it represented. In turn, this cannot be understood without a clear picture of what the first Intifada (1987–1994) as well as Al-Aqsa Intifada (2000) meant to this society, which itself cannot be understood without a clear conception of life under occupation.

In the literature the recovery from trauma has always been described from a protective and supportive perspective. In the Gaza situation the

Disasters and Mental Health. Edited by Juan José López-Ibor, George Christodoulou, Mario Maj, Norman Sartorius and Ahmed Okasha.
©2005 John Wiley & Sons Ltd. ISBN 0-470-02123-3.

whole community, even the traditional sources of protection (e.g., parental authority) had been undermined. It is unknown how a recovery process develops under these circumstances. Gaza has a relatively large number of young individuals (age $<20 = 60\%$): it is unknown what the long-term consequences are for the development of an individual when a whole generation has been traumatized. Furthermore, in the first Intifada, children and adolescents were *actors*, and it is especially this fact which makes the situation of the Gaza community different from combat situations in the West.

In facing and confronting the repeated and ongoing various forms of trauma and violence, Palestinians were to resort to the basic security structures which have helped them historically to survive. The cohesion of the family, the tribal structure, and a high degree of political involvement have helped the population's adaptive mechanisms and its capacity for resilience. In recent years the rise of Islam as a political movement of resistance has further sharpened their resolve, although it has politically radicalized increasing segments of the population.

It is a tragic fact that children have become laboratories for the study of the relationship between trauma and violence, conflict, and well-being during war. Wars and battles have been fought without interruption in the region for 50 years. None of these wars, however, have brought a solution to the conflict between Jews and Arabs. Since the war area is small, it is difficult to protect children from the sights of destruction or to protect them from the dangers of war and insecurity. Many of these children have taken part in their national struggle. Even if they were not actively fighting in the streets, as so many were, they still could not help but experience the national struggle on an emotional level. The atmosphere of insecurity, danger, violence, and hostility that prevailed during the two Intifada inevitably left scars on the mental health of the Palestinian children.

Owing to the difficulties in conducting nationwide research and service projects in the West Bank and Gaza Strip, we in the Gaza Community Mental Health Programme have focused on the population of Gaza. The results of our work, however, could also be applied to the Palestinians living in the West Bank, since both populations live under similar conditions and share the same cultural and socioeconomic life.

THE ONGOING TRAUMA IN GAZA: RESEARCH FINDINGS

Trauma in Gaza is ongoing and is both direct and indirect. Direct trauma refers to the episodes of organized violence during the first and present Intifada. Indirect trauma refers to the long-term consequences of the direct trauma. The Palestinian Human Rights Information Centre estimates that during the period of the first Intifada (from December 9, 1987, to December 31, 1993), Palestinians suffered 130,472 injuries and 1,282 deaths, of which 332 were deaths of children. Among these victims are those who were shot, beaten, tear-gassed, or burned to the extent that they are suffering from permanent disability. Approximately 57,000 Palestinians were arrested, many of whom were subjected to systematic physical and psychological torture. Records show that over 481 were deported, and 2,532 had their house demolished during the first Intifada. The psychosocial and financial costs for the affected families in terms of medical and psychosocial care, loss of productive time, chronic disability, loss of function, and loss of life and property were enormous [1]. Most children living in the Occupied Palestinian Territory (OPT) have directly experienced physical or psychological violence or have witnessed this violence directed towards their families and friends. Also, it is important to note that the atmosphere of political violence creates a state of disorganization inside the Palestinian family. Especially frightening is the fact that parents are unable to protect their children and are perceived to be helpless victims by their own children. The image of a young boy being shot at and killed while his father stands and screams to stop the storm of bullets has a lasting impact on viewers, especially children.

Losing one's home means more than acute disaster for Palestinians, as it evokes the memories of the traumatic experiences associated with being a refugee. In fact, the current shelling and house demolitions evoke memories associated with the loss of historic Palestine in the 1948 war, which have been a central source of fear and insecurity and deeply affect the inner layers of the Palestine psyche [2]. When a family is witness to the destruction of its own home by enemy soldiers, the psychological effect is immense. The home is not only a shelter, but also the heart of family life. There are memories of joy and pain as well as attachment to familiar objects. Home is associated with feelings of security and consolation [3]. Moreover, shelling or demolition often happens suddenly, without prior notice. It is this unpredictability that is considered to be the most traumatic factor for human beings. Finally, shelling and demolition have meant that families are forced to live in tents or in the houses of relatives, which not only is reminiscent of the situation in 1948 but also causes many practical and social problems, and puts people in more danger. In a study exploring psychological symptoms in children whose homes were demolished or who witnessed the demolition of other houses, we found that the former were significantly more symptomatic than the latter and a control group (Table 16.1).

Another issue is that of curfew. Curfews are considered as a collective punishment, turning every home into a prison. Under the curfews all

TABLE 16.1 Psychological symptoms in children whose houses were demolished, in children witnessing the demolition of other houses and in a control group

Symptom	Loss group ($n = 38$)	Witness group ($n = 36$)	Control group ($n = 50$)	χ^2 value
Dread of the army	97.4	77.8	70.0	10.63**
Lack of concentration	84.2	19.4	0.0	74.41***
Constant weeping	65.8	19.4	12.0	32.39***
Easily irritated	63.2	37.0	32.0	8.95**
Re-experiencing trauma	60.5	27.8	8.0	28.56**
Night terror	60.5	41.7	4.0	33.63***
Loss of interest	60.5	11.1	12.0	32.27***
Sleeping difficulties	57.9	16.7	6.0	32.89***
Explosive and touchy	55.3	52.0	20.0	9.98**
Clinging behavior	52.6	33.3	2.0	29.51***
Disobedience	50.0	30.6	18.0	10.27**
Afraid of going out	47.4	22.9	4.0	23.10**
Sad mood	42.1	5.6	0.0	34.13***
Aggressive behavior	42.1	16.7	16.0	9.59**
Feeling suffocation	39.5	8.3	2.0	25.28***
Bedwetting	31.6	17.1	12.0	5.44*
Social withdrawal	23.7	2.8	2.0	14.89***
Sucking thumb	21.1	5.6	2.0	10.38**
Biting nails	21.6	11.1	2.0	8.67**
Beating siblings	21.0	5.6	2.0	13.34***
Bullying peers	15.8	8.3	4.0	3.73
Eating difficulties	15.8	2.8	0.0	5.72*
Involuntary movements	15.8	5.6	6.0	3.25
Telling lies	15.8	8.3	4.0	3.73
Speech problems	10.5	2.8	2.0	3.88
Somnambulism	7.9	0.0	0.0	6.88*
Encopresis	5.3	0.0	0.0	4.55
Stealing	5.3	8.3	2.0	1.84

*$p < 0.05$, **$p < 0.01$, ***$p < 0.001$.

aspects of daily life are paralyzed; the result is the total breakdown of normal patterns of social and economic interactions. Curfews create frustration, and one of the main common responses to frustration is active aggression. If the stressful condition continues, and the individual is unable to cope with it, apathy may deepen into depression [4]. During the 5 years of the first Intifada, the population in the Gaza Strip was confined to their homes during curfews every night from 7 p.m. to 4 a.m. Furthermore, curfews were imposed around the clock on many occasions for various periods. During the Gulf War, curfew was imposed for a continuous 42 days. In the study of collective punishments and mental health, we tried to assess the effects of curfews on the behavior of children: results show that 66.1% of children began to fight each other, 54% were afraid of new things,

38% started to develop aggressive behavior, 18.9% started to suffer from bedwetting and 2.3% had speech difficulties [4].

Experiences related to political violence and war constitute a serious risk for the well-functioning of family [5,6]. War and political conflict disrupt some of the basic parental functions, such as protecting children and enhancing trust in security and human virtues. Palestinian families in the Gaza Strip are large, and people show strong affiliation to them. "El Hamula" (the extended family) continues to play an important protective role in modern life. Traditionally, children submit to the authority of their parents, and older members of the family enjoy special respect. The constant enemy threat and the collective trauma of losing their homeland in 1948 have further increased social cohesion in Palestinian society. However, the Intifada created a situation that apparently shook traditional parent–child relations and family hierarchy. First, the increased influence of political parties decreased the social role of the extended family. Second, children and youths played a very active role in the national struggle. They were an essential element in the initiation, planning, and organizing of demonstrations against and confrontations with Israeli soldiers [7].

Palestinians have expressed serious concerns about the future consequences of these shattered parental bonds. There is a common belief that children who threw stones and fought against the occupation army may also challenge their parents' authority. Children living in conditions of political violence and war have been described as "growing up too soon", "losing their childhood", and taking political responsibilities before maturation [8]. This development is predicted to result in negative psychological consequences [9].

Research focusing on the associations between traumatic events, children's gender and political activity, and parenting styles showed that the more the children were exposed to traumatic events, the more they perceived both their parents as strictly disciplining, rejecting, and hostile, and their mothers as more negatively evaluating (Tables 16.2 and 16.3). Traumatic events increased perceived parental rejection and hostility only among boys, and perceived strict discipline only among girls. In the families exposed to a high level of traumatic events, passive boys perceived their fathers as more rejecting and hostile than active boys did. It is suggested that mothers and fathers rear girls restrictively and with greater attention, and boys with rejection, when the family faces traumatic events. In exposed families, fathers also tend to discourage boys' political passivity and apparently encourage activity. Children who enjoyed good parenting have the ability to adapt and achieve better mental health than children who had poor parenting [10].

After 3 years of reduced military violence, the children who had responded actively to that violence suffered less from post-traumatic stress

TABLE 16.2 Mothers: relation between traumatic events, child's gender and political activity, and perceived parenting styles ($n = 56$)

Independent variables	Strict discipline		Intimacy and love		Lax control		Negative evaluation		Rejection and hostility	
	Beta	r	Beta	r	Beta	r	Beta	r	Beta	r
Traumatic events	0.14	0.22	0.03	0.00	0.07	0.4	0.23	0.32	0.10	0.23
Gender	0.28	0.32	0.01	0.02	0.10	0.8	0.34	0.40	0.32	0.37
Political activity	0.01	0.11	0.00	0.01	−1.8	−1.2	−0.04	0.14	0.9	0.21
R^2	0.12		0.00		0.3		0.21		0.16	
F (6,56)	4.71		0.01		1.20		9.06		6.72	
p	<0.04		ns		ns		<0.0001		<0.003	

TABLE 16.3 Fathers: relation between traumatic events, child's gender and political activity, and perceived parenting styles ($n = 56$)

Independent variables	Strict discipline		Intimacy and love		Lax control		Negative evaluation		Rejection and hostility	
	Beta	r	Beta	r	Beta	r	Beta	r	Beta	r
Traumatic events	0.17	0.28	0.02	−0.04	0.15	0.1	0.07	0.06	0.25	0.31
Gender	0.37	0.42	0.09	0.05	0.15	0.14	0.11	0.08	0.40	0.44
Political activity	0.00	0.16	−1.0	−0.08	−2.3	−1.3	−0.05	−0.5	−1.3	0.07
R^2	0.02		0.01		0.6		0.02		0.24	
F (6,56)	8.90		0.53		2.40		0.58		11.14	
p	<0.0001		ns		0.7		ns		<0.0001	

disorder (PTSD) and emotional disorders than the passive children. Conversely, in the midst of Intifada violence, these active children had showed the highest levels of psychological symptoms. The result thus confirms that children's political activity serves different mental health functions in acutely dangerous conditions than in safe ones.

Parental relationships were very important determinants of the children's post-Intifada adjustment. Results expand on the simple assumption that good and loving parenting is beneficial, and rejective and hostile parenting is harmful, by showing that it was rather the perceived discrepancy between the mothering and fathering that was malfunctioning. The children turned out to be especially vulnerable to PTSD and emotional disorders (self-reported) if they felt that their mothers showed positive and their fathers negative attitudes towards them. Harmful effects of parental discrepancy may arise from three sets of circumstances. First, mothers may be especially attached to and protective of children who suffer from symptoms and disorders, whereas fathers may show less caring attitudes.

Second, the perceived discrepancy may reveal conflicting marital relations, involving a disagreement about child-rearing practices, which, in turn, is associated with children's poor psychological adjustment. Third, we measure parenting, which could mean that children with severe symptoms tend to favor one parent over the other.

We have an accumulated knowledge about the children's responses to air-raids, bombardment shelling, loss of family member and being target of and witnessing killing and destruction. Children's responses to danger and life-threat include anxiety, somatization and withdrawal symptoms and, especially among younger children, regression to the earlier stages of development and clinging to parents. Family ties are considered one of the most important protectors of the child's mental health in war conditions. The results of a recent study [11] indicate that both children and their mothers are suffering from various psychological symptoms and that direct exposure to trauma as well as witnessing trauma constitute traumatic experiences. These results confirm that the population of Palestinian children and their mothers have a high prevalence of both types of trauma (exposure and witnessing). 55.1% of the children suffered from severe PTSD. The variation of the PTSD symptoms was a function of the child's and the mother's characteristics and the mother's responses to trauma, and only marginally the function of the level of trauma exposure. Most vulnerable to the intrusion symptoms were girls whose mothers were educated and showed a high level of PTSD symptoms, whereas most vulnerable to avoidance symptoms were children who personally experienced violence and whose mothers were educated and showed a high level of PTSD symptoms.

Palestinian militant groups have recently resorted to suicide bombing killing of civilian Israelis. Suicide bombing is a complex phenomenon and can be seen as a reflection of despair on the one hand and a desire for defiance and revenge on the other. One of the essential elements to understand is the tribal mentality which urges individuals to avenge defeat to the bitter end, even across generations. They will continue to fight forever if needed as long as their dignity is injured. They will only stop if the aggressor will publicly acknowledge his guilt and assume responsibility for his aggression. They will then enter the honorable *Solha* or peace. To be a martyr is highly glorified and places one on the highest level of respect, almost that of prophets. Politically, suicide bombing is an act of absolute despair and a very serious stage in the perception of the seemingly perpetual Arab–Israeli conflict. One of the most significant observations is that an increasing number of children are identifying with martyrdom. In a recent research project of the Gaza Community Mental Health Programme, 34% of boys aged 12–14 years reported they considered that the best thing to do in life is to die as a martyr.

CONCLUSIONS

The history of Palestinians is composed of a series of disasters which took place in different periods of time, with serious impact on their psyche. The mood of Palestinian people is still fluctuating between hope and despair.

In the Gaza Community Mental Health Programme we have embarked since 1990 on a mission to try and help as many people as we can. We have 11 community centers which provide mental health services particularly geared to the needs of children, women and victims of torture. We have reached around 18% of the population, directly helping over 15,000 victims of violence, and have trained hundreds of doctors, nurses and teachers in basic counseling.

In the last 3 years alone, and through a special project of crisis intervention, we have reached around 6,000 people. We apply debriefing, supportive counseling, group therapy, child and family therapy and individual programs of therapy. Our team strives to reach people in the areas where Israeli army actions result in demolishing homes or killing and injuring civilians. On many occasions our teams were not able to reach the people who needed services due to Israeli blockade of roads. Some areas in the Gaza Strip are still unreachable by medical or other teams.

Nations are like individuals: each tries to be the master of its destiny. Like many other groups, Palestinians are victims of their history, discrimination, and persecution. Palestinians are struggling to assert their identity and to heal their injured dignity. Their suffering and forced subjugation cause more anger, hate, and distrust. Yet, the world was not responding to their crisis. Justice was being denied, and hope was being destroyed. And within this context, neither individual mental health nor regional peace can exist.

REFERENCES

1. Khamis V. (1995) Coping with stress. Palestinian families and Intifada-related trauma. Unpublished manuscript.
2. El Sarraj E., Tawahina A.A., Abu Hein F. (1991) The Palestinian: the story of uprooting. Presented at The First International Conference on the Mental Health of Refugees and Displaced Persons, Stockholm, October 6–11.
3. Qouta S., El Sarraj E. (1997) House demolition and mental health: victims and witnesses. *Journal of Social Distress and the Homeless*, **6**: 3.
4. Qouta S., El Sarraj E. (1994) Palestinian children under curfew. *Psychol Studies*, **4**: 1–12.
5. Garbarino J., Kostelny K. (1993) Children's response to war: what do we know? In L.A. Leaved, N.A. Fox (Eds.), *The Psychological Effects of War and Violence on Children*, pp. 23–39. Lawrence Erlbaum, Hillsdale, NJ.

6. Hobfoll S., Spielberger C., Breznitz S., Figley C., Folkman S., Lepper-Green B., *et al.* (1991) War-related stress: addressing the stress of war and other traumatic events. *Am Psychol*, **46**: 848–855.
7. Kuttab D. (1988) A profile of the stone throwers. *Journal of Palestinian Studies*, **17**: 14–23.
8. Boothby N., Upton P., Sultan A. (1992) *Children of Mozambique: The Cost of Survival*. US Committee for Refugees, Washington, DC.
9. Garbarino J., Kostelny K., Dubrow N. (1991) What children can tell us about living in danger? *Am Psychol*, **46**: 376–383.
10. Punamaki R.-L., Qouta S., El Sarraj E. (1997) Relationship between traumatic events, children's gender and political activity, and perceptions of parenting styles. *Int J Behav Develop*, **21**: 91–109.
11. Qouta S., El Sarraj E., Punamaki R. Prevalence of PTSD among Palestinian mothers and children exposed to shelling and loss of home. Submitted for publication.

The Experience of Bosnia-Herzegovina: Psychosocial Consequences of War Atrocities on Children

Syed Arshad Husain

University of Missouri, Columbia, MO, USA

INTRODUCTION

Violence exploded in Bosnia when it declared independence from Yugoslavia in March 1992. Until this time Bosnia-Herzegovina (B-H) was one of the six republics of Yugoslavia (Croatia, Macedonia, Montenegro, Slovenia and Serbia being the other five). Slovenia was the first to declare independence. The population of B-H consists of 40% Muslim, 30% Orthodox Serbs, and 18% Roman Catholics, and a significant percentage of Jews. Ethnic tension became a dominant factor in the region. Bosnians, Serbs and Croats had fears of under-representation and possible persecution. In this atmosphere of ethnic tension, the war broke out in B-H and the capital city of Sarajevo was put under siege by the Serbian forces. Although Bosnian Croats and Muslims fought together against the Serbs in 1992 and liberated a big portion of territory around Mostar, several months later new conflicts broke out setting the two groups against each other. The three-party conflict soon gave rise to horrible atrocities, most of them aimed at Bosnian Muslims in an effort to kill them or drive them out of Bosnia.

Before the war, Sarajevo was a prosperous, sophisticated city, often nicknamed "Paris of the Balkans", and was the site of the 1984 Winter Olympics. During the war, Sarajevo was under siege for approximately 4 years and was bombarded on a daily basis from the surrounding hills. The destruction the city saw was massive. Half of the city inhabitants, roughly 300,000 people, fled to safety. Those who remained moved to the basements

Disasters and Mental Health. Edited by Juan José López-Ibor, George Christodoulou, Mario Maj, Norman Sartorius and Ahmed Okasha.
©2005 John Wiley & Sons Ltd. ISBN 0-470-02123-3.

of their houses or camped out in the dark hallways, as far away from windows as possible to avoid direct hits or sniper fire. Obtaining food and water was a daily struggle. Many people were killed while standing in long lines for water, by sniper fire from the high-rise buildings. Repeated mass killings of residents gathered at marketplaces made finding food even more difficult and dangerous. Throughout most of the siege, the citizens of Sarajevo had to endure the long winters without heat or electricity. By the end of the war, the death toll in Sarajevo reached 11,000 people, and 61,000 were wounded. The figure for B-H, with a pre-war population of 4.3 million, was 242,000 killed, 175,000 wounded and 1.3 million refugees.

In the war in B-H, children were specially targeted. The snipers would take aim at them first if they were walking with adults. When you kill an adult you kill the present and the past, but when you kill children, you kill the future. Children were sometimes used as human shields by the Serbian soldiers as they advanced toward the front line. Girls as young as 6, 7 or 8 were gang-raped and some girls who got pregnant were forced to bear the child. The intended goal was to demoralize the family, create discord and destroy the family unit.

According to the statistics released by the Institute of Public Health of B-H, 16,854 children were killed during the war. 1,601 children were killed in Sarajevo and 14,946 (25% of child population of Sarajevo) were wounded.

Many of the children's growth was stunted by the severe trauma they had endured. One 7-year-old girl's hair turned gray after she witnessed the torture and murder of her father. We discovered that some children developed a fear of light and preferred dark. Light meant that the snipers could take aim and shoot at them. Darkness, on the other hand, provided a protective shield from the snipers.

RESEARCH DATA

During the siege of Sarajevo, we collected data on 791 children randomly selected from 10 schools of one school district [1]. The students were administered the following instruments: the Children Post Traumatic Stress Reaction Index, the Impact of Events Scale, the Children Depression Inventory (CDI) and the General Information Questionnaire. The sample was divided into two groups, using a cut-off age of 13 years, to determine whether adolescents as a group respond differently to the events around them by reason of their being in a different stage developmentally and cognitively.

The age of children ranged from 7 to 15 years, approximately half males and half females. 85% of the students had experienced sniper attacks. 665 children (84.1%) had lost an immediate member of their family during the war. These children showed more avoidance and re-experiencing symptoms than the group that did not have loss of a family member. This group was also more depressed. 76% of students felt deprived of food, 48% felt deprived of clothes, 29% felt deprived of water and 10% reported that they were deprived of shelter. The rate of post-traumatic stress disorder (PTSD) as a whole was higher in the deprived group when compared with the non-deprived group. The former group also reported more avoidance and re-experiencing symptoms.

We assessed the presence of PTSD in two ways: by using the Post Traumatic Stress Reaction Index alone and by combining Post Traumatic Stress Reaction items and Impact of Events Scale items to produce a composite score which was consistent with DSM-IV criteria. On the Post Traumatic Stress Reaction Index, the PTSD rate was 40%, while on the composite scale only 18% fulfilled the criteria for PTSD. This finding indicates that the DSM-IV criteria are more stringent.

This study also showed that a higher percentage of the older age group had symptoms of PTSD as compared to the younger age group and more females had PTSD than males in both the older and younger age groups.

The finding that only 18% of children developed PTSD merits a discussion of factors which may make a child vulnerable or resistant to the effects of traumatic events.

Much has been written about the vulnerability of children to the various stressors often present in their environments. That children by and large grow up to become strong, productive adults may be surprising to most of us in seemingly dire times. However, resistance and resilience are qualities that children possess that function like an antidote to the many poisons life has to offer. Vulnerability and resistance are like opposite ends of a continuum counterbalancing one another in a delicate dance that at any given time may be weighted more heavily on one side than the other. Variations would occur because of differences in experiences, temperaments, intelligence, knowledge and even upbringing.

One characteristic that is built into childhood, and which may protect the children from the effect of trauma, is the capacity for magical thinking. I came across an example of the power of magical thinking among some young boys in Sarajevo who had become self-styled experts in artillery. They were used to hearing the sounds of different guns used by snipers in different parts of the city and surrounding hills and had learned the characteristic noise that each gun made, differentiating one gun from another by its sound. The boys knew the guns, the size and the location. They could even tell from shrapnel or the exploded parts of a shell what kind of weapon had launched it. They used this knowledge to reassure themselves. When they heard the report of a particular gun they would say to each other: "He's all the way across town, he can't get us here". I was not able to tell how accurate the boys' knowledge was, but I do know their knowledge tied into magical thinking that gave them a feeling of control over their lives. Making a game of the voices and personalities of the guns transformed their fear into play. As they became experts at this game, it reduced the negative psychological impact of living in fear.

Play is another strength for children. Play is an elemental part of childhood, and it is not surprising that children's healing after trauma often occurs through play, a fact that mental health professionals take advantage of when they use play therapy in their practice.

One important factor in Bosnian children's resilience to trauma has been family. In Bosnia, the family unit is very strong. Children grow up with aunts, uncles, cousins and grandparents as members of a large and loving extended family. During the war, other family members were immediately available when parents were separated from their children or killed. Most orphaned children continued to receive love and protection from someone they knew and trusted.

Children in Bosnia also benefited from the attitude of the adults around them. Studies have indicated that, especially among younger children, children's responses to traumatic events are largely mediated by the responses of their parents and other important adults. It is through these adults that children learn the meaning of what is happening. During my trips to Bosnia during the war, I often noticed that many Bosnians avoided referring to enemy soldiers as Serbs or, early in the war, as Croats. Instead they were always called "aggressors". Adults who had grown up side by side with Serbs and Croats knew that not all of the people in these ethnic groups supported the war. They consciously avoided giving children the message that people could be labeled as good or bad by their ethnicity. In addition, teachers discouraged children from talking about or valuing revenge, explaining that this was the kind of thinking that had started the war. Some research has indicated that children focused on revenge fantasies following armed conflict do not do as well as children who have a more positive outlook. This attitude on the part of teachers very possibly bolstered some of the children's resilience and provided moral guidelines.

One other factor I believe may help some children do well after they have experienced trauma and loss is having a sense of purpose. This is important: unlike many other factors apparently buffering children from trauma (such as family support, intelligence, and temperament), which children generally either have or do not have, a sense of purpose can be acquired, even after the traumatic event. Engendering a sense of purpose in children is one of the core goals of the therapeutic interview that I teach to Bosnian teachers during seminars.

Children who have survived trauma can be helped to see the future as an opportunity to live out the interests and talents that make each one of them unique. Survivor guilt is helped by knowing that they are not betraying a loved one by living life to its fullest, but instead carrying on the trust that is implicit in having survived. Possibly the most hopeful change I have seen among war-traumatized children who reclaim their sense of purpose, is the way they can suddenly let go of this destructive guilt and begin to live their own lives again. Some children have beliefs that may add a religious interpretation to their sense of purpose. In any case, the idea seems to provide meaning, comfort, and hope to many children who have been exposed to wartime stress and extreme losses.

Helping a child gain a sense of purpose after a traumatic event is one of the primary ways they can be helped to recreate a future for themselves. Wartime trauma, especially when accompanied by loss of a family member, is so devastating because it takes away not only a child's past and present, but the future as well. Each of these three losses must be addressed. This is why, during my seminars, I teach Bosnian teachers and mental health professionals to help children focus on good memories and remember a loved one during happy times, rather than during times close to the loss when memories are dominated by that person's injury, fear, or pain. The happy memories are the ones that help them regain their past. Overcoming symptoms of flashbacks, withdrawal, and hyperarousal is part of regaining the present and the potential of each moment as it unfolds for the traumatized individual. And, finally, the future can also be retrieved, especially if teachers and mental health professionals help children reconstruct their dreams for the lives ahead of them. Some children inevitably find that there are pieces missing from the dreams they used to have.

A CASE HISTORY

A mother from a refugee camp near the city of Tuzla consulted me about her 10-year-old son who, since his displacement from his hometown, had become very withdrawn and depressed. "He used to be a lively, outgoing and happy-go-lucky child", his mother told me with tears in her eyes. Since his migration to the refugee camp, this child had become sad, as if he had no wish to live. I talked to this boy through the help of an interpreter. He sat slouched in his chair with poor eye contact. He told me that he had always dreamed of being a professional soccer player. "But now I cannot. I am here in the refugee camp. The nearest soccer field is in Tuzla 12 miles away. My father is unemployed; he can't take me to the soccer field. He says I have to wait. If I don't practice I can't be a soccer player." Suddenly the story of

Pelè, the great soccer player, came to my mind and I told the boy that story. "Have you heard of Pelè?", I asked. He knew of Pelè. I said "Pelè was born very poor. He couldn't afford a soccer ball. There were no playing fields around his neighborhood. He asked his mother to make him a ball of rags. He then hung that ball off a limb of a tree behind his house and started practicing dribbling, heading and ball control. For leg strength he used skipping techniques. He overcame the lack of a playing field and a soccer ball through ingenuity and improvising." As I was telling this story to this boy, his eyes started to twinkle and his ears began to perk up and his posture straightened. "Did he really do that?", the boy asked. I said, "Yes, indeed he did that." "I can do that too", the boy said with a resolute voice. He stood up with glee on his face and hugged me. As I hugged him back I could sense that a flame of hope had rekindled in the heart of this young man. I also did another thing. I went to Tuzla and bought a couple of soccer balls and gave them to the young boy and suggested that he start a soccer team in the refugee camp. A few days later when I met with his mother again, she asked me, "What did you say to my boy? He is happy, he is back to normal."

TEACHERS AS THERAPISTS

According to reports of the Ministry of Health of B-H, only approximately 100 mental health professionals remained in the city of Sarajevo to serve its 60,000 children who were exposed to war trauma. This disproportion between the number of mental health professionals and the children needing psychological help created a necessity to train lay therapists. Consequently, we developed a model to train teachers in diagnosing and treating children suffering from PTSD and comorbid conditions.

The selection of teachers to train as therapists was based on the observation that the teachers in Sarajevo were recognized as the ones who had intuitively and effectively provided psychological help to their students during the war. The literature on the subject has repeatedly advocated the use of teachers as interventionists for the children after trauma. Most children trust their teachers and spend a significant amount of their wakeful hours with their teachers. Teachers have extensive experience in relating with children, they have exposure to children in crisis and they often have intuitive mental health care skills that allow them to acquire therapeutic skills rapidly.

During the siege of Sarajevo, it was estimated that approximately 5,000 teachers remained. They provided an effective pool of sophisticated workers who could be trained in detecting and treating PTSD and other comorbid conditions.

Since February 1994, the team led by this author made 16 trips to the besieged city of Sarajevo and trained 2,000 teachers and over 200 mental health professionals who, in turn, helped over 20,000 children.

The "teachers as therapists" model has now been used effectively in Kosova, Russia, Afghanistan, Pakistan, Chechenya, Palestine, India, and, most recently, in Iraq.

CONCLUSIONS

As alarming as the statistics presented above are, they cannot tell the full story of the Bosnian children's plight during the war and the turbulence the war atrocities caused in their lives. Many children I had the opportunity to know, expressed their confusion and dismay at the carnage perpetrated around them by the hands of the people who once were their neighbors.

Sometimes the pain and confusion are too great, causing children to lose the ability to feel and express emotions. One 13-year-old girl revealed to me: "I feel so empty, sometimes I feel I am not alive, I am just here." Some children give up their childhoods too early, like one boy who said: "I am bored playing games that my friends play." Many children who saw their parents or loved ones killed are tormented by guilt, blaming themselves for having done nothing while the parent or loved one was murdered.

Possibly the worst scenario is when children turn their pain and anger into aggressive acts against other children, creating further isolation for them. One 13-year-old boy was quarrelsome at school, often getting into fights. He was attracted by sharp objects and concerns grew that he might pose a danger to his peers. During the interview it was revealed that this boy experienced unbearable pain and loss. His father was beaten and killed in his presence. He and his sister were often forced to leave their home while the aggressor soldiers raped their mother. When I met him, he was still having recurrent nightmares about some of his terrible experiences. With therapy, this young man stopped fighting, dropped his interest in sharp objects and knives, and resumed his interest in art "to become a famous artist one day". Many children lose their ability to hope for the future. Most children I met could not talk about their future plans. They developed a foreshortened sense of the future.

Hearing these stories, it is difficult to believe that any one could survive such devastating emotional wound. However, in B-H, I not only learned about the destructiveness of war, I also learned about the resilience of children. I learned of the importance of adults, such as teachers making an effort to help and protect the most precious gift to mankind, the children. I saw the humanitarian workers extending a helping hand to the war-traumatized children and their families and offering them hope. Above all, I learned that hope is an amazingly powerful force, even in the face of the worst cruelty and tragedy.

REFERENCE

1. Husain S.A., Nair J., Holcomb W., Reid J.C., Vargas V., Nair S.S. (1998) Stress reactions of children and adolescents in war and siege conditions. *Am J Psychiatry*, **155**: 1718–1719.

The Serbian Experience

Dusica Lecic-Tosevski and Saveta Draganic-Gajic

University of Belgrade, Belgrade, Serbia and Montenegro

INTRODUCTION

The population of Serbia and Montenegro (former Yugoslavia) has been struck by repeated traumas of severe intensity during the last 12 years: wars in the region, United Nations (UN) sanctions, bombardments. These traumas caused acute and chronic stress, which produced significant psychological sequelae, especially to vulnerable people, as well as significant social consequences. The range of responses of affected individuals and groups have been important lessons and a challenge to mental health professionals, prompting self-education and education of other professionals and para-professionals, specific treatment action and preventive programs, as well as research into psychiatric morbidity following disasters.

THE STRESS OF WAR AND EXILE

At the beginning of the 1990s, the republics of former Yugoslavia were involved in a civil conflict that had disastrous consequences. 700,000 people from Bosnia and Croatia were forced to leave their homes and find exile in Serbia. At the beginning, most of these refugees were staying in host families, while 5% lived in collective centers. However, when a new wave of about 250,000 refugees from Croatia arrived in August 1995, the number of those living in collective centers increased to 30%. A further 250,000 refugees, or so-called internally displaced persons, were forced to leave Kosovo after the bombardment in 1999.

War, the relocation process, the experience of violence and of detention led to degradation, poverty, dehumanization, violence, illness and the death

Disasters and Mental Health. Edited by Juan José López-Ibor, George Christodoulou, Mario Maj, Norman Sartorius and Ahmed Okasha.
©2005 John Wiley & Sons Ltd. ISBN 0-470-02123-3.

of many. Most of the refugees reported severe traumatic experiences which made this population at a high risk for developing psychiatric psycho-pathology. A substantial proportion of refugees experienced post-traumatic stress reactions after adversities [1,2].

VICTIMS OF TORTURE

Many thousands of individuals were detained during the civil war in Croatia and Bosnia, of whom about 5,000 live in Serbia now. The detention camps were characterized by extremely poor living conditions, use of prisoners as human shields, executions and deaths due to torture or neglect. Physical, psychological and sexual violence were frequent and extreme, which caused post-traumatic and other stress disorders in the victims of torture.

UN SANCTIONS

The sanctions of the UN Security Council were imposed against the Federal Republic of Yugoslavia on June 1, 1992, and lasted for 3.5 years. By these sanctions most of the citizens have been put in almost complete isolation from the rest of the world. Not only economic, but also scientific, cultural and sports cooperation has been interrupted and forbidden. Even the import of pharmaceutical preparations and raw material for pharmaceutical products and other medical supplies, as well as other goods for basic needs (heating oil, food), was prevented by the sanctions. The sanctions have inflicted great damage on the economy and prompted a drastic drop in the standard of living and the quality of life. The inflation rate was the highest registered in the world since the 1930s. The average salary was 5 dollars per month, and due to the galloping inflation the morning money would become totally worthless in the evening.

Reactions of citizens to the extraordinary circumstances caused by the sanctions were various. The extremely high rate of unemployment and lack of basic needs caused diffuse anxiety, helplessness, hopelessness, low self-esteem, and lost perspectives in life [3]. Part of the population exhausted its adaptive forces under the effects of chronic stress with constant new "daily stresses".

Under the UN sanctions, mental health services in the Federal Republic of Yugoslavia have been hit by the following problems: shortage of medication and other essentials, increased patient load and stress on mental health care providers. Some psychosocial consequences of the stress of the sanctions will be mentioned here, according to data of the Republic Committee for Psychiatry, reports of World Health Organization (WHO)'s experts [4] and humanitarian organizations, as well as from the observations from our own clinical practice [5].

There was a significant increase of the number of patients with anxious and depressive reactions, substance abuse, and psychosomatic disorders. Owing to a lack of medication for the treatment of psycho-organic and somatic diseases of the chronic psychiatric patients, mortality in hospitals increased considerably. During 1993, 250 patients died in the psychiatric hospital in Kovin, which was twice the usual mortality rate. In the psychiatric hospital in Gornja Toponica, 70 new cases of tuberculosis have been registered. Only about 30% of the medication required by patients was covered, and the available psychotropic drugs were scarce, thus making target pharmacotherapy impossible. There was an increasing number of patients with resistant depression, and relapses of psychotic disorders were on the rise since specific antidepressants and depot preparations could not be used.

Most of the population was suffering from impoverished nutrition. The rate of anemic students increased from 3.4% to 36.7% during the period of the UN sanctions. In 1993 the incidence of tuberculosis increased fourfold. The prevalence of coronary diseases increased, as well as the mortality from malignant diseases. About 10% patients died waiting for the pacemaker operation. Mortality of patients with renal insufficiency rose by 20% since they could not be put on dialysis. Mortality of diabetic patients doubled, owing to a lack of insulin, and the incidence of the diabetic gangrene increased tenfold. Especially difficult was the situation of the pregnant women and newborn children. In addition to a decreased birth rate, premature births were increasing as well as severe complications during pregnancy. There was an increase of risky pregnancies, of the number of operative interventions and of infants with disturbed psychophysical development. The total mortality rate in Yugoslavia rose by 13% in 1993.

THE STRESS OF BOMBARDMENT

The bombardment which was called air strikes or the "merciful angel" campaign lasted 11 weeks in spring 1999, from 24 March until 10 June. Targets were in densely inhabited urban areas, which resulted in casualties among civilians throughout the country. In continuous day and night air attacks, terrifying sounds of air raids and explosions were heard and many people spent nights in shelters. Estimates of casualties among civilians range around 1,500. A few thousand people were injured, some of them became invalids. The bombardment caused intense acute stress, which was superimposed to the already existing chronic one. During that time people became anxious, angry, helpless and hopeless.

Many industrial targets were destroyed and damaged, as well as schools, health centers, media and cultural monuments. The damage was estimated to be around 30 billion dollars. Bombs filled with depleted uranium destroyed the natural environment in the country.

SOCIAL TRANSITION

The democratic changes of October 5, 2000 brought hope to people after many years of stress and tension. However, social transition, as in other countries of the region, is rather painful. The quality of life of the people is still very low. The cultural disintegration due to prolonged stress and a continuous political upheaval resulted in anomie and alienation. The feelings of helplessness and uncertainty prevail among the people.

Disastrous events in our country and in the region caused a steady increase of mental and behavioral disorders over the years. According to the Institute of Public Health, the number of registered mental disorders increased from 271,944 in 1999 to 309,281 in 2002, thus making them the second largest public health problem (after cerebro-vascular diseases). The prevalence of stress-related disorders is great, but other mental health problems are also on the increase, such as depression, suicide rate, substance abuse, psychosomatic disorders, delinquency and violence, as well as the burnout syndrome among physicians who shared the destiny of their patients and worked hard under adverse circumstances.

OUR ACTION

Care for patients suffering from post-traumatic stress is a challenge to health services. What follows are the activities we undertook in order to protect the mental health of the population during the years of stress. The scope of action had three levels – treatment, education and research.

Treatment

In order to take care of the traumatized people, we have established the Stress Clinic within the Institute of Mental Health (Belgrade) in 1994. The predominant activity of the Clinic was treatment of individuals who experienced acute and chronic stress reactions, as well as primary, secondary and tertiary prevention of the psychosocial consequences of war and exile-related trauma [6]. Most of the other clinics and hospitals all over the country had also to treat traumatized people. In order to educate the professionals and para-professionals we have translated a few WHO books on disaster and the mental health of refugees and have published our own books, manuals and articles.

Psychosocial Programs

We have developed many programs during the last 12 years. One of them was the Mental Health Assistance of Refugees. The program started in 1991 and lasted until 2000 [1]. Since 1993 it was supported by the United Nations High Commissioner for Refugees (UNHCR). A network of 100 teams was organized which covered the whole country. After the training in the field of trauma and stress, the teams consisting of a psychiatrist, a psychologist and a social worker were involved in helping the refugees in counseling services. Mobile teams regularly visited collective centers for refugees. Through a series of seminars supported by the Swiss Disaster Relief, several hundreds of para-professionals and laymen were provided with a basic knowledge of stress disorders. We also trained primary care physicians, about 1,000 Red Cross volunteers, commissioners for refugees, and social workers, as well as refugees in order to enable them to organize self-help groups. Within the program a close cooperation has been established with the Red Cross and other humanitarian agencies, centers for social work, primary health care centers, governmental institutions and mass media.

The Centre for Rehabilitation of Torture Victims was established in 2000 within a non-governmental organization (NGO), the International Aid Network, and supported by the European Commission. So far more than 1,000 torture victims have been helped. The staff of the Centre comprises a multidisciplinary team of experts (psychiatrists, psychologists, lawyers, etc.) [7].

Research

The available epidemiological evidence suggests that although 38% of the population is exposed to severe stresses, only about 9.2% ever experience post-traumatic stress disorder (PTSD)-like reactions [8]. The PTSD construct is rather complex and still controversial, and complicated by the issue of vulnerability.

In our study of stress and PTSD, we found that the latter disorder was diagnosed in 29.2% of refugees [2]. Most of the refugees examined had multiple traumas, such as combat, injury, loss of a family member, forced labor, witnessing of torture, sexual abuse or imprisonment. In addition to

PTSD, other disorders were also registered, such as adjustment disorder (18.6%), mixed anxious-depressive disorders (11.3%), and depressive episodes (5%). The highest prevalence of PTSD was found among the group of refugees who experienced sexual abuse (56%) and severe forms of torture during detention (74.8%) [9].

According to another study [10], a significant number of civilians (11%) had psychological symptoms of post-traumatic stress, such as intrusion and avoidance, 1 year after being exposed to air attacks.

It has been suggested that previous experience of trauma may qualitatively change the way subjects respond to further traumatic events [11]. We found that experience of previous non-war-related stress seems to enable individuals to cope better with low exposure to trauma. But, with high exposure, this protection appears insufficient.

According to a study conducted among the student population 1 year after the air attacks [12], personality traits, previous stressful experiences, and exposure to traumatic events had an independent and direct influence on developing post-traumatic stress. However, the effect of these factors cannot just be added up. Rather, the factors interact in their impact on post-traumatic stress symptoms.

Studying associations of post-traumatic stress symptoms and personality traits in civilians 1 year after air attacks, we found that the more disturbed the personality is, the more it is prone to the development of intrusion, the most difficult symptom of post-traumatic stress, owing to impaired cognition and less successful coping strategies [12,13].

Among the students examined 1 year after the air attacks, "talking and gathering" was the most prevalent strategy which was used during the time of bombardment, followed by "leisure activities" and "sport and walks" [14]. Social support activities were almost ubiquitous in the examined population. The students that predominantly used "leisure activities" had the lowest scores of intrusive symptoms 1 year after the attacks, which might suggest that this strategy has been successful. In this way, leisure activities at the time of exposure to an uncontrollable external stressor could be a form of "healthy denial" [15] reflecting resilience in extremely difficult situations. The quality of life also decreased in all areas of life 1 year after air strikes [16].

In 2002 we started a multicentric research on "The Treatment Behavior and Outcomes of Treatment in People with Post-Traumatic Stress Following Conflicts in ex-Yugoslavia". This study is supported by the European Commission and includes trauma centers in two EU countries (the UK and Germany) and in ex-Yugoslav republics (Croatia, Bosnia and Serbia) [17]. It is hoped that the study will answer some controversial questions regarding the concept of PTSD and help in the process of reconciliation.

LESSONS LEARNED

After Disaster – a Need for Mental First Aid

Mental first aid after a disaster might reduce the psychosocial effects of traumatic experiences. The psychosocial support should be adapted to each individual's needs. Since stress reactions are normal reactions to abnormal situations, what is needed is information and normalization of symptoms. Medicalization of problems should be avoided and the traumatized person empowered so that personal autonomy can be maintained.

Training in stress and coping strategies of traumatized individuals is also important, as is the organization of self-help groups. Practical support should be mobilized, especially of children, orphans, single mothers and victims of torture. Such an approach may prevent poor adjustment and chronic consequences.

Preventive action after a disaster should be carried out by the collaborative efforts of many agencies. Partnership for mental health after disasters, i.e. collaboration between psychiatrists, primary care physicians, para-professionals, humanitarian agencies and NGOs is a sine qua non. A network of teams of professionals and para-professionals should be developed.

Research into psychiatric morbidity after a disaster is also necessary. Systematic screening of children and adults for PTSD can provide critical information for rational public mental health programs after a disaster. Early detection of post-traumatic reactions is important, since timely intervention may prevent poor adjustment and a chronic outcome. Research into psychiatric morbidity following disasters can provide a more general insight into the process of coping and the etiology and course of psychiatric illness in general. It also extends our knowledge and improves clinical care in this field of human distress. However, since trauma and disasters often strike suddenly and unexpectedly, we should be prepared before disaster strikes.

Before Disaster Strikes – Outreach Programs

Extensive outreach programs should be developed and pre-disaster education carried out. Systematic education of health care workers and their associates is necessary, and disaster psychiatry should be included in the medical curricula. There should be a unified approach to disaster and trauma. National programs for the prevention and mitigation of the psychosocial consequences of disasters should be developed in each country, as requested by the WHO since 1987. The effects of such an approach would be better preparedness for disasters, management of victims, improved survival and decreased post-disaster morbidity, and improved health and adaptation.

CONCLUSIONS

Dealing with the consequences of disasters is a challenge to mental health professionals, whose work during the years of stress has to be outside their traditional roles. Professionals should attempt to investigate the chain of interactions between personality, environment and behavior initiated by trauma. Moreover, they should work hard to prevent the maintenance of malignant memories and their pernicious effects in traumatized people, such as lasting scars on the psyche and personality changes. The process of reconciliation should be initiated which, it can be hoped, will prevent a transgenerational transmission of trauma.

REFERENCES

1. Kalicanin P., Bukelic J., Ispanovic-Radojkovic V., Lecic-Tosevski D. (1993) *The Stresses of War*. Institute for Mental Health, Belgrade.
2. Lecic-Tosevski D., Draganic S., Jovic V., Ilic Z., Drakulic B., Bokonjic S. (1999) Posttraumatic stress disorder and its relationship with personality dimensions. In G.N. Christodoulou, D. Lecic-Tosevski, V. Kontaxakis (Eds.), *Issues in Psychiatric Prevention*, pp. 95–102. Karger, Basel.
3. Lecic-Tosevski D., Kalicanin P. (1994) Effects of the United Nations sanctions on the mental health of the Yugoslav population. *Psychiatriki*, 1–2: 59–65.
4. Wig N.N. (1993) *The Present State of Mental Health Institutions and Services in the Countries of the Former Yugoslavia*. World Health Organization, Geneva.
5. Kalicanin P., Lecic-Tosevski D., Bukelic J., Ispanovic-Radojkovic V. (1994) *The Stresses of War and Sanctions*. Institute for Mental Health, Belgrade.
6. Lecic-Tosevski D., Drakulic B., Ilic Z., Jovic V., Florikic D., Bokonjic S. (1997) The Stress Clinic, Institute for Mental Health. *Torture* 1: 23–24.
7. Lecic-Tosevski D., Bakalic J. (in press) Centre for rehabilitation of torture victims. In Z. Spiric, G. Knezevic, G. Opacic, V. Jovic, D. Lecic-Tosevski (Eds.), *Against Torture*. IAN, Belgrade.
8. Breslau N., Davis G.C., Andreski P. (1991) Traumatic events and post-traumatic stress disorder in an urban population of young adults. *Arch Gen Psychiatry*, 48: 216–222.
9. Ilic Z., Jovic V., Lecic-Tosevski D. (1998) Post-traumatic stress disorder among prisoners of war. *Psychiatry Today (Psihijatrija Danas)*, 30: 87–106.
10. Gavrilovic J., Lecic-Tosevski D., Knezevic G., Priebe S. (2002) Predictors of posttraumatic stress in civilians 1 year after air attacks: a study of Yugoslav students. *J Nerv Ment Dis*, 190: 257–262.

11. Breslau N., Chilcoat H.D., Kessler R.C., Davis G.C. (1999) Previous exposure to trauma and PTSD effects of subsequent trauma: results from Detroit Area Survey of Trauma. *Am J Psychiatry*, **156**: 902–907.
12. Lecic-Tosevski D., Gavrilovic J., Knezevic G., Priebe S. (2003) Personality factors and posttraumatic stress: association in civilians one year after air attacks. *J Person Disord*, **17**: 537–549.
13. Draganic S., Lecic-Tosevski D., Calovska-Hercog N. (1997) Relationship between borderline personality disorder and posttraumatic stress. *Psychiatry Today (Psihijatrija Danas)*, **29**: 49–59.
14. Gavrilovic J., Lecic-Tosevski D., Dimic S., Pejovic-Milovancevic M., Knezevic G., Priebe S. (2003) Coping strategies in civilians during air attacks. *Soc Psychiatry Psychiatr Epidemiol*, **38**: 128–133.
15. Druss R.G., Douglas C.J. (1988) Adaptive responses to illness and disability: healthy denial. *Gen Hosp Psychiatry*, **10**: 163–168.
16. Lecic-Tosevski D., Susic V., Dimic S., Jankovic J., Colovic O., Priebe S. (2003) Quality of life in the years of stress. In V. Sulovic, D.J. Jakovljevic (Eds.), *Medicine and Quality of Life*, pp. 103–118. Serbian Academy of Science and Arts, Belgrade.
17. Priebe S., Gavrilovic J., Schuetzwohl M., Lecic-Tosevski D., Ljubotinja D., Bravo Mehmedbasic A., *et al.* (2002) Rationale and method of the STOP study – study on the treatment behavior and outcomes of treatment in people with posttraumatic stress following conflicts in ex-Yugoslavia. *Psychiatry Today (Psihijatrija Danas)*, **34**: 133–160.

19

The Croatian Experience

Vera Folnegović Šmalc

Vrapče Psychiatric Hospital, Zagreb, Croatia

INTRODUCTION

The war in Croatia started in 1991, very shortly after the establishment of the independence of the country. It started without announcement, at first only in some regions. Even when the first victims fell, the majority of Croats did not seriously realize that this was the beginning of a war that would last for years. But very soon war horrors started, from individual killings, attacks on police vehicles, road barricades, intimidation, to mass expulsion of Croatian population from almost one-third of the Croatian territory, with all the aspects of ethnic cleansing, and to the demolition of hospitals and killing of patients. Such and similar highly stressful phenomena came suddenly and unexpectedly.

Up to the beginning of the war, the Croatian population had been unarmed. With the development of defense, a lot of firearms arrived in Croatia, and a great percentage of the population could obtain a weapon. This later brought the increase in suicides using firearms, that previously had been very rare in the country.

The war in Croatia led to intense migrations. First, migrations started within Croatia itself, i.e., Croats were expelled from occupied regions of the country. In the period 1991–1995, the number of exiles and refugees amounted to 600,000 [1,2]. Numerous exiles found jobs in larger towns, sometimes in the USA or in Western European countries, and did not return to their previous residence after the liberation of Croatia. After the occupation of Bosnia and Herzegovina, many Croats and Bosnians escaped to Croatia and a proportion of them stayed permanently. After the liberation of the whole of Croatia, a part of the Serbian population moved to Bosnia and Serbia.

Besides the usual war traumatic events, the population of Croatia during the war years was also frequently confronted with specific types of

Disasters and Mental Health. Edited by Juan José López-Ibor, George Christodoulou, Mario Maj, Norman Sartorius and Ahmed Okasha.
©2005 John Wiley & Sons Ltd. ISBN 0-470-02123-3.

psychotrauma, for example, mass raping of women and men (both in Croatia and in Bosnia-Herzegovina, from where they moved to Croatia in large numbers). A large number of people were taken to war detention camps; many patients were moved from hospitals (e.g., from the hospital in Vukovar), and their fate remained unknown for a long period.

The phenomenon of postponed grieving was very frequent among family members of missing and imprisoned persons. The fate of these "missing" persons was at first uncertain; later on, they were found dead (usually exhumed from common graves), and some of their family members developed a severe psychic breakdown, often with psychotic symptoms, and some developed clinical features of psychotic denial.

The occupiers deported the majority of psychiatric patients from the hospitals in the occupied Croatian territories, regardless of their nationality. For example, 200 mental patients were transported from the hospital in Pakrac in one day, most of whom were in a state of very severe psychic and physical dysfunction, urgently needing lodging and general medical care.

Since 1973, a long-term follow-up of a representative sample of patients with schizophrenia has been carried out in Croatia. The sample was taken from all over the country [3]. After the war, a significant proportion of these patients were "lost", i.e. they were no longer at their addresses and no information was available about their move or their possible death.

The incidence of substance abuse increased dramatically during the war period. In 1990, the number of newly registered opiate-dependent patients was 79, while in 2000 it reached 347 [4]. Analogously, the number of examined patients dependent on psychoactive drugs increased from 14 in 1991 to 1,584 in 1999 [4].

Almost overnight Croatia found itself in a situation of rapid reduction in psychiatric facilities and staff resources, also because part of them remained on the occupied territory. One of the most urgent tasks of psychiatrists was to educate professionals and common people on war-related issues. In 1990, under the supervision of E. Klain (Head of the Mental Health Department of Medical Corps Headquarters of the Republic of Croatia), the leading psychiatrists and psychologists in Croatia had already produced a handbook entitled "Introduction to War Psychology and Psychiatry" [5]. This handbook contained guidelines and expert texts, as well as experiences from foreign literature. A year later the School of Medicine of the University of Zagreb published a comprehensive handbook entitled "Psychology and Psychiatry of War" [6], in both Croatian and English. This handbook contains several chapters describing the Croatian experiences, e.g. the development of a pharmacotherapeutic algorithm for "the physician's bag at the battle field" [7], and the experience at the Manjača prisoner of war camp [8].

POST-TRAUMATIC STRESS DISORDER

The data from the largest psychiatric institution in Croatia (the Vrapče Psychiatric Hospital) show significant changes in psychiatric morbidity in hospitalized psychiatric patients before, during and after the war (in 1989, 1994 and 2000) (Table 19.1), with a dramatic increase in the number of patients with post-traumatic stress disorder (PTSD) and other stress-related disorders in 1994 and a sharp decrease in the year 2000.

Persons who received psychosocial support from the environment developed PTSD symptoms less frequently than persons deprived of such help. That is to say, persons of the same sex, after experiencing similar traumatic events (expulsion from their own homes and places, feeling of life threat, witnessing the killing and raping of others, with the possibility of being raped oneself) differed in the frequency of PTSD symptoms whether they had received psychosocial help (from professionals) or not. In the group of persons who got professional help, 43% developed PTSD [8], while among those without help after trauma, 64% developed the disorder. The prevalence of PTSD also differed depending on the type of traumatic event: in persons who witnessed killing or raping of a close family member (children, parents, siblings or spouse), PTSD occurred in 100% of the cases.

We tried to apply both ICD-10 and DSM-IV criteria in our routine clinical work. In a short while it became obvious that these two classifications did not always produce the same diagnosis. Therefore we performed a clinical research among patients who got the clinical diagnosis of PTSD upon discharge. Included were 250 patients without any other concomitant psychiatric diagnosis. These patients were diagnosed anew by two psychiatrists who had previously completed a training course for the application of both ICD-10 and DSM-IV, and had achieved a satisfactory

TABLE 19.1 Patients discharged from the Vrapče Psychiatric Hospital in Zagreb before, during and after the war

	Years		
Diagnosis (ICD-10)	1989	1994	2000
Organic mental disorders	638	756	1019
Mental disorders due to substance use	1337	1279	1791
Schizophrenia and other psychoses	1504	1538	1945
Mood disorders	264	311	562
Personality disorders	158	291	209
Reaction to severe stress and adjustment disorders; enduring personality change after catastrophic experience	38	1365	365
Others	868	883	482
Total	4807	6423	6373

level of reliability. Out of the total of 250 patients with the clinical diagnosis of PTSD, 186 received this diagnosis according to DSM-IV, and 217 according to ICD-10. Only 183 patients had PTSD according to both classifications.

As emphasized in the DSM-IV, when making a diagnosis of PTSD in people who have experienced some form of physical violence, malingering must be ruled out. This is very relevant to the Croatian situation, because, in accordance with our regulations, people with the diagnosis of PTSD who had served in the Homeland War have the right to certain material benefits. In contrast to the people who are inclined towards exaggeration of symptoms, there are persons who are prone to avoid retelling the traumatic event and to deny the PTSD symptoms. These are mostly people who developed PTSD after a rape, particularly women who got pregnant.

The prognosis of PTSD depends not only on treatment, but also on the continuous support of the family and community, the fulfillment of expectations after the war, previous (premorbid) personality structure, comorbidity, the feeling of belonging to a society with positive evaluation of an individual and his/her merits, as well as the absence of new stressful situations. Unfortunately, in Croatia a very large number of people are unemployed. Even healthy people can hardly get a job, while psychically handicapped persons find it even more difficult. Because of that, a large number of persons with PTSD are unemployed, often without any income; they lack self-confidence, and they feel cheated and useless. Often their own life seems worthless; they often avoid treatment and tend to self-treatment, sometimes with alcohol. Moreover, they often develop symptoms of increased arousal, such as: irritability and outbursts of anger and agitation; hypervigilance and markedly decreased threshold when frustrated; incapacity to wait; impatience; and an inclination towards acting out reactions. Very often they have sleep disturbances and present suicidal behavior. The majority of these patients no longer fulfil the criteria for PTSD, either according to ICD-10 or to DSM-IV. If we did not have medical records and good history data, we could hardly diagnose them according to DSM-IV. However, exactly for this (unfortunately large) group of patients who previously had fulfilled the criteria for PTSD, ICD-10 foresees a diagnostic category even today, 10 years after they had fallen ill. It is called "enduring personality change after catastrophic experience", code F62.0. Typical symptoms are inflexibility, maladjustment and intolerance, leading to deep personality changes and damage to family, interpersonal and social functioning.

On the basis of our experience with a large number of people with PTSD, we have reached the conclusion that the ICD-10 diagnostic criteria are much more suitable for diagnosing chronic patients, while in acute states DSM-IV is more adequate.

CONCLUSIONS

The war in Croatia has left severe and often long-lasting sequels on psychic and physical health in a great proportion of traumatized persons. Some of these consequences will be transgenerational, because PTSD has often occurred in children as well, but has been recognized in few of them. On the other hand, with their disturbed behavior, psychotraumatized persons often cause mental disturbances in their children.

The war has led to significant changes in psychiatric morbidity and to the decrease in the number of hospitalized patients with the diagnosis of schizophrenia, other psychoses and dementia. Several tens of thousands of persons in Croatia had or still have PTSD. In some of these people, PTSD has turned into a chronic form, which according to ICD-10 is called "enduring personality change after catastrophic experience". We believe that ICD-10 is more applicable for clinical use than DSM-IV, particularly in chronic states. The frequency of occurrence of PTSD depends on the type of traumatic event experienced, on the support received from the environment after psychotrauma, and on the type of premorbid personality, as well as on the type and timeliness of treatment.

REFERENCES

1. Kostović I., Judaš M. (Eds.) (1992) *Mass Killing and Genocide in Croatia 1991/92. A Book of Evidence.* Sveučilišna Naklada, Zagreb.
2. Kostović I., Judaš M., Henigsberg N. (1993) Medical documentation of human rights violations and war crimes on the territory of Croatia during the 1991/93 war. *Croat Med J*, **34**: 285–293.
3. Folnegović-Šmalc V., Folnegović Z. (1985) *Evaluacija Terapije Shizofrenih Bolesnika.* U: Rad, Jugoslavenska Akademija Znanosti i Umjetnosti, Zagreb.
4. Sakoman S. (2001) *Društvo bez Droge. Hrvatska Nacionalna Strategija.* Institute of Social Sciences I, Pilar, Zagreb.
5. Klain E. (1991) *Uvod u Ratnu Psihologiju i Psihijatriju.* Odjel za Psihijatriju i Psihologiju GSS RH, Zagreb.
6. Klain E. (Ed.) (1992) *Psychology and Psychiatry of War.* Faculty of Medicine, University of Zagreb.
7. Folnegović-Šmalc V., Jakovljević M., Hotujac Lj. (1992) Psychopharmacotherapy in war conditions. In E. Klain (Ed.), *Psychology and Psychiatry of War.* Faculty of Medicine, University of Zagreb.
8. Folnegović-Šmalc V. (1997) Posttraumatic stress disorder in Eastern Europe: the Croatian experience – psychiatric and personal perspectives. Presented at the 10th Congress of the European College of Neuropsychopharmacology, Vienna, 13–17 September.

APPENDIX:
Statement by the World Psychiatric Association on Mental Health Implications of Disasters (approved by the General Assembly on August 26, 2002)

The World Psychiatric Association would like to draw the attention of psychiatrists and other mental health professionals, health authorities, decision-makers and the general public to the serious and potentially catastrophic psychological and psychopathological effects of disasters. These effects can be diverse in character, intensity and potential for chronicity, but acute stress reactions, post-traumatic stress disorder (PTSD), mood, anxiety and psychotic disorders, and permanent changes in the personality are the ones that, if left untreated, may have the most serious consequences.

Disasters can result from a variety of causes such as earthquakes, floods, hurricanes, fires, naval and plane accidents and terrorist attacks, but also from acts and consequences of war and negative conditions affecting important groups of population like famine, sanctions, forced migrations and similar deprivations. All of them produce very serious effects on the population and particularly on children, having a negative impact on the social structure and systems, which increases the effect of the disaster on individuals and population.

Reliable diagnostic methods and effective treatments exist for the behavioral effects of disasters. For every individual physically damaged during a disaster there are three psychologically damaged. Among them relatives and rescue personnel should get priority. Early, on-site intervention, integrated with the rescue teams and health care personnel, is essential.

Disasters and Mental Health. Edited by Juan José López-Ibor, George Christodoulou, Mario Maj, Norman Sartorius and Ahmed Okasha.
©2005 John Wiley & Sons Ltd. ISBN 0-470-02123-3.

Disasters are not fatal events and the distinction between natural and man-made disasters is not a clear cut one. Even in disasters unchained by natural forces, human factors play a significant role. Among those, poor living and social conditions and lack of preventive and intervention plans.

On an individual basis, identification, preparation and protection of vulnerable individuals and social groups should be taken care of. This is the responsibility of mental health workers and must be carried out in collaboration with, among others, the family, the school and employing agencies.

On a general population basis, mental health professionals have a significant role to play (a) as consultants to the health authorities on how to prevent and treat the behavioral consequences of disasters in the community; (b) as advisors to decision-makers with an aim to inform them on the catastrophic behavioral consequences of disasters and exert their influence to prevent man-made and other disasters from occurring and (c) as advisors to the general public on ways to minimize the behavioral consequences of disasters.

Two important components of the World Psychiatric Association, the Sections and more specifically the Section on Military and Disaster Psychiatry, the Section on Preventive Psychiatry and the Section on Anxiety and Obsessive Compulsive Disorders, as well as the Special Program on Disasters (headed jointly by Prof. G.N. Christodoulou and Prof. J.J. López-Ibor) are at present working on these issues and seek collaboration with the psychiatric community, health and state authorities and the general public, being convinced that this collaboration is essential for the positive outcome of their efforts.

The World Psychiatric Association urges its member societies and its scientific sections, the World Health Organization and other appropriate associations and organizations to join forces in promoting acquisition of new information on the behavioral effects of disasters through research, dissemination of this information through education, and prevention and management of these behavioral consequences, by the creation of networks of experts who can advise, educate and even intervene in cases of disasters.

Index

Note: page numbers in *italic* refer to tables; PTSD = post-traumatic stress disorder

Disasters and Mental Health. Edited by Juan José López-Ibor, George Christodoulou, Mario Maj, Norman Sartorius and Ahmed Okasha.
©2005 John Wiley & Sons Ltd. ISBN 0-470-02123-3.

LaVergne, TN USA
05 May 2010
181679LV00001B/31/P